Exam Preparatory Manual for Undergraduates
Obstetrics and Gynecology

Exam Preparatory Manual for Undergraduates
Obstetrics and Gynecology

As per the Competency Based Medical Education Curriculum (NMC)

Third Edition

Punit S Bhojani
MS DNB FICOG FCPS DGO DFP
Consultant Obstetrician and Gynecologist
Mumbai, Maharashtra, India
Founder: www.drmentors.com

Forewords
Geeta M Niyogi
Vinita S Salvi
Nozer K Sheriar

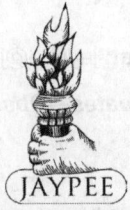

JAYPEE BROTHERS MEDICAL PUBLISHERS
The Health Sciences Publisher
New Delhi | London

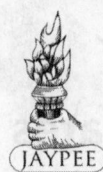

Jaypee Brothers Medical Publishers (P) Ltd.

Headquarters
Jaypee Brothers Medical Publishers (P) Ltd
EMCA House
23/23-B, Ansari Road, Daryaganj
New Delhi - 110 002, India
Landline: +91-11-23272143, +91-11-23272703
+91-11-23282021, +91-11-23245672
Email: jaypee@jaypeebrothers.com

Corporate Office
Jaypee Brothers Medical Publishers (P) Ltd
4838/24, Ansari Road, Daryaganj
New Delhi 110 002, India
Phone: +91-11-43574357
Fax: +91-11-43574314
Email: jaypee@jaypeebrothers.com

Overseas Office
J.P. Medical Ltd
83 Victoria Street, London
SW1H 0HW (UK)
Phone: +44 20 3170 8910
Fax: +44 (0)20 3008 6180
Email: info@jpmedpub.com

Website: www.jaypeebrothers.com
Website: www.jaypeedigital.com

© 2023, Jaypee Brothers Medical Publishers

The views and opinions expressed in this book are solely those of the original contributor(s)/author(s) and do not necessarily represent those of editor(s) and publisher of the book.

All rights reserved. No part of this publication may be reproduced, stored or transmitted in any form or by any means, electronic, mechanical, photocopying, recording or otherwise, without the prior permission in writing of the publishers.

All brand names and product names used in this book are trade names, service marks, trademarks or registered trademarks of their respective owners. The publisher is not associated with any product or vendor mentioned in this book.

Medical knowledge and practice change constantly. This book is designed to provide accurate, authoritative information about the subject matter in question. However, readers are advised to check the most current information available on procedures included and check information from the manufacturer of each product to be administered, to verify the recommended dose, formula, method and duration of administration, adverse effects and contraindications. It is the responsibility of the practitioner to take all appropriate safety precautions. Neither the publisher nor the author(s)/editor(s) assume any liability for any injury and/or damage to persons or property arising from or related to use of material in this book.

This book is sold on the understanding that the publisher is not engaged in providing professional medical services. If such advice or services are required, the services of a competent medical professional should be sought.

Every effort has been made where necessary to contact holders of copyright to obtain permission to reproduce copyright material. If any have been inadvertently overlooked, the publisher will be pleased to make the necessary arrangements at the first opportunity.

Inquiries for bulk sales may be solicited at: jaypee@jaypeebrothers.com

Exam Preparatory Manual for Undergraduates—Obstetrics and Gynecology

First Edition: 2016

Second Edition: 2019

Third Edition: 2023

Reprint : **2024**

ISBN: 978-93-5696-229-3

Printed at Nutech Print Services - India

Dedicated to
My teachers, students and family

FOREWORD

Today, with the pattern of examination system changing from descriptive form to more precise subject-specific short answers and MCQs, it is important for the students not only to have complete knowledge of the subject including recent advances but also about how to write an answer within the limited frame of time in an examination. Dr Punit S Bhojani has done a wonderful job in his book *Exam Preparatory Manual for Undergraduates—Obstetrics and Gynecology*, where he has precisely addressed the above issues. The line drawings and flowcharts are simple and easy to reproduce in the answer paper.

I am sure this book will be of immense help to the students preparing not only for the undergraduate but also for the postgraduate examinations; and, it should also have a place in the libraries of the medical colleges.

I wish Dr Punit S Bhojani all the success with this book and in his future endeavors.

Geeta M Niyogi
Ex-Dean and Professor
Department of Obstetrics and Gynecology
KJ Somaiya Medical College,
Hospital and Research Centre
Mumbai, Maharashtra, India

FOREWORD

Every MBBS student approaches the university examinations with apprehension and anxiety. There is much to read and remember. The subject is vast and it is difficult to revise the entire syllabus on short notice. *Exam Preparatory Manual for Undergraduates—Obstetrics and Gynecology* fulfils the need of every undergraduate student who wishes to have a quick but thorough revision of the subject prior to the examinations. The book discusses various topics in a lucid and precise fashion.

Common questions asked in the papers are clubbed together and answers given. The diagrams are clear and easy to understand. The answers are written in a point-format, which makes them easy to remember.

Students will certainly like the format of the book as it will help them to approach the examinations with confidence.

Vinita S Salvi
MD DNBE FCPS DGO DFP (Obs & Gyne)
MPhil (Sports Science)
Consultant Obstetrician and Gynecologist
Ex-Professor and Unit Head
Seth GS Medical College and KEM Hospital
Ex-Officer In-charge
Indian Council of Medical Research
Mumbai, Maharashtra, India

FOREWORD

"If we encounter a man of rare intellect, we should ask him what books he reads."
—*Ralph Waldo Emerson*

For a student, a book is the most convenient form of collective human intellect and a teacher, allowing the readers to benefit from knowledge, work and understanding of experts in any selected field. It is the starting point of building one's own viewpoint and professional foundation. Today, there has been a veritable explosion in scientific information, which often leaves students preparing for an examination overwhelmed and confused.

This book *Exam Preparatory Manual for Undergraduates—Obstetrics and Gynecology* is formatted to address the special need of the undergraduate medical students. While it is particularly useful for preparing for the examinations, in my opinion, the information which is presented with clarity and lucidity could be of use to any practitioner of obstetrics and gynecology.

I have known Punit S Bhojani as a student and seen him grow and evolve into being an inspiring teacher and successful practitioner. He seems to have developed a deep understanding for the requirements of medical students and is passionate about teaching and imparting knowledge.

I wish the students reading this book the very best and hope that they achieve academic and professional success while also enjoying the journey.

Nozer K Sheriar
MD DNB FICOG FCPS DGO
Consultant Obstetrician and Gynecologist
Breach Candy Hospital, Hinduja Hospital
Holy Family Hospital and Masina Hospital
Mumbai, Maharashtra, India
Postgraduate Teacher for DNB

PREFACE TO THE THIRD EDITION

It gives me immense pleasure to present the third edition of *Exam Preparatory Manual for Undergraduates—Obstetrics and Gynecology*. A big thanks to all my readers for making the second edition a huge success and a highly popular book among the exam-going students. As per the feedback received, the second edition was extremely helpful for all university examinations.

The focus is to cover majority of the topics in the subject with an emphasis on how to present the answers in the examinations. Simple, yet highly effective, diagrams and flowcharts are presented, which the students will be able to reproduce in the examinations to secure higher marks and, thus, achieve success. Few important short notes and recent advances (including recent changes in the MTP ACT) have been added in the third edition.

This book is mainly targeted to the MBBS students. Even though this is not a substitute for the standard textbooks, I am pretty much confident that even the postgraduate students will find it extremely useful for rapid revision before their examinations.

Wishing you all the success for the final examinations and your postgraduate career!!

Punit S Bhojani

PREFACE TO THE FIRST EDITION

It gives me immense pleasure to present to you the first edition of the book *Exam Preparatory Manual for Undergraduates—Obstetrics and Gynecology*.

Ever since I started teaching the undergraduate students, I realized that there was a heartfelt need for a simplified, yet detailed, book devoted to the subject for the students of the final MBBS course.

The focus is to cover majority of topics in the subject with an emphasis on how to present the answers in the examinations. Simple, yet highly effective, diagrams and flowcharts are presented, which the students will be able to reproduce in the examinations to secure higher marks and, thus, achieve success.

Extreme care has been taken to authenticate each statement made in this book based not only on the undergraduate-level but also on the postgraduate-level textbooks.

The guidelines and recent advances are also covered, which are generally not taught to the undergraduate students.

This book is mainly targeted to the MBBS students. Even though this is not a substitute for the standard textbooks, but I am pretty much confident that even the postgraduate students will find it extremely useful for rapid revision before their examinations.

Suggestions, queries and corrections are always welcome. You can personally contact me at *drpunit@hotmail.com*.

Wishing you all the success for the final examinations and your postgraduate career!!

Punit S Bhojani

ACKNOWLEDGMENTS

Big thanks to Dr Radhika Sheth for contributing to the chapters on *Placental Functions*, *Male Infertility* and *Genital Tuberculosis*.

I take this opportunity to thank all my teachers for molding my career.

Very special thanks to my teachers Dr Geeta M Niyogi, Dr Vinita S Salvi and Dr Nozer K Sheriar, for writing the forewords.

Sincere thanks to all my dear students who have been a great motivational force.

I would like to thank my publishers M/s Jaypee Brothers Medical Publishers (P) Ltd, New Delhi, India, for their efforts and suggestions, especially Shri Jitendar P Vij (Group Chairman), Mr Ankit Vij (Managing Director), Mr MS Mani (Group President), Dr Madhu Choudhary (Director–Educational Publishing), Ms Pooja Bhandari (Director–Production), Ms Sunita Katla (Executive Assistant to Group Chairman and Publishing Manager), Ms Samina Khan (Executive Assistant to Director–Educational Publishing), Dr Aditya Tayal (Team Lead–UG Publishing), Mr Rajesh Sharma (Production Coordinator), Ms Seema Dogra (Cover Visualizer), Mr Laxmidhar Padhiary (Proofreader), Mr Akshay Thakur (Typesetter), Mr Gopal Singh Kirola (Graphic Designer) and their team members for their hard work.

Last but not least, I express profound sense of gratitude to my parents and my wife Dr Resham Bhojani, for their unconditional love, help and support, without whom this book would not have seen the light of the day.

LIST OF REFERRED BOOKS

1. *Williams Obstetrics*, 25th Edition
2. Speroff. *Clinical Gynecologic Endocrinology and Infertility*, 7th Edition
3. *TeLinde's Operative Gynecology*, 9th Edition
4. *Novak's Gynecology*, 14th Edition
5. Chaudhuri SK. *Practice of Fertility Control*, 7th Edition
6. Dutta DC. *Textbook of Obstetrics*, 10th Edition
7. Dutta DC. *Textbook of Gynecology*, 8th Edition
8. Callen. *USG in Obstetrics and Gynecology*, 4th Edition

IMPORTANT INSTRUCTIONS FOR THE STUDENTS

Please send me a Whatsapp message with your name on 09404634654 to get my guidance.
- Always structure and classify your answers
- Every answer should begin with introduction/definition
- Draw line diagrams and figures wherever possible
- Draw flowcharts wherever possible
- Answers should be to the point
- Do not write just to fill the pages
- Read this book throughout the year (and not only before the examinations)
- After reading this book first, read from the standard textbooks and then again read this book

Most important high-yield topics of this book (and frequently asked in the examinations) are as follows:

Gynecology	Obstetrics
Infertility	Preeclampsia and eclampsia
Contraception	Medical and surgical disorders
Prolapse	APH and PPH
Fibroids	Labor and malpresentations
Oncology	Ectopic pregnancy
Menstrual disorders	

- One short note of pediatrics is generally always asked in the obstetrics paper
- You can mail me your doubts on *drpunit@hotmail.com*.

Punit S Bhojani

LIST OF ABBREVIATIONS

ACOG	American College of Obstetricians and Gynecologists
A/W	Associated with
B/W	Between
BOH	Bad obstetric history
CPD	Cephalopelvic disproportion
DOC	Drug of choice
FHR	Fetal heart rate
FHS	Fetal heart sound
IUFD	Intrauterine fetal death
IUGR	Intrauterine growth restriction
LSCS	Lower segment cesarean section
MC	Most common
MSAF	Meconium-stained amniotic fluid
MSAFP	Maternal serum alpha-fetoprotein
NST	Nonstress test
O/E	On examination
PV	Per vaginam

CONTENTS

Chapter No.	Chapter Name	NMC Competency No.	Page No.
	Section 1: Gynecology		
1.	Infertility	OG28.1 to OG28.4	3
2.	Infections	OG27.1 to OG27.4	29
3.	Menstrual Disorders	OG25.1	45
4.	Fibroids	OG29.1	58
5.	Prolapse	OG 31.1	67
6.	Polycystic Ovarian Syndrome and Endometriosis	OG30.1, OG30.2	81
7.	Hysterolaparoscopy	OG34.4	91
8.	Oncology	OG33.1 to OG33.4, OG34.1 to OG34.4	96
9.	Contraception	OG21.1, OG21.2	119
10.	Miscellaneous	—	137
	Section 2: Obstetrics		
11.	Placental Functions and Physiological Changes	OG4.1, OG7.1	151
12.	Antenatal Care and Tests for Fetal Well-being	OG8.1 to OG8.8	157
13.	Labor	OG13.1 to OG13.5	167
14.	Malpresentations and Malposition	OG14.1 to OG14.4	180
15.	Abortions/Miscarriages	OG9.1 to OG9.3	190
16.	Ectopic Pregnancy	OG9.3	200
17.	Preeclampsia/Eclampsia	OG12.1	208
18.	Antepartum Hemorrhage and Postpartum Hemorrhage	OG10.1, OG10.2, OG16.1	221
19.	Medical and Surgical Disorders	OG12.1 to OG12.8	232
20.	Preterm, Intrauterine Growth Restriction and Postdatism	OG13.2	244
21.	Puerperal Sepsis	OG19.1	257
22.	Obstructed Labor and Rupture Uterus	OG14.3	264
23.	Vesicular Mole and Liquor Disorders	OG9.4	271
24.	Twins	OG11.1	280
25.	Induction of Labor and Operative Delivery	OG13.1, OG15.1, OG15.2	288

Chapter No.	Chapter Name	NMC Competency No.	Page No.
26.	Previous Lower Segment Cesarean Section/Vaginal Birth After Cesarean	OG8.2	297
27.	Miscellaneous	—	301
Section 3: Pediatrics Short Notes			
28.	Pediatrics Short Notes • Manual Method • APGAR Score • Asphyxia Neonatorum • Care of the Newborn at Birth • Causes of Convulsion in Neonate • Down Syndrome • Kernicterus • Neonatal Jaundice	OG18.1 to 18.4	325
Index			345

SECTION 1

Gynecology

Section Outline

1. Infertility
2. Infections
3. Menstrual Disorders
4. Fibroids
5. Prolapse
6. Polycystic Ovarian Syndrome and Endometriosis
7. Hysterolaparoscopy
8. Oncology
9. Contraception
10. Miscellaneous

CHAPTER 1

Infertility

Q. Define infertility. What are the causes of infertility?
Q. Causes of female infertility.
Q. Causes of male infertility.

DEFINITION
Infertility is defined as the failure to conceive after **one year** of **regular unprotected** intercourse.

INCIDENCE
10–20% of reproductive ages couples.

TYPES OF INFERTILITY
- **Primary:** Patient has never conceived.
- **Secondary:** Previous pregnancy but failure to conceive subsequently (irrespective of outcome of that pregnancy).

CAUSES OF INFERTILITY
- Male factor: 30–40%
- Female factor: 35–50%
- Both male + female factors: 20%
- Unexplained: 10%

Female Factors
- Ovarian: 30–40%
- Tubal and peritoneal factors: 30–40%
- Uterine: 5–10%
- Cervical: 5%
- Unexplained: 10–15%

Worldwide ovarian factors are the most common cause of female infertility, but in India tubal factors are equally or more common.

Ovarian Factors

- **Anovulation** *or* **oligo-ovulation:** Examples are **polycystic ovary syndrome (PCOS)**, ovarian failure (primary or secondary), thyroid dysfunction, adrenal dysfunction, hyperprolactinemia.
  WHO Category for Anovulation
     I: Hypothalamic pituitary failure
    II: Hypothalamic pituitary disturbance/PCOS
   III: Ovarian failure
   IV: Hyperprolactinemia
- **Diminished ovarian reserve or premature ovarian failure:** Increasing age leads to diminished ovarian reserve. Ovarian reserve means the quality and quantity of oocytes in the ovary.
  Causes of premature ovarian failure:
  - Idiopathic (unknown)
  - Genetic disorders (fragile X syndrome and Turner syndrome)
  - Autoimmune diseases (thyroiditis and Addison's disease)
  - Chemotherapy or radiation therapy
  - Metabolic disorders (e.g. galactosemia)
  - Toxins (such as cigarette smoke, chemicals, and pesticides)
  - Surgical alteration of ovarian blood supply
  - Savage syndrome (gonadotropin-resistant ovary syndrome)
  - Infections.
- **Luteal phase defect (LPD):** Inadequate function of corpus luteum leading to progesterone deficiency which hinders implantation. LPD is mainly due to defective folliculogenesis. PCOS, ovulation induction, thyroid dysfunction, hyperprolactinemia, endometriosis, and decrease in follicle stimulating hormone (FSH) and/or luteinizing hormone are important causes.
- **Luteinized unruptured follicle (LUF):** Ovum is trapped inside follicle which gets luteinized. It is along with hyperprolactinemia, endometriosis.

Tubal and Peritoneal Factors

Tubal obstruction/blocks due to:
- Pelvic inflammatory disease (PID); chlamydia, gonococci, etc.
- Genital tuberculosis
- Endometriosis
- Previous tubal surgery or sterilization
- Pelvic adhesions.

Uterine Factors (Prevent Implantation)

- Fibroids (submucous and intramural which distort the cavity)
- Polyps
- Endometritis especially tuberculosis
- Synechiae (Asherman's syndrome)

Chapter 1: Infertility

- Uterine hypoplasia
- Uterine anomalies (septate uterus, unicornuate uterus).

Cervical

- Cervical stenosis
- Prolapse
- Scanty cervical mucus
- Viscous or purulent discharge (chronic cervicitis)
- Antisperm antibody cervical mucus.

Vaginal

- Vaginal atresia
- Transverse vaginal septum.

Male Factors

- Pretesticular (hypothalamic-pituitary disorder): 1–2%
- Testicular disorder: 30–40%
- Post-testicular disorder (sperm transport problem): 10–20%
- **Idiopathic: 40–50% cases**

Pre-testicular	Testicular	Post-testicular
Hypogonadotropic hypogonadism	Varicocele, orchitis, trauma, torsion	Obstruction (infection)
Idiopathic	Heat/irradiation/chemotherapy	Kartagener syndrome/Young syndrome
Kallmann syndrome (deficient gonadotropin-releasing hormone secretion associated with anosmia)	Bilateral cryptorchidism	Postvasectomy
Erectile dysfunction/ejaculatory failure	Klinefelter syndrome, Yq11 microdeletion	Congenital bilateral absent vas deferens (associated with cystic fibrosis)
	Idiopathic	Inguinal hernia repair (accidental damage to vas deferens)

Idiopathic variety is considered to be the most common cause of male infertility. Varicocele is the most common surgically correctable cause of male infertility.

I. Congenital

- *Undescended testes:* Spermatogenesis is affected because the scrotal temperature should be 1–2°F lesser than the body temperature
- Congenital absence of vas deferens
- *Kartagener syndrome:* Loss of ciliary function and sperm motility
- *Epispadias/hypospadias*: Failure to deposit sperms in the vagina.

II. Thermal Factors

Scrotal temperature is raised in conditions such as varicocele, big hydrocele, filariasis, tight undergarments, working in hot atmosphere.

III. Infection

- Mumps orchitis after puberty
- Chronic systemic illnesses such as bronchiectasis
- *Mycoplasma* or *Chlamydia trachomatis* or viral infection of seminiferous tubules or prostate depresses sperm count.

IV. General Factors

Chronic debilitating illnesses, malnutrition, heavy smoking, alcohol (inhibit spermatogenesis by suppressing Leydig cell function and gonadotropin levels).

V. Endocrine

- *Kallmann syndrome*: Deficient gonadotropin-releasing hormone (GnRH) secretion, hypogonadotropic hypogonadism associated with anosmia
- *Sertoli-cell-only-syndrome*: FSH is raised in idiopathic testicular failure with germ cell hypoplasia
- *Hyperprolactinemia*: Associated with impotence.

VI. Genetic

- Klinefelter syndrome (47 XXY)
- Yq11 microdeletion

These would lead to azoospermia or severe oligospermia.

VII. Iatrogenic

Radiation, cytotoxic drugs, cimetidine, beta-blockers, antihypertensives, anticonvulsants and antidepressants can hinder spermatogenesis.

VIII. Immunological

Antibodies against spermatozoal surface antigens clumping of spermatozoa after ejaculation.

IX. Obstruction of Efferent Ducts

Due to tuberculosis (TB), gonococcal infection, surgical trauma (herniorrhaphy, vasectomy), congenital (Young's syndrome).

X. Failure to Deposit Sperms High in the Vagina (Coital Problems)

- Erectile dysfunction
- Hypospadias
- Ejaculatory defect—premature, retrograde or absence of ejaculation.

XI. Errors in Seminal Fluid

- Low fructose
- High prostaglandin content
- High viscosity.

Factors Affecting Both Sexes

- Environmental and occupational factors
  - Male infertility has been associated with exposure to lead, other heavy metals, and pesticides
  - Excessive radiation can also damage the germinal cells in both
- Smoking, recreational drugs and alcohol have been associated with infertility in both males and females
- Exercise: Compulsive heavy, over strenuous exercise is deleterious and leads to ovulatory disorders and luteal phase dysfunction and can cause oligospermia in males
- Inadequate diet associated with extreme weight loss or gain:
  - Weight has an impact on fertility at either extreme
  - Weight loss associated with anorexia nervosa or bulimia induces hypothalamic amenorrhea
  - Obesity may be associated with anovulation and also has been associated with decreased sperm quality.

Q. Methods of diagnosing ovulation.

Various methods used to detect ovulation are:

Indirect methods
- Menstrual history
- Evaluation of end organ changes:
  - Basal body temperature (BBT)
  - Cervical mucus study
  - Vaginal cytology
  - Hormonal estimation
    - Serum (Sr) progesterone
    - Sr estradiol
    - Sr luteinizing hormone
    - Urinary luteinizing hormone
  - Endometrial biopsy
- Ultrasonography (USG) follicular study [transvaginal sonography (TVS) preferred]

Direct method
- Laparoscopy

Conclusive method
- Pregnancy

INDIRECT METHODS

Menstrual History

The following features are strong evidence of ovulation:
- Regular cycles
- **Mid-menstrual pain (ovulation pain—Mittelschmerz)** or excessive mucoid vaginal discharge or spotting
- Features of primary dysmenorrhea or premenstrual syndrome (PMS).

Evaluation of End Organ Changes

Basal Body Temperature (BBT)
- **Rarely done nowadays**
- **Biphasic pattern** of temperature variation in ovulatory cycle
- In anovulatory cycle there is no rise of temperature throughout the cycle.

Principle

Progesterone and norepinephrine both are thermogenic and therefore there would be rise in temperature following ovulation.

Procedure

The patient takes daily oral temperature in morning before rising out of bed.

Interpretation

The temperature is raised by 0.5–1°F (0.2–0.5°C) following ovulation and remains high throughout the second half of cycle and falls about 2 days prior to the next period—**'biphasic pattern'.**

There may be a drop in temperature of about 0.5°F before the rise and that almost coincides with luteinizing hormone surge or ovulation.

It helps in determining ovulation and helps the couple to determine the most fertile period.

Limitations
- BBT indicates ovulation retrospectively and cannot predict precisely with time.
- Rarely, ovulation has been observed though BBT is monophasic.

Cervical Mucus Study

From 7th to the 8th day of the menstrual cycle, a fern-like pattern of dried cervical mucus is seen. Disappearance of this fern-like pattern beyond twenty-second day of the cycle is suggestive of ovulation.

The fern pattern is due to sodium chloride. Progesterone causes dissolution of sodium chloride crystals and hence ferning will not occur.

Also following ovulation, there is **loss of Spinnbarkeit** present in the mid cycle.

Vaginal Cytology

Rarely done nowadays.

Maturation index shifts to left from preovulatory phase to the secretory phase due to the effect of progesterone. Single smear on day 25/26 reveals effect of progesterone if ovulation has taken place.

Hormonal Estimation
- **Serum progesterone:** Done on day 8 (<1 ng/mL) and **day 21 (>6 ng/mL) indicates ovulation.**
- **Serum estradiol:** It attains a peak rise about 24 hours prior to luteinizing hormone surge.

- **Serum luteinizing hormone:** Daily estimation at midcycle period can detect the luteinizing hormone surge. Ovulation occurs 36 after the onset of luteinizing hormone surge and 12 hours after the luteinizing hormone peak.
- **Urinary luteinizing hormone:** Luteinizing hormone kits are available. The patient does the test at home on daily basis. It is started 2–3 days before the expected surge. Ovulation occurs 14–26 hours of detecting urinary luteinizing hormone.

Endometrial Biopsy

Rarely done nowadays for the purpose of detecting ovulation.
- Endometrial sampling can be done on OPD basis with Pipelle
- Dilatation and curettage (D/C) reserved for cases if more sample needed (cases of suspected endometrial TB)
- **Done on 21st–23rd day of cycle** (contraception used in the cycle to prevent pregnancy)
- **Evidence of secretory endometrium** (progesterone action on estrogen primed endometrium) indicates ovulation
- **Subnuclear vacuolation is the earliest evidence (36–48 hours following ovulation).**

Sonography (Very Commonly Done)

- **Serial sonography (TVS, follicular study) can measure the Graafian/dominant follicle just prior to ovulation (18–20 mm).**
- It is very useful following ovulation induction for timing of intrauterine insemination (IUI)/planned relations and also for ovum pick up in *in vitro fertilization (IVF)*.
- **Collapsed follicle and free fluid in pouch of Douglas (POD) are features of recent ovulation.**
- Also, the endometrium in proliferative phase has triple stripe echotextural pattern and following ovulation under progesterone influence **endometrium becomes more hyperechoic and homogeneous, and continues to thicken during the luteal phase.**

■ DIRECT METHOD

Laparoscopy

- Only for the purpose of detecting ovulation, laparoscopy is almost never done.
- However, when it is done for evaluation of tubal or peritoneal factors or other indications, microscopic detection of ovum from aspirated fluid from POD or visualization of recent corpus luteum is the direct evidence of ovulation.

■ CONCLUSIVE METHOD

Pregnancy is the surest and conclusive evidence of ovulation.

Q. What is ovarian reserve? What are the tests for ovarian reserve?

■ INTRODUCTION

Female reproductive aging is a process in which over time, oocytes decrease in quantity and quality and do not regenerate.

Factors such as genetics, lifestyle, environment, and medical issues, including endometriosis, ovarian surgery, and chemotherapy, and radiation, can influence the quantity and quality of a woman's oocytes.

■ DEFINITION

The concept of 'ovarian reserve' defines a woman's **reproductive potential** as a function of the **number and quality of her remaining oocytes**.

The purpose is to assess the quality and quantity of the remaining oocytes in an attempt **to predict reproductive potential.**

■ TESTS

Available tests of ovarian reserve include biochemical markers (i.e., FSH, estradiol, anti-Müllerian hormone, and inhibin B) and ovarian ultrasound imaging (i.e., antral follicle count and ovarian volume). These screening tests have been best studied as predictors of IVF outcome, oocyte yield from ovarian stimulation and rate of pregnancy.

Test	Cutpoint
FSH (international units/L)	10–20
AMH (ng/mL)	0.2–0.7
AFC (n)	3–10
Inhibin B (pg/mL)	40–45
CCCT, day 10 FSH (international units/L)	10–22

Ovarian reserve testing should be performed for women **older than 35 years** who have not conceived after 6 months of attempting pregnancy and women at higher risk of diminished ovarian reserve, such as those with a history of **cancer treatment,** pelvic irradiation, those with medical conditions who were treated with gonadotoxic therapies; or those who had **ovarian surgery** for endometriomas and smokers.

Basal Follicle-Stimulating Hormone (Day 3 FSH)

With advancing reproductive age, basal serum FSH concentrations increase on day 2 or day 3 of the menstrual cycle.

High values (greater than 10–20 International units/L) are associated with diminished ovarian reserve and poor response to ovarian stimulation.

Basal Estradiol

The estradiol level is usually low (less than 50 pg/mL) on days 2–4 of the menstrual cycle. However, an elevated value (greater than 60–80 pg/mL) in the early follicular phase can indicate reproductive aging and hastened oocyte development. Through central negative feedback, a high estradiol level can suppress an elevated FSH concentration into the normal range, so the value of obtaining an estradiol level is that it allows the correct interpretation of a normal basal FSH level. Basal estradiol has low predictive accuracy for poor ovarian response and failure to conceive; therefore, this test should not be used in isolation to assess ovarian reserve.

Anti-Müllerian Hormone (AMH)

- Anti-Müllerian hormone is a glycoprotein produced by the **granulosa cells of primary, preantral, and antral follicles 2–6 mm in diameter; thus, it reflects the size of the primordial oocyte pool.**
- **Anti-Müllerian hormone test can be done on any day of a woman's cycle** unlike FSH level test, which has to be done on day 2 or 3 of the menstrual cycle.
  - As the number of ovarian follicles decreases with age, a concomitant decrease in AMH levels occurs
  - Undetectable and **low AMH levels (0.2–0.7 ng/mL) indicate diminished ovarian reserve.**

Inhibin B

Inhibin B is a glycoprotein hormone secreted primarily by preantral and antral follicles. The serum concentration of **inhibin B decreases with the age-related decrease in the number of oocytes**. Inhibin B has central negative feedback that controls FSH secretion; therefore, a decrease in inhibin B levels leads to increased FSH secretion and higher early follicular FSH levels.

Clomiphene Citrate Challenge Test

- The test is performed by measuring serum FSH on cycle day 3, administering 100 mg clomiphene citrate daily on cycle days 5–9, and again measuring serum FSH on cycle day 10.
- After taking the last dose of clomiphene, the **FSH level should return to a normal level by the next day—menstrual cycle day 10.**
- If the ovaries are not functioning normally, the **FSH level will still be elevated on day 10.**
- In women with a reduced number of ovarian follicles, lower estradiol and inhibin B production leads to less central negative feedback of FSH secretion and an elevated FSH level after clomiphene stimulation.
- Therefore, an elevated FSH level on day 10 of the clomiphene citrate challenge test is suggestive of diminished ovarian reserve.

ULTRASOUND EVALUATION OF OVARIAN RESERVE

Antral Follicle Count (AFC)

The AFC records the number of visible ovarian follicles (2–10 mm mean diameter) that are observed during transvaginal USG in the early follicular phase (cycle days 2–5). The number of antral follicles correlates with the quantity of remaining follicles. **A low AFC is considered 3–6 total antral follicles and is associated with poor response** to ovarian stimulation during IVF.

Ovarian Volume

Ovarian volume on TVS decreases with progressive follicular loss. Low ovarian **volume <3 mL** predicts poor response to ovarian stimulation during IVF.

Q. Tests for tubal patency.

■ INTRODUCTION

- ❖ Tubal and peritoneal factors account for 30–40% cases of female infertility.
- ❖ At least one fallopian tube should be structurally and functionally normal to achieve a pregnancy.

The anatomical patency of the fallopian tubes can be assessed by following tests:
1. Rubin's test (obsolete now)
2. Hysterosalpingography (HSG)
3. Saline infusion sonography (SIS)/saline infusion sonohysterography
4. Hysterosalpingo contrast sonography (HyCoSy)
5. Laparoscopy and chromopertubation
6. Falloposcopy
7. Salpingoscopy.

Rubin's Test/Insufflation Test

Obsolete now, not done

Principle

Entry of air or CO_2 into peritoneal cavity when pushed transcervically under pressure gives evidence of tubal patency.

When to do? In postmenstrual phase, 2 days after stoppage of bleeding.

Observation

Pressurized CO_2 is pushed through cervix into uterus via cannula. The test is considered positive and the tubes are patent if:
- ❖ Fall in pressure occurs when raised beyond 120 mm Hg
- ❖ Gas passes out of the tubes into the abdomen to produce hissing sounds that can be heard on auscultation
- ❖ It causes referred shoulder pain
- ❖ It gives false negative findings due to cornual spasm in one-third cases
- ❖ It cannot detect the site and side of block.

HSG (Short Note)

- ❖ HSG is a radiographic diagnostic study of the uterus and fallopian tubes to assess the uterine cavity and tubal patency **(Fig. 1.1)**
- ❖ Considered as the **first line/initial investigation** of choice for tubal factors.

Indications

HSG is helpful in detecting:
- ❖ **Tubal patency** in cases of infertility or following tuboplasty surgery. **It can detect the side and site of block**
- ❖ It can detect tubal pathologies like hydrosalpinges, salpingitis isthmica nodosa (SIN), and peritubal adhesions

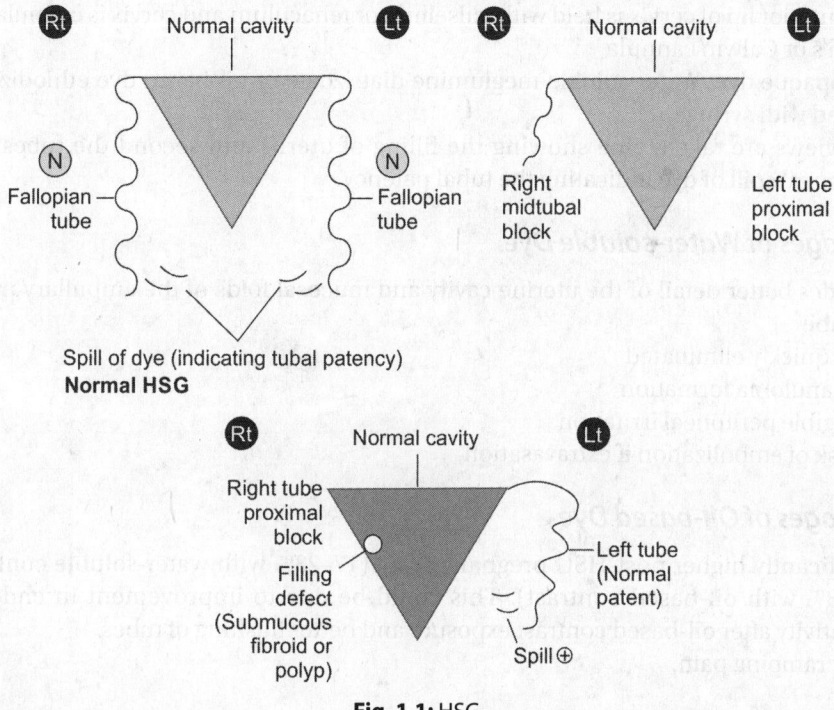

Fig. 1.1: HSG.

- Uterine cavity pathologies like polyps, submucosal leiomyomas (filling defects)
- Asherman's syndrome (intrauterine synechiae) multiple filling defects
- Müllerian anomalies like unicornuate/bicornuate/septate uterus or any variation in cavity shape like 'T' shaped uterine cavity
- After metroplasty operation (septal resection/lateral metroplasty for T-shaped uterus) to verify the success of surgery.

When is it done?

The procedure should be performed on day 8 or day 9 of the menstrual cycle to ensure that the patient is not pregnant and to prevent false-positive intrauterine filling defects and proximal tubal occlusion due to endometrial thickening and to avoid radiation to the ovum.

Pre-procedure

- Antibiotic prophylaxis: Doxycycline, 100 mg orally twice daily, beginning the day before the HSG and continuing for 5 days
- Consent taken
- Preprocedure atropine given; antispasmodics/pain killer advisable.

Steps

- Hysterosalpingography is performed by instilling radiopaque contrast into the uterine cavity while using fluoroscopy
- Performed in radiology department **without anesthesia** (major advantage over laparoscopy)

- The anterior lip of cervix is held with vulsellum or tenaculum and cervix is cannulated with Rubin's or Calwin cannula
- Radiopaque dye: Water soluble meglumine diatrizoate or oil-based dye ethiodized, oil is pushed with syringe
- Two views are taken: One showing the filling of uterus and second the tubes and the peritoneal spill of dye indicating the tubal patency.

Advantages of Water-soluble Dye

- Provides better detail of the uterine cavity and mucosal folds of the ampullary portion of the tube
- More quickly eliminated
- No granuloma formation
- Negligible peritoneal irritation
- No risk of embolization if extravasation.

Advantages of Oil-based Dye

- Significantly higher post-HSG pregnancy rate (17–23% with water-soluble contrast and 24–38% with oil-based contrast). This could be due to improvement in endometrial receptivity after oil-based contrast exposure and better flushing of tubes.
- Less cramping pain.

Contraindications

Absolute contraindications to the procedure:
- Known contrast allergy
- Pregnancy
- Active pelvic infection.

Complications (Rare)

- Pelvic pain
- Vasovagal reaction with bradycardia and hypotension, potentially resulting in syncope
- Flair up of pelvic infection
- Allergic reaction to the dye
- Extravasation of dye may result in embolism with an oil contrast agent.

Hysterosalpingography has sensitivity and specificity of **65% and 85%,** respectively, for fallopian tube assessment and sensitivity and specificity of approximately **80%** incorrectly identifying uterine cavity pathology with both false-positive and false-negative rates approximately 10–20%.

Saline Infusion Sonography (SIS)

Steps

- A transcervical catheter with balloon or pediatric Foley's catheter is placed in uterine cavity and balloon inflated at the level of ostium.
- Saline is injected into the uterine cavity.
- The cavity is evaluated for filling defects.

Chapter 1: Infertility

- Finally, small amount of air bubbles are injected to assess tubal patency.
- USG can follow the fluid through the tubes into the POD indicating tubal patency.

When to Do?

- The SIS should be performed during cycle days 6–10 (like HSG) as the endometrium is thin, allowing better detection of intrauterine lesions. In addition, this ensures that an undiagnosed pregnancy is not disrupted.
- Antibiotic prophylaxis: Same as HSG.
- If the patient has a history of genital tract infection or pelvic inflammatory disease, antibiotics may be given before the procedure. If hydrosalpinges are noted, antibiotics are given after the procedure.

Advantages

- It provides a simple and inexpensive means by which to evaluate the uterine cavity and assess tubal patency.
- It is well-tolerated and can be done in the OPD.
- Additionally, it **eliminates the risks associated with the use of dye and radiation required by the HSG**.
- Saline infusion sonography has been shown to reveal a substantial percentage of infertile patients with intracavitary abnormalities like synechiae or polyps (superior to HSG) and uterine anomalies.

While the SIS can confirm tubal patency, it does not provide information about the contour of the tubes. Thus, if a patient has a history of endometriosis or other tubal disease, an HSG would be preferred.

Hysterosalpingo Contrast Sonography (HyCoSy)

- It is an effective tool for tubal patency and uterine cavity evaluation.
- It is considered safe, well-tolerated, rapid, easy to perform, and inexpensive.
- HyCoSy is a transvaginal sonography in which a galactose solution containing galactose microbubbles is injected into the uterine cavity using a cervical catheter.
- Studies have shown that HyCoSy displays high specificity and sensitivity in tubal patency and uterine cavity assessment.

Laparoscopy and Chromopertubation (with a methylene blue dye)

- It is the **gold standard (definitive) method** for evaluation of tubal and peritoneal factors for infertility.
- It is also the investigation of choice for diagnosing endometriosis.
- It is both diagnostic and therapeutic.
- It is generally combined with hysteroscopy to evaluate the uterine cavity.

Steps

Generally done **postmenstrually**.

- Laparoscope is introduced into the peritoneal cavity to view the pelvic structures (uterus, tubes, ovaries, POD).

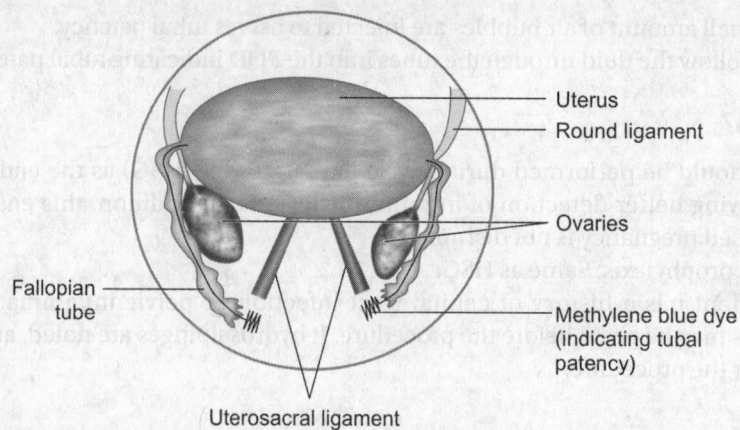

Fig. 1.2: Laparoscopy and chromopertubation.

- Methylene blue dye is injected into the uterus through the cervix. The dye passes through the tubes into the peritoneal cavity and can be seen coming out of the fimbrial end indicating tubal patency (spill of the dye) **(Fig. 1.2)**.
- Thus, the side and the site of the block are visualized.

In infertile patients, laparoscopy **(diagnostic)** can evaluate:
- **Tubes:** Tubal blocks, tubal patency (with chromopertubation), peritubal adhesions, hydrosalpinges, genital tuberculosis
- **Uterus:** Uterine anomalies, fibroids
- **Peritoneal factors:** Endometriosis, adhesions, PID
- **Ovaries:** PCOD, chocolate cyst of endometriosis.

Therapeutic: In the same sitting
- **Tubes:** Adhesiolysis, tuboplasty, tubal ligation (TL) reversal
- **Uterus:** Myomectomy
- **Ovary:** Cystectomy, oophorectomy, cyst aspiration, laparoscopic electrocoagulation of the ovarian surface (LEOS) for PCOS
- **Endometriosis.**

Indications
- Abnormal HSG
- Failure to conceive after reasonable period (6 months) of normal HSG
- Unexplained infertility
- Suspected endometriosis, chronic PID
- Infertility with advanced age (>35 years).

Falloposcopy
- Very rarely performed.
- A flexible microendoscope (through the hysteroscope) is inserted into the tube through its uterine opening to study the lumen of entire length of tube.
- Initially a hysteroscope is introduced into the uterus to identify the proximal tubal ostium. Once the ostium is identified the falloposcope can be inserted through the operative channel of the hysteroscope and advanced.

Chapter 1: Infertility

- The patient needs general anesthesia or conscious sedation.
- Obstructions, adhesions, polyps within the tubal canal, and debris can be identified.
- Complication: Fallopian tube perforation.

Salpingoscopy

- Very rarely done.
- Tubal lumen is studied introducing a rigid endoscope through the fimbrial end of the tube. It is performed through the operative channel of a laparoscope.

Q. Evaluation of uterine factors of infertility.

INTRODUCTION

Uterine factors are responsible for around 10% cases of female infertility.

Uterine factors (prevent implantation) which can lead to infertility or recurrent pregnancy loss are:

- Fibroids (submucous and intramural which distort the cavity)
- Polyps
- Endometritis especially tuberculosis
- Synechiae (Asherman's syndrome)
- Uterine hypoplasia
- Uterine anomalies (septate uterus, unicornuate uterus).

EVALUATION

- Ultrasonography (USG)
    - USG imaging is an effective, easy to use, safe, and readily available noninvasive method. Three-dimensional USG is also now available
    - It can detect **fibroids, polyps, uterine anomalies**
    - Also, it can measure **endometrial thickness (ET) and vascularity** which is very important factor for implantation
    - Endometrium in proliferative phase has **triple stripe echotextural pattern** (estrogenic action) and following ovulation under progesterone influence endometrium becomes more hyperechoic and homogeneous, and continues to thicken during the luteal phase.
- HSG: As in previous answer.
- SIS: As in previous answer
- Hysterosalpingo contrast sonography (HyCoSy): As in previous answer
- Laparoscopy can evaluate the uterus from outside and is helpful in cases of intramural fibroids, uterine anomalies (unicornuate/bicornuate uterus). **It cannot diagnose intracavitary pathology and septate uterus.**
- Hysteroscopy:
    - **Most useful investigation to evaluate any intracavitary pathology**
    - It is both diagnostic and therapeutic
    - Increases accuracy in diagnosing the cause of intrauterine filling defects detected on HSG
    - Intracavitary lesions (fibroids, septum, and adhesions) implicated as causes of infertility can be visualized and treated
    - In unexplained infertility, hysteroscopy may be performed simultaneously with laparoscopy to evaluate the uterine cavity.

Indications of Therapeutic/Operative Hysteroscopy

For all intracavitary pathologies **hysteroscopy is the gold standard for treatment.**
- **Polyps and fibroids:** Endometrial polyps and submucous fibroids are known to cause infertility and can be removed with hysteroscopy (polypectomy, myomectomy)
- Intrauterine adhesions: Asherman's syndrome
- Are often associated with amenorrhea or infertility
- Hysteroscopy is the gold standard used to diagnose and treat these adhesions. Benefits include visually directed lysis of adhesions
- **Lateral wall Metroplasty** in cases of T-shaped uterus and **septal resection** in cases of septum
- It can also help in taking endometrial biopsy for genital TB (histopathology and TB-PCR).

Q. Evaluation of male partner in an infertile couple.

INTRODUCTION

Infertility is defined as the failure to conceive after one year of regular unprotected intercourse. Male is directly responsible in 30–40% of cases and both male and female could be responsible in about 20% cases.

DETAILED HISTORY

- Age, duration of marriage, any previous marriage and proven fertility to be enquired
- Medical history including history of sexually transmitted diseases (STDs), infections such as **mumps orchitis** after puberty, TB, recurrent chest infection **(Young's syndrome)**, diabetes
- *Any recent febrile illness* (can depress spermatogenesis up to 6 months)
- H/o surgeries, e.g. herniorrhaphy, operation on the testis, genital area (orchidopexy, scrotal, urethral surgery, retroperitoneal surgery)
- Undescended testes, testicular trauma or torsion
- *Occupational history*: To note if there is excessive exposure to heat/radiation or h/o chemotherapy or radiotherapy
- Sexual history: Erectile or ejaculatory dysfunctions, frequency of coitus
- Impotence, loss of libido, diminution in beard growth and decrease frequency of shaving are suggestive of testosterone deficiency
- Use of any antiandrogen drugs (cimetidine, spironolactone) or anabolic steroids
- Headache, visual disturbances, galactorrhea (pituitary tumors, hyperprolactinemia) and anosmia (Kallmann's syndrome)
- History of addictions: smoking, alcohol.

PHYSICAL EXAMINATION

General

- Body proportions
- Beard growth
- Anosmia
- Gynecomastia

Penile Examination

- Urethral meatus
- Ulcers/discharge
- Scars

Scrotal/Testes

- Testes volume **(Prader orchidometer). Average testicular volume = 18 mL (range 12–30 mL)**
- Small testes indicative of pre-testicular or testicular causes
- In pretesticular causes testes size generally is 5–12 mL with soft consistency
- Consistency of testes [in **Klinefelter's syndrome (KF) syndrome small, firm testes, <3 mL each**]
- Position
- Presence of varicocele.

Epididymal

- Nodules/irregularity
- Tenderness
- Palpable cystic distention of caput epididymis (Bayle's sign) indicates epididymal obstruction.

Vas Deferens

- Presence/absence
- Nodules/irregularity
- Tenderness.

INVESTIGATIONS

1. Routine Tests

Blood sugars
- Thyroid stimulating hormone (TSH)
- Urinalysis

2. Semen Analysis

The first and the most important investigation (asked as a separate short note).

Methods of Semen Collection

- Masturbation and collecting the sample into a sterile container. This is the most common way to collect a semen sample
- Sexual intercourse in a special type of condom known as a collection condom (made from silicone or polyurethane, as latex is somewhat harmful to sperm). Such samples are inferior to the ones collected by masturbation in clean cup

- Coitus interruptus (withdrawal). The man removes his penis from his partner near the end of intercourse and ejaculates into a wide-necked container
- Sample sent to laboratory as soon as possible
- Penile vibratory stimulation and electroejaculation are two other alternatives for men with an ejaculation due to spinal cord injury.

The ideal specimen for examination is after **3–5 days of abstinence**. More prolonged period does not yield better results.

Accepted Reference Values for Semen Analysis (WHO, 2010)

	Reference value
Ejaculate volume	1.5 mL or more
pH	7.2–7.8
Sperm concentration	15 million/mL (20 million/mL is the old criteria)
Motility (within 1 hour of collection)	
Total motility (progressive + nonprogressive)	40% or more (50% or more is old criteria)
Progressive motility	32% or more
Normal morphology	4% or more (70% or more old criteria)
Vitality (live spermatozoa)	58% or more
Leukocytes	Less than 1 million/mL
Viscosity	<2 cm thread post-liquefaction

Recent Advances

WHO 2020 Semen Analysis Values

Comparing 2010 and 2020 WHO manual semen analysis:

Semen parameters	WHO 2010	WHO 2020
Semen volume	1.5 mL	1.4 mL
Sperm concentration	15 million/mL	16 million/mL
Total motility	40%	42%
Progressive motility	32%	30%
Viability	58%	54%
Morphology (normal forms)	4%	4%

Abnormal Semen Analysis (Nomenclature)

- Aspermia: Absence of semen
- Azoospermia: Zero sperm count
- Asthenospermia: Less than 42% motile spermatozoa
- Oligozoospermia: Count less than 16 million/mL
- Teratospermia: Less than 4% normal forms
- Necrozoospermia: Dead or immobile sperms
- Oligoasthenoteratospermia: Disturbance in all three variables.

3. Hormonal Evaluation

Serum FSH, luteinizing hormone, testosterone, prolactin, TSH.
- Testicular dysfunction causes an increase in FSH and luteinizing hormone.
- Serum FSH level estimation helps determine the site of pathology:
    1. A very high FSH would indicate a **testicular cause**
    2. A very low FSH would indicate pretesticular (hypothalamic/pituitary) cause
    3. A **normal FSH** would indicate a **post-testicular** cause.
        - Low FSH and luteinizing hormone are seen in hypogonadotropic hypogonadism
        - Low testosterone, high luteinizing hormone are noted in Leydig cell dysfunction
        - Elevated prolactin may be seen in pituitary adenoma leading to impotency.

4. Fructose Content in Seminal Fluid

Absent fructose suggests congenital absence of seminal vesicles or part of ductal system or both.

5. Testicular Biopsy

- Done in cases of azoospermia to differentiate testicular failure from post-testicular pathology. The tissue to be sent in Bouin's solution and not in formol saline.
- The testicular tissue may be cryopreserved for future intracytoplasmic sperm injection (ICSI).

6. TRUS (Transrectal Ultrasound)

To visualize the seminal vesicles, prostate and ejaculatory ducts obstruction.

Indications for TRUS

- Azoospermia
- Severe oligospermia with normal testicular volume
- Abnormal digital rectal examination
- Ejaculatory duct abnormality (cysts, dilatation).

Distention of seminal vesicles on TRUS is suggestive of ejaculatory duct obstruction.

7. Scrotal Ultrasonography

It is used to evaluate the anatomy of the testis, epididymis, and spermatic cord. It is a useful adjunct for evaluating testicular volume, testicular and paratesticular masses, and color Doppler for the presence or absence of varicoceles.

8. Vasogram

Radiographic study to evaluate ejaculatory duct obstruction. Mostly replaced by TRUS.

9. Chromosome and Genetic Analysis

- To be done in cases of azoospermia with testicular causes (raised FSH)
- **Klinefelter's syndrome** (XXY) is the most common abnormality

- ❖ **Yq11 microdeletions** (microdeletions in long arm of Y chromosome) can also be detected (male children of these men will carry same microdeletions and exhibit infertility in adulthood).

10. Sperm Function Tests

- ❖ In selected case, biochemical tests of creatine phosphokinase (CPK) and reactive oxygen species (ROS) are done as sperm function tests.
- ❖ CPK helps in sperm transport and ROS interfere with sperm function.

Q. Various treatment options for male infertility.

Q. ART (IUI, IVF, ICSI).

■ INTRODUCTION

Male is directly responsible in 30–40% of cases of infertility and both male and female could be responsible in about 20% cases.
- ❖ The treatment will depend on the cause and the semen analysis report.
- ❖ The treatment is often difficult and unsatisfactory.

■ TREATMENT

General

Lifestyle Modification

- ❖ **Improvement in general health, weight loss in cases of obesity,** and patients should be encouraged to **stop smoking cigarettes** and alcohol and to limit environmental exposures to harmful substances and/or conditions
- ❖ **Control of sugars in cases of diabetes mellitus and correction of thyroid disorders if present**
- ❖ Stress-relief therapy and consultation of other appropriate psychological and social professionals may be advised
- ❖ Infections should be treated with appropriate antimicrobial therapy.

Specific

Impotence

- ❖ Psychosexual treatment may help
- ❖ Dopamine agonist (**cabergoline, bromocriptine**) in cases of hyperprolactinemia
- ❖ **Sildenafil 50–100 mg or tadalafil (10–20 mg)** is recommended one hour before sexual activity
- ❖ In unresponsive cases IUI can be done.

Retrograde Ejaculation

- ❖ Phenylephrine (alpha-agonist) to improve the tone of internal urethral sphincter
- ❖ **Postejaculatory urine sample** can be used to recover the sperms and **IUI** can be done.

Chapter 1: Infertility

Hypogonadotropic Hypogonadism

The following is tried with varying success:
- **Injection HCG** 5,000 IU, IM given once or twice a week (to increase endogenous testosterone production)
- **Injection HMG or FSH** (75–150 IU) twice or thrice a week is added if no response
- **Pulsatile GnRH** therapy is also helpful especially in cases of Kallman's syndrome. It is given by minipumps infusion
- **Clomiphene citrate**: 25 mg once a day for 2–3 months increases FSH, luteinizing hormone and testosterone and can increase the sperm count.

Hypergonadotropic Hypogonadism/Testicular Failure

- Medical treatment has no role
- Treatment options include (depending on the sperm count)
- IUI
- IUI-donor [artificial insemination donor (AID)]
- IVF/ICSI
- Adoption.

Genetic Abnormality

In cases of genetic abnormality like KF syndrome, Yq11 microdeletions, Sertoli-cell-only syndrome, testicular atrophy, the only options are:
- AID
- Adoption

Medical Management

In cases of oligoasthenospermia due to idiopathic causes, various medical management can be tried with variable success.

The following are thought to improve sperm count/motility:
- Antioxidants like astaxanthin
- Multivitamin (specially vitamin E and C)
- Coenzyme Q
- Levocarnitine
- Zinc, selenium
- Glutathione
- L-arginine.

Clomiphene citrate: 25 mg once a day for 2–3 months increases FSH, luteinizing hormone and testosterone and can increase the sperm count.

   IUI or IVF (depending on the count) will be needed in cases where the medical management fails.

Surgeries

Varicocele
- Varicocele is the most common surgically correctable cause of male infertility
- Successful surgery results in improvement in semen parameters in 60–70% of patients

- ❖ The repair also typically halts further testicular damage and improves Leydig cell function
- ❖ Semen analysis may show improvement as early as the 3-month follow-up visit.

Obstruction of Vas or Epididymis

In cases with normal FSH and azoospermia, i.e., post-testicular pathology:
- ❖ Microsurgery: Vasoepididymostomy or vasovasostomy
- ❖ Patency can be obtained in up to 80% cases and pregnancy rate is 50%.

Transurethral Resection of the Ejaculatory Ducts

Patients with a known or suspected obstruction of the ejaculatory ducts may be eligible for transurethral resection of the ejaculatory ducts (TURED), which improves semen quality in these patients.

Assisted Reproductive Technology (ART)

ART encompasses all procedures that involve manipulation of gametes and embryos outside the body for treatment of infertility.

It mainly includes:
- ❖ IUI
- ❖ IVF-ET
- ❖ ICSI

Gamete intrafallopian transfer (GIFT) and zygote intrafallopian transfer (ZIFT) are no longer done.

1. IUI (Intrauterine Insemination)

Mainstay treatment and most commonly used treatment for male infertility.

Indications:
- ❖ Male factor infertility (sperm counts between 5 million/mL and 15 million/mL). **If sperm count is less than 5 million/mL, IUI is ineffective**
- ❖ Unexplained infertility (treatment of choice is superovulation plus IUI)
- ❖ Antisperm antibody in cervical mucus
- ❖ Erectile dysfunction or impotency
- ❖ Semen deposition problem (epispadias/hypospadias/penile deformities)
- ❖ Vaginismus
- ❖ Retrograde ejaculation (immediate postcoital urine is collected. Semen is then separated from urine)

Patent fallopian tube is prerequisite. Fallopian tubes have to be patent for IUI to be successful. If fallopian tubes are blocked, IUI should not be done.

Procedure:
- ❖ In IUI, the semen sample is washed or prepared (swim-up technique/swim-down technique/density gradient technique).
- ❖ The dead sperms or debris and immotile sperms are removed; only highly motile good-quality sperms are taken in the catheter.
- ❖ 0.5–0.7 mL washed sample is injected into the uterine cavity at the time of ovulation.
- ❖ Follicular study is done and injection HCG 5,000 IU, IM is given when the dominant follicle is **18–20 mm**.
- ❖ Intrauterine insemination is generally done 36 hours after HCG injection.

- The success of IUI in one cycle is about 15–20%. Total 3–6 cycles may be needed (50–60% success).

IUI with donor semen is done in cases of:
- Genetic disorders
- Azoospermia due to testicular causes (sperms not available at all for ICSI)
- Oligoasthenospermia requiring IVF/ICSI in nonaffording patients.
  - The donor should be healthy with same blood group and ethnic group as the husband
  - Free from venereal diseases including human immunodeficiency virus (HIV) and hepatitis
  - Consent of both the partners is required.

If the sperm count is less than 5 million/mL, the options are:
- IVF/ICSI
- IUI-D (donor) in patients not affording IVF/ICSI
- Adoption

2. In vitro Fertilization and Embryo Transfer (IVF-ET)

Indications:
- Tubal pathology/blocks
- Male factor: Count less than 5 million/mL
- More than or equal to 6 IUI failures
- Unexplained infertility
- Ovarian failure (donor oocyte IVF)
- Surrogacy.

Basic Steps of IVF:
- Ovarian stimulation with gonadotropins and follicular monitoring
- Oocyte retrieval (ovum pickup) done through TVS—guided needle
- *Fertilization*: 50,000 sperms are put on each oocyte retrieved
- Embryos kept in incubator for 48–72 hours
- Embryo transfer done on day 2 or day 3 (48–72 hours) after oocyte retrieval
- Generally 2–4 embryos are transferred in the uterine cavity via catheter and deposited 1 cm below the fundus
- Success rate of IVF per cycle is 35–40%.

3. Intracytoplasmic Sperm Injection (ICSI) (micromanipulation)

Indications:
- Severe oligoasthenoteratospermia
- Azoospermia (provided testes are producing sperms)
- Repeated fertilization failure in IVF

The steps are identical to IVF (oocyte retrieval and embryo transfer), but for fertilization, one sperm is mechanically injected into one oocyte.

Success rate of ICSI per cycle is 35–40%.

Sperm retrieval techniques in case of azoospermia before doing ICSI:
- PESA= percutaneous epididymal sperm aspiration
- MESA= microscopic epididymal sperm aspiration
- TESA= testicular sperm aspiration
- TESE= testicular sperm extraction (testicular biopsy).

Q. Treatment of female infertility.

■ INTRODUCTION

Female factor accounts for 35-50% cases of infertility and in 20% cases both partners have a problem.

■ TREATMENT

General

Lifestyle Modification

- **Improvement in general health, weight loss in cases of obesity**, and patients should be encouraged to **stop smoking cigarettes** and alcohol and to limit environmental exposures to harmful substances and/or conditions
- Control of sugars in cases of diabetes mellitus and correction of thyroid disorders if present
- Stress-relief therapy and consultation of other appropriate psychological and social professionals may be advised
- Infections should be treated with appropriate antimicrobial therapy.

Specific

Specific treatment depends on the cause of infertility.

Anovulation

Ovulation Induction (Medical and Surgical): Refer to PCOS answer.

Diminished Ovarian Reserve (DOR)

Options are:

- **Dehydroepiandrosterone (DHEA) 25 mg three times a day for 3 months** has been reported to improve pregnancy chances in patients with DOR.
- DHEA is a naturally existing hormone that the female body converts into androgens, mainly testosterone. Even though androgens are male hormones, they are essential in the female body for the production and development of healthy eggs.
- DHEA's beneficial effects on female fertility include:
  - Increased IVF pregnancy rates
  - Increased chance of spontaneous conceptions
  - Increased quality and quantity of eggs and embryos
  - Decreased risk of miscarriage and chromosomal abnormalities in embryos
  - Improved cumulative pregnancy rates in patients under fertility treatment.
- **IVF:** As in previous answer
- **IVF with donor oocyte**.

Luteal Phase Defect (LPD)

Progesterone gels or natural micronized progesterone 100-200 mg, 2-3 times a day vaginally or orally can be used from day of ovulation for 10-14 days.

If the patient conceives, it should be continued till 10 weeks of gestation.

Endometriosis

Refer to answer of endometriosis.

Tubal Factor

- ❖ Tuboplasty
- ❖ IVF (as in previous answer) if tuboplasty fails or is unsuccessful
- ❖ Adoption.

Tuboplasty Operation

Adhesiolysis (salpingo-ovariolysis)	Separation or division of adhesions
Fimbrioplasty	Separation of the fimbrial adhesions to open up the abdominal ostium
Salpingostomy	That creates a new opening at the abdominal ostium in a completely occluded tube. It is called **terminal or 'cuff' salpingostomy**. The eversion of the neo-ostium is maintained by few stitches of 6-0 Vicryl
Tubotubal anastomosis	When the segment of the diseased tube following tubectomy operation is resected and end to end anastomosis is done
Tubocornual anastomosis	When there is cornual block, the remaining healthy tube is anastomosed to the patent interstitial part of the tube

Cornual Cannulation

- ❖ 10–20% of all tubal blocks are in the proximal part of the fallopian tube.
- ❖ Management with IVF or microsurgical tubocornual anastomosis is more expensive, invasive, and less successful.
- ❖ Cornual cannulation can be one under fluoroscopy, USG or hysteroscopic guidance.
- ❖ With the introduction of operative hysteroscopy, **cannulation of fallopian tube ostia is now the procedure of choice to treat proximal tubal blocks.**
- ❖ Hysteroscopic proximal tube cannulation can be performed for proximal blocks and is generally accompanied with laparoscopy so that any distal tubal disease if present can be evaluated and simultaneously the tubal patency can be confirmed with chromopertubation.

Advantages:
- ❖ Laparotomy and IVF are avoided
- ❖ High success rates
- ❖ Day-care surgery
- ❖ Safe and highly cost effective.

Results: Hysteroscopic tubal cannulation can result in a **patency rate of up to 90%** in at least 1 tube and a pregnancy rate in the range of **50–60%**.

Reversal of Tubal Ligation

- ❖ The remaining length of the tube is one of the most important factors influencing reversal. The more the length, the more successful the results. **Minimum length of reconstructed tube should be 4 cm and the ampullary part should be at least 2 cm**.
- ❖ Isthmo-isthmic anastomosis has maximum chance of success.
- ❖ Most suitable for reversal is clips followed by silastic bands.

- The patient should be informed of the 10 times higher chance of ectopic pregnancy (risk of ectopic pregnancy is 3–9%), with danger to the life of the woman herself, following the reversal procedure.

Results of microsurgical reconstructive surgery after sterilization procedures

Sterilization procedure	Term pregnancy (range%)
Spring-loaded clip	88 (75–100)
Ring occlusion (silastic bands)	75 (44–95)
Pomeroy ligation	59 (45–70)
Electrocoagulation	43 (26–58)

Uterine Factors

For all intracavitary pathologies hysteroscopy is the gold standard for treatment.
- **Polyps and fibroids:** Endometrial polyps and submucous fibroids are well-known to cause infertility and can be removed with hysteroscopy **(polypectomy, myomectomy)**.
- Intrauterine adhesions (Asherman's syndrome):
    - The intrauterine adhesions are often associated with amenorrhea or infertility.
    - **Hysteroscopy is the gold standard** used to diagnose and treat these adhesions. Benefits include visually directed lysis of adhesions.
    - After adhesiolysis an IUCD or pediatric Foley's catheter is inserted to keep the cavity distended to prevent recurrence. Oral contraceptive (OC) pills or estrogen and progesterone tablets are used for 1–3 months to regenerate the endometrium.
- **Lateral wall metroplasty** in cases of T-shaped uterus and **septal resection** in cases of septum.

Cervical Factors

- Cervical mucus quality can be increased by estrogen supplementation
- Also **N-acetyl cysteine** makes cervical mucus thin and improves sperm penetration
- Infections if any are to be treated
- **IUI** is very commonly used.

Unexplained Infertility

- **Superovulation + IUI** treatment of choice
- **IVF** in cases where the above treatment fails.

Immunological Factors

In cases of antisperm antibodies in cervical mucus: Steroids can be given to female and male partner can use condoms. However, the benefit is limited and so IUI is the preferred treatment.

In Cases of Normal Ovaries and Absent Uterus

Surrogacy (gestational surrogacy = IVF surrogacy)

Examples:
- Congenital absence of the uterus [Mayer-Rokitansky-Küster-Hauser (MRKH) syndrome]
- Postpartum hysterectomy
- Hysterectomy done for any reasons (cancer, menorrhagia, etc.)
- TB endometritis with dense intrauterine adhesions.

CHAPTER 2

Infections

Q. Describe the pathogenesis, clinical features management and treatment of genital tuberculosis.

Q. Genital tuberculosis.

■ INCIDENCE

Genital tuberculosis (TB) is seen in 1% of outpatients in developing countries. About 5-10% of patients with infertility have genital TB.

■ PATHOGENESIS

Causative organism: *Mycobacterium tuberculosis* (human type):
- ❖ It is **almost always secondary** to primary infection in extragenital sites like lungs (most common), lymph nodes, urinary tract or bones and joints.
- ❖ In the genital tract, the **fallopian tubes are usually the first and most common to get infected**.

Mode of Spread

- ❖ *Bloodstream:* It is the **most common route of spread**. In 90% of cases, the pelvic organs are involved by hematogenous spread from any primary site. If the postprimary hematogenous spread coincides with the growth spurt of puberty, the genital organs are affected. If the spread is earlier than the growth phase, the genital organs are spared. The infection remains dormant for 4-6 years before clinical features appear.
- ❖ *Lymphatic/direct:* The genital organs are involved directly or by lymphatics from infected organs like peritoneum, bowel or mesenteric lymph nodes.
- ❖ *Ascending (very rare):* Sexual transmission from a male with urogenital TB is possible in vulval, vaginal or cervical lesions.

Pathology of Pelvic Organs

Fallopian Tube (100% cases)

- ❖ **Most common organ involved.**
- ❖ **Ampullary part** most commonly affected.

The initial site of infection is the **submucosal part** of the ampullary part of the fallopian tube.
- The infection spreads medially along the wall to destroy the muscles which are replaced by fibrous tissue.
- The walls get thickened at times in segments, calcified or ossified.
- The infection may spread inwards; the mucosa gets edematous and destroyed.
- The fimbria gets everted. The elongated and distended distal tube with the patent abdominal ostium causes the appearance of '**tobacco pouch.**' At times, adhesions may cause occlusion of the ostium.
- The tubercles burst pouring caseous material inside the lumen producing tubercular pyosalpinx which many adhere to the ovaries and other adjacent structures. The infection may spread outwards producing **perisalpingitis** with exudation causing dense adhesions with the surrounding structures, thus forming a **tubo-ovarian mass (TO mass)**.
- At times, miliary tubercles may be seen on the serosal surface of the tubes, uterus, peritoneum or bowels. These are often seen with TB peritonitis.
- At times, the tubes may look normal or nodular at places. These nodules may be present in the isthmic part of the tubes due to proliferation of the tubal epithelium within the hypertrophied muscle layer. This is known as salpingitis isthmica nodosa (SIN). It is seen radiologically as a small diverticulum. SIN is also seen in pelvic endometriosis.

Uterus (60% cases)

- Second most common organ involved.
- The infection may spread from the tubes by lymphatic spread or directly through proximity.
- **Cornual endometrium** is commonly affected due to their dual blood supply as well as their anatomical proximity to the tubes.
- Infection starts from the basal endometrium and reaches the surface premenstrually and gets shed off with menses. Reinfection again starts from the basal layer of the endometrium.
- Endometrial ulceration may result in adhesions—*'Asherman's syndrome.'* This may lead to secondary amenorrhea, infertility and recurrent abortion.
- Rarely the infection spreads to the myometrium and if caseation occurs it may lead to pyometra.

Cervix (20% cases)

- Not commonly affected
- May be ulcerative or nodular type
- It may present as contact bleeding
- On gross appearance, it may appear like carcinoma (CA) cervix.

Vulva/Vagina: Rare (1%)

- The lesion may be ulcerative with undermined edges
- Rarely hypertrophic variety.

Ovary (30% cases)

It may present as surface tubercles, adhesions, capsular thickening or caseating abscess.

Pelvic Peritoneum (40–50% cases)

- TB peritonitis may be wet or dry

- Wet peritonitis presents with ascites (straw-colored fluid) and tubercles on peritoneal surfaces
- In the dry peritonitis, there are dense bowel adhesions due to fibrotic sequelae when the wet peritonitis heals.

■ MICROSCOPY

Granuloma consists of infiltration of **Langhan's cells**, chronic inflammatory and epithelioid cells surrounding a central area of **caseation necrosis**.

■ CLINICAL FEATURES

80% of the affected patients are of childbearing age (20–40 years). Genital TB occurs in 10–20% of patients who have pulmonary TB in adolescence.

Symptoms

- Many patients are **asymptomatic** and accidently detected during infertility work up.
- Infertility:
  - Most common presenting feature, present in 70–80% cases
  - It may be primary or secondary
  - It is mainly due to tubal blockage
  - Adhesions in endometrial cavity or ovulatory dysfunction also contribute.
- Menstrual abnormality: Menorrhagia → oligomenorrhea → secondary amenorrhea.
  - In early stages, menorrhagia due to ovarian involvement, pelvic congestion or endometrial proliferative lesion. It is a rare cause of puberty menorrhagia.
  - In later stages, oligomenorrhea and then secondary amenorrhea are common. This may be due to **endometrial destruction due to uterine synechiae formation** or ovarian suppression due to tuberculin toxin.
- Chronic pelvic pain: In 20–30% cases. Often associated with TO mass.
- Vaginal discharge: Cervical or vaginal TB along with postcoital bleeding or blood stained discharge
- Constitutional symptoms such as weight loss, fever, anorexia.

Signs

General: General health usually unaffected. May be low grade fever, anemia. There may be evidence of active or healed tubercular lesion.

Per abdomen: Negative findings or doughy feel due to matted intestines. TB ascites when encysted resembles an ovarian cyst.

Per vaginum: Negative findings in 50% cases.
- Vulval or vaginal ulcers with undermined edges
- Palpable thickened tubes felt through lateral fornices
- Pelvic masses
- Nodules through posterior fornix.

■ INVESTIGATIONS

- Blood: Increased erythrocyte sedimentation rate (ESR), leukocytosis.

- ❖ Mantoux test.
- ❖ Chest X-ray for healed or active pulmonary TB.
- ❖ Dilatation and curettage: **Preferably 1 week prior to menses.**

Endometrium to be sent in formalin for **histopathology** to detect the giant cell and caseation and in normal saline for: acid-fast bacilli (AFB) microscopy by **Ziehl-Neelsen stain, culture in Lowenstein-Jensen media.**

- ❖ **PCR:** Samples also send for detection of *M. tuberculosis* by polymerase chain reaction (PCR) for nucleic acid amplification. PCR is more sensitive (85–95%) than microscopy and culture. It can detect less than 10 organisms in specimens compared to 10,000 needed for smear positivity.
- ❖ Menstrual blood collected with a pipette and sent AFB stain/culture/PCR.
- ❖ Sputum and urine culture for TB bacillus.
- ❖ Biopsy from lymph nodes, lesions in the cervix, vagina or vulva.
- ❖ **In a proven case of tuberculosis, hysterosalpingography (HSG) is contraindicated** for the risk of reactivation and spread. But HSG done for routine work up of infertile female may reveal the following suggestive features **(Fig. 2.1)**:
  - ➢ Lead pipe tubes
  - ➢ Tobacco pouch appearance
  - ➢ Beaded tubes
  - ➢ Hydrosalpinx
  - ➢ Cornual blocks
  - ➢ Intravasation of the dye
  - ➢ Golf club tube
  - ➢ Sperm head tube

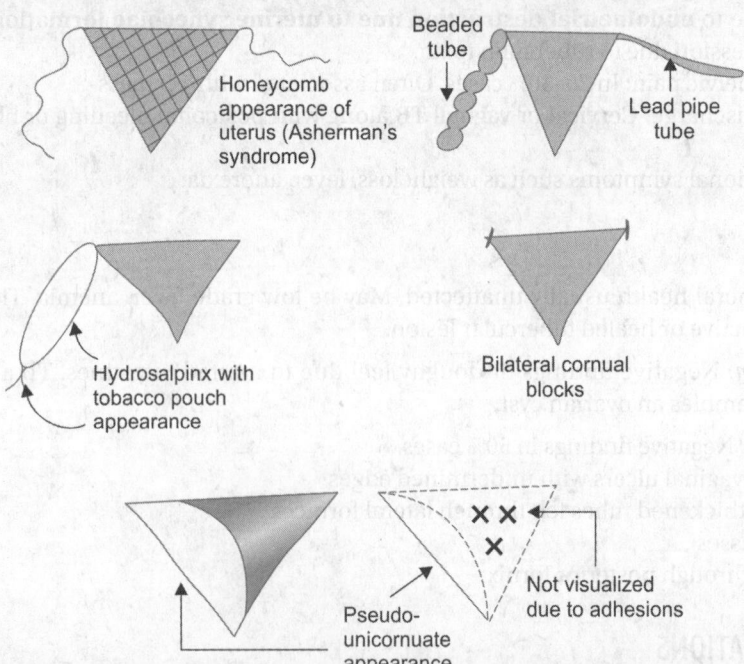

Fig. 2.1: Various hysterosalpingography (HSG) findings in case of genital TB.

- Uterus—honeycomb appearance (Asherman's syndrome)
- Pseudo-unicornuate appearance.
- ❖ Ultrasonography or computed tomography (USG/CT) scans in case of pelvic mass or ascites.
- ❖ **Laparoscopy:** If no endometrial evidence, laparoscopy may be done. This may reveal tubercles and beaded tubes and TO masses. Biopsy can be taken from peritoneal tubercles. Peritoneal fluid may be sent for culture and **adenosine deaminase (ADA) levels**.

DIFFERENTIAL DIAGNOSIS

- ❖ Pyogenic tubo-ovarian mass
- ❖ Pelvic endometriosis
- ❖ Adherent ovarian cyst
- ❖ Chronic ectopic pregnancy.

TREATMENT

General

Hospitalization only for active infection. Correction of anemia and healthy diet to improve resistance is essential. The husband should use a condom during active infection to prevent possibility of contracting urogenital TB.

Chemotherapy

Anti Koch treatment (AKT) is the treatment of choice.

As per RNTCP, GOI and WHO

A. **Initial phase:** Four drugs (2HRZE) are used daily for 2 months to reduce bacterial load. The drugs are as below:

Drug	Daily adult dose	Type	Toxicity	Points to note
Isoniazid	5 mg/kg max 300 mg	Bactericidal	Hepatitis, peripheral neuropathy	Add pyridoxine 50 mg/day, check liver function tests (LFTs)
Rifampicin	10 mg/kg max 600 mg	Bactericidal	Hepatitis, orange discoloration of urine, febrile reaction	Check LFTs, Avoid oral contraceptive pills (OCPs)
Pyrazinamide	20–25 mg/kg max 2 g	Bactericidal	Hepatitis, hyperuricemia, gastrointestinal (GI) upset, arthralgia	Check LFTs, active against intracellular dividing forms of *Mycobacterium*
Ethambutol	15–20 mg/kg max 2.5 g	Bacteriostatic	Optic neuritis, visual disturbances	Ophthalmoscopy prior to therapy

B. **Continuation phase:** Isoniazid, rifampicin and ethambutol (4HRE) are continued daily for 4 more months.

After 1 year of treatment, endometrium should be sampled. If histological or bacteriological examination is positive, the treatment must be continued further. If negative, it should be rechecked after 6 months. A patient may be considered cured if at least 2 histological reports come negative.

For Infertility

- Intrauterine insemination (IUI) should not be done as tubes are damaged
- In vitro fertilization (IVF) **after completion of AKT** is the treatment for infertility (provided the uterine cavity is normal)
- If the endometrium is cicatrized, then **IVF and surrogacy should be recommended.**

Surgical

Surgery is not routinely indicated.

Indications

- Unresponsive active disease despite adequate chemotherapy
- TB pyosalpinx, ovarian abscess or pyometra
- Chronic pelvic pain.

Surgery for restoration of fertility (corrective tuboplasty) is contraindicated in genital TB.

Contraindications

- Active TB in extragenital site
- Good response to AKT with decrease in size of pelvic mass
- Incidental finding of tubercular tubo-ovarian mass on laparotomy in young patient. After taking tissue for biopsy, the abdomen should be closed.

Surgery

- Total abdominal hysterectomy with bilateral salpingo-oophorectomy
- In young women, at least one ovary should be preserved
- In selected cases, isolated excision of tubo-ovarian mass, drainage of pyometra or fistula repair may be done.

■ PROGNOSIS

Pregnancy is rare (5–10%). If the patient conceives, there is 40% chance of ectopic pregnancy and high probability of spontaneous abortion. Higher pregnancy rates are noted with the help of assisted reproductive technology after completion of AKT (provided the uterine cavity is normal). If the endometrium is cicatrized, then IVF and surrogacy should be recommended.

Q. Describe the pathogenesis, clinical features and management of acute pelvic infection.

Q. Acute PID: Clinical features and treatment.

■ DEFINITION

Pelvic inflammatory disease (PID) is a spectrum of infection and inflammation of the upper genital tract involving the endometrium, fallopian tubes, ovaries, pelvic peritoneum and surrounding structures.

Chapter 2: Infections

■ INCIDENCE

One to two percent per year among sexually active women, 85% of these are spontaneous infections in sexually active women and the remaining 15% are due to procedures that favor ascending infection [e.g. procedures such as D and C, intrauterine contraceptive device (IUCD) insertion, hysterosalpingogram (HSG), etc]. Two-thirds of cases are seen in young women less than 25 years of age.

The incidence is on rise due to rise in sexually transmitted diseases (STDs).

■ RISK FACTORS

- Multiple sexual partners
- IUCD users
- Previous history of acute pelvic inflammatory disease (PID)
- High prevalence of STDs
- Surgical procedures like D/C, HSG
- Menstruating teenagers.

■ PROTECTIVE FACTORS

Contraception
- Barrier methods like condom and spermicidals containing nonoxynol-9 (bactericidal and viricidal)
- Oral contraceptive pills—they make the cervical mucus thick thereby preventing sperm ascent and bacterial penetration, also decrease in duration of blood flow, create shorter interval of bacterial colonization of the upper tract
- Women with monogamous partner who has had a vasectomy
- Pregnancy
- Menopause
- Azoospermic husband.

■ MICROBIOLOGY

Polymicrobial Ascending Infection

Primary Organisms—Sexually Transmitted

- *Neisseria gonorrhoeae*: 30%
- *Chlamydia trachomatis*: 30%
- *Mycoplasma hominis*: 10%.

Secondary Organisms

- Aerobic: Nonhemolytic *Streptococcus, Escherichia coli*, group B *Streptococcus* and *Staphylococcus*
- Anaerobic: *Bacteroides fragilis* and *bivius, Peptostreptococcus* and *Peptococcus*.

■ MODE OF AFFECTION

- *Gonococcus* ascends up to the tubes through mucosal contiguity and continuity, facilitated by vectors such as sperms and trichomonads

- Reflux of menstrual blood with gonococci into the fallopian tubes
- *M. hominis* spreads across the parametrium to affect the tube
- Secondary organisms affect the tube through lymphatics
- Direct infection from the gut.

■ PATHOLOGY

- Fallopian tubes are involved bilaterally
- The process initiated in endosalpinx
- Damage of cells and cilia and also invades in all layers of tubes
- Exudate pours in lumen, both the openings of tube are closed due to congestion and adhesions
- Exudate may be watery producing hydrosalpinx or purulent forming pyosalpinx
- Occasionally the exudate pours into abdomen → pelvic peritonitis or abscess or affects ovary → ovarian abscess.
- A tubo-ovarian mass or abscess is thus formed.

■ CLINICAL FEATURES OF ACUTE PID

Symptoms

Wide range of nonspecific symptoms:
- Symptoms usually appear at and immediately following menses
- Bilateral lower abdominal and pelvic pain, rapid and acute in gonococcal infection (3 days) than in chlamydial infection (5–7 days)
- Fever
- Irregular excessive vaginal bleeding (along with endometritis)
- Purulent or copious vaginal discharge (due to associated lower tract infection)
- Nausea, vomiting
- Dyspareunia
- Pain in right hypochondrium due to perihepatitis (Fitz-Hugh-Curtis syndrome). 5–10% cases of acute salpingitis liver is affected by transperitoneal or vascular spread.

Signs

- Rise of temperature more than 38°C
- Lower abdominal tenderness, liver may be enlarged and tender
- Purulent vaginal and cervical discharge, congested cervix
- Congested external urethral meatus or opening of Bartholin's duct, through which pus may be seen
- Tenderness on movement of the cervix (CMT+)
- Bilateral tenderness on fornix palpation
- Adnexal mass felt through fornices.

■ INVESTIGATIONS

Gram staining and culture (aerobic and anaerobic) of discharges. Discharges collected from:
1. Urethra, Bartholin's glands

2. Cervical canal
3. Fallopian tube (laparoscopy), cul-de-sac.
    - *Blood:* Leukocytosis more than 10,000/mm3 and **C-reactive protein (CRP) raised**, erythrocyte sedimentation rate (ESR) raised more than 15 mm/hour
    - Serological test for syphilis and other STDs in both partners
    - *Laparoscopy:* **Most reliable (gold standard)** but reserved only in nonresponding cases or in cases where differential diagnosis is acute appendicitis or ruptured ectopic or torsion or hemorrhage or rupture of ovarian cyst
        - The tubes would appear edematous and congested
        - Hydrosalpinx or pyosalpinx or TO mass may be seen
        - Exudates can be collected from fimbrial ends and pouch of Douglas (POD) for studies
        - **Violin string adhesions** in pelvis and around liver suggest chlamydial infections
        - **Endometrial biopsy** is warranted for women undergoing laparoscopy who do not have visual evidence of salpingitis because endometritis is the only sign of PID for certain women.
    - Culdocentesis with purulent fluid having white cell count more than 30,000/mL
    - *Sonography:* Dilated tubes, fluid in POD and tubo-ovarian mass, Doppler studies showing tubal hyperemia are suggestive of PID
    - *Male partner:* Smears and cultures from urethral secretions.

STAGES OF PID (GAINESVILLE)

Stage 1: Acute salpingitis without peritonitis
Stage 2: Acute salpingitis with peritonitis
Stage 3: Acute salpingitis with tubal occlusion or tubo-ovarian complex
Stage 4: Ruptured tubo-ovarian abscess
Stage 5: Tubercular salpingitis.

DIFFERENTIAL DIAGNOSIS

- Acute appendicitis
- Ruptured ectopic
- Torsion/hemorrhage/rupture of ovarian cyst
- Endometriosis
- Diverticulitis
- Urinary tract infection (UTI).

COMPLICATIONS

Immediate

- Pelvic peritonitis, pelvic abscess
- Septicemia, septic shock.

Late

- Chronic PID, pelvic adhesions and formation of tubo-ovarian mass
- Chronic pelvic pain

- Infertility (12% with one episode, 25% with 2 episodes and 50% with 3 episodes)
- Ectopic pregnancy (6–10 fold increase risk)
- Fitz-Hugh-Curtis syndrome
- Dyspareunia.

TREATMENT

- Adequate rest, analgesics and anti-inflammatory drugs to be prescribed
- Sexual partner also to be treated appropriately
- Antibiotics started even before the reports are available.

CENTERS FOR DISEASE CONTROL AND PREVENTION GUIDELINES FOR TREATMENTS OF PELVIC INFLAMMATORY DISEASES (2021)

Recommended Parenteral Regimens for Pelvic Inflammatory Disease

- Ceftriaxone 1 g IV every 24 hours
    PLUS
- Doxycycline 100 mg orally or IV every 12 hours
    PLUS
- Metronidazole 500 mg orally or IV every 12 hours
    OR
- Cefotetan 2 g IV every 12 hours
    PLUS
- Doxycycline 100 mg orally or IV every 12 hours
    OR
- Cefoxitin 2 g IV every 6 hours
    PLUS
- Doxycycline 100 mg orally or IV every 12 hours

After clinical improvement with parenteral therapy, transition to oral therapy with doxycycline 100 mg 2 times/day and metronidazole 500 mg 2 times/day is recommended to complete 14 days of antimicrobial therapy.

Alternative Parenteral Regimens

- **Ampicillin-sulbactam** 3 g IV every 6 hours
    PLUS
- **Doxycycline** 100 mg orally or IV every 12 hours
    OR
- **Clindamycin** 900 mg IV every 8 hours
    PLUS

Gentamicin loading dose IV or IM (2 mg/kg body weight), followed by a maintenance dose (1.5 mg/kg body weight) every 8 hours; single daily dosing (3–5 mg/kg body weight) can be substituted

Recommended Intramuscular or Oral Regimens for Pelvic Inflammatory Disease

- **Ceftriaxone** 500 mg IM in a single dose*
    PLUS
- **Doxycycline** 100 mg orally 2 times/day for 14 days
    WITH
- **Metronidazole** 500 mg orally 2 times/day for 14 days
    OR
- **Cefoxitin** 2 g IM in a single dose and **Probenecid** 1 g orally administered concurrently in a single dose
    PLUS
- **Doxycycline** 100 mg orally 2 times/day for 14 days
    WITH
- **Metronidazole** 500 mg orally 2 times/day for 14 days
    OR
- Other parenteral third-generation **cephalosporin** (e.g., ceftizoxime or cefotaxime)
    PLUS
- **Doxycycline** 100 mg orally 2 times/day for 14 days
    WITH
- **Metronidazole** 500 mg orally 2 times/day for 14 days

*For persons weighing >150 kg (~300 lbs.) with documented gonococcal infection, 1 g of ceftriaxone should be administered.

Indications of Inpatient Antibiotic Therapy

- Suspected pelvic abscess
- Severe illness, temperature >38°C
- Uncertain diagnosis—where surgical emergencies, e.g., ectopic pregnancy cannot be excluded
- Unresponsive to outpatient therapy for 48 hours
- Intolerance to oral antibiotics
- Coexisting pregnancy
- Patient is known to have HIV infection.

Indications for Surgery

- Generalized peritonitis
- Pelvic abscess (which does not respond to drainage and antibiotics)
- TO abscess (which does not respond to antibiotics).

To Prevent Reinfections

- Patient education (avoid multiple partners, use of condoms)
- Partner treatment.

The only unequivocal proof of successful treatment after salpingitis is an intrauterine pregnancy.

Q. Bacterial vaginosis or vaginitis (BV).

INTRODUCTION

Bacterial vaginosis (BV) is a common vaginal infection. **The term vaginosis is preferred over vaginitis as there is no vaginal inflammation.**

ETIOLOGY

In BV the number of the normal *Lactobacilli* (*Doderlein's bacilli*) decreases with simultaneous increase in concentration of other types of bacteria, especially anaerobic bacteria.

It is caused by an imbalance and decrease in the naturally occurring bacteria of the vagina.

The causative organisms which act synergistically are:
- *Gardnerella vaginalis*
- *Ureaplasma urealyticum*
- *M. hominis*
- *Peptococcus* and *Mobiluncus*.

CLINICAL FEATURES

- Moderate, malodorous, grayish white homogenous discharge, adherent to vaginal wall
- No evidence of vaginal inflammation.

DIAGNOSIS

- **Amsel's criteria** are used.
- **Any three out of four** should be present:
  1. Grayish white discharge
  2. Vaginal pH more than 4.7 (alkaline)
  3. **Drop of discharge mixed with 10% KOH = Fishy odor** (due to release of amines, acridine, and putredine) = **Whiff test**
  4. Smear prepared with normal saline: **Clue cells** (vaginal epithelial cells covered with *Coccobacilli and the cells appear as stippled or granular*). Clue cells are diagnostic of BV.

COMPLICATIONS OF BV IN PREGNANCY

- Preterm labor
- PROM (Premature rupture of membranes)
- Chorioamnionitis.

TREATMENT

- **Metronidazole** 400 mg thrice a day for 5–7 days is the drug of choice
- Locally clindamycin and metronidazole gel can be used
- **Probiotics** to be given to increase the number of *Lactobacilli* in the vagina
- **Lactic acid wash** to maintain the pH of vagina to prevent recurrence.

Q. Trichomoniasis

■ INTRODUCTION

Vaginal trichomoniasis is the most common and important cause of vaginitis in child bearing age period.

■ CAUSATIVE ORGANISM

Actively motile parasite *Trichomonas vaginalis*, a pear-shaped parasite, 20 ×10 microns.

■ MODE OF TRANSMISSION

- Predominantly by sexual contact
- Also possible by toilet articles from one woman to another or rarely through examining gloves
- Incubation period 3–28 days.

■ PATHOLOGY

- The favorable vaginal pH for trichomonads to thrive is **5.5–6.5**
- In 25% women the parasite is present in vagina in asymptomatic state
- During and after menses, after sexual stimulation and following illness, the pH is raised to 5.5–6.5
- In 75% cases the organism can be isolated from urethra, Skene's tubercles or Bartholin's glands.

■ CLINICAL FEATURES

Symptoms

- Profuse offensive vaginal discharge (often dating from last menstruation)
- Itching and irritation
- Dysuria and frequency.

On Examination

- **Greenish-yellow frothy** offensive discharge
- Vulval and vaginal inflammation
- **Strawberry appearance** of cervix and vagina (multiple punctate hemorrhagic spots on cervix and vagina).

■ DIAGNOSIS

- Flagellate motile organism **(Hanging drop preparation)**
- The confirmation is by culture of discharge in **Kupferberg's media or Feinberg-Whittington media.**

TREATMENT

- Both partners need to be treated
- **Metronidazole** 400 mg thrice a day for 5–7 days is the drug of choice for both husband and wife. A second course may be required
- To use barrier contraception until wife is cured
- *To prevent recurrence:* Both partners, metronidazole for 7 days, following menstruation for 3 consecutive cycles
- Locally clindamycin and clotrimazole pessaries and metronidazole gel can be used
- Probiotics to be given to increase the number of *Lactobacilli* in the vagina
- **Lactic acid wash** to maintain the pH of vagina to prevent recurrence.

Q. Moniliasis or Candida vaginitis.

INTRODUCTION

- It is a very common vaginal infection.
- It is caused by *Candida albicans,* gram positive yeast like fungus.

ETIOPATHOLOGY

The organism thrives on carbohydrates and likes an acid medium (pH 4.0–5.5). Hence, candidal vaginitis is associated with a pH of less than 4.5.

RISK FACTORS

- Oral contraceptive or steroids use.
- Young age at first intercourse
- Diabetes (increased glycogen and glucosuria)
- HIV or other immunocompromised states
- Broad spectrum antibiotic use (destroy the good *Lactobacilli*)
- Pregnancy (increased glycogen and renal glycosuria).

During and following menses the vaginal pH is elevated and there is relief of symptoms.

CLINICAL FEATURES

Symptoms

- Vaginal discharge
- Intense pruritus, out of proportion to discharge
- Dyspareunia due to local soreness.

On Examination

- Vaginal erythema with adherent thick, **curdy white or cottage-cheese-like vaginal discharge**
- Cervix usually appears normal
- Vulva may be red and swollen
- Removal of white flakes reveals multiple oozing spots.

DIAGNOSIS

- Direct smear of the discharge-pseudohyphae and spores
- Culture media for *Candida*—Sabouraud's agar or Nickerson's media.

In cases of repeated attacks diabetes mellitus to be ruled out. Fasting blood sugar (FBS) and post lunch blood sugar (PLBS) to be done.

TREATMENT

- Both partners need to be treated
- To use barrier contraception until wife is cured
- Nystatin or clotrimazole, miconazole pessaries for local use. One pessary to be inserted in vagina high up for 7–14 days.
- **Fenticonazole is a new drug for resistant cases**
- Oral: Fluconazole or itraconazole is also highly effective
- Husband should also be treated with clotrimazole or nystatin ointments and oral fluconazole if needed.

Q. Leukorrhea.

DEFINITION

It is strictly defined as excessive normal vaginal discharge. It is inappropriate to include vaginitis as a cause of leukorrhea.

CRITERIA

- Excess secretion is evident from persistent vulval moistness or brownish yellow stains on drying or need to use pads
- Nonpurulent
- Nonoffensive
- Nonirritant
- Never causes pruritus.

ETIOLOGY

The excess secretion is due to:
- Physiologic excess
- Cervical cause
- Vaginal cause.

Physiologic Excess

Along with increase in estrogen:
- **During puberty:** Increased endogenous estrogen may also lead to cervical erosion
- **Menstrual cycle**
    - *Around ovulation:* Peak in estrogen
    - *Premenstrual pelvic congestion:* Increase mucus secretion from cervix and endometrial glands

❖ **Pregnancy:** Increase in estrogen and vascularity. Increased vaginal transudate and cervical gland secretions
❖ **During sexual excitement:** Secretions from Bartholin's glands.

Cervical Cause

Noninfective lesions
❖ Cervical erosions
❖ Chronic cervicitis
❖ Mucus polyps
❖ Ectropion.

Vaginal Cause

❖ Increased pelvic congestion → vaginal transudation
❖ Prolapse
❖ Chronic PID
❖ Birth control pills
❖ Ill health: Excess exfoliation of superficial cells.

■ DIAGNOSIS

❖ The discharge is nonpurulent, nonoffensive, and nonirritant
❖ General examination may reveal ill health (leukorrhea does not lead to ill health, reverse is true)
❖ Vulval examination reveals white or creamy discharge and no evidence of pruritus
❖ Bimanual and speculum examination: Normal or conditions mentioned above causing cervical and vaginal leukorrhea
❖ To rule out infections the discharge is subjected to microscopic examination for pus cells
❖ If pus cells detected further investigations like hanging drop preparation, gram stain, culture, etc., to be done.

■ TREATMENT

❖ Improve general health
❖ To have sympathetic attitude and anxiety state should be removed
❖ Cervical lesions may require electrocautery, cryosurgery or trachelorrhaphy
❖ Appropriate treatment for lesions producing vaginal leukorrhea
❖ Pill users may require to stop the pill temporarily
❖ Local hygiene.

CHAPTER 3

Menstrual Disorders

Q. Cryptomenorrhea.

Q. Imperforate hymen.

INTRODUCTION

Crypto = hidden
It is a condition in which there is periodic shedding of endometrium (menstruation) but the blood fails to come out of the genital tract due to outflow tract obstruction.

CAUSES

Congenital

- *Imperforate hymen*: It is due to failure of disintegration of the central cells of Müllerian eminence that project into urogenital sinus.
- Transverse vaginal septum.
- Atresia of vagina, cervix.

Acquired

Cervical stenosis (following surgeries like conization, amputation or cancer).

PATHOLOGY

The blood fails to come out of hymen → distends the vagina → hematocolpos → then uterus distends (hematometra) → hematosalpinx.

CLINICAL FEATURES

- *In congenital variety*: The girl is around 14–16 years of age, presents with primary amenorrhea.
- In acquired cases there would be secondary amenorrhea.
- Periodic lower abdominal pain.

- Urinary complaints like frequency, dysuria or retention of urine (hematocolpos leads to elongation of urethra).

■ EXAMINATION

- Abdominal examination reveals globular mass (distended uterus or full bladder) in suprapubic region.
- *Vulval examination*: Tense bulging hymen with bluish coloration.
- Rectal examination reveals bulged vagina and uterine mass.

■ MANAGEMENT

Ultrasonography (USG) makes the diagnosis of hematometra and hematocolpos **(Fig. 3.1)**.
- *Imperforate hymen*: **Cruciate incision on hymen**.
- Antibiotics.
- Head end elevated postsurgery.
- Dilatation of cervix in cases of cervical stenosis.
- Reconstructive surgery in cases of transverse septum of vagina, and vaginal and cervical atresia.

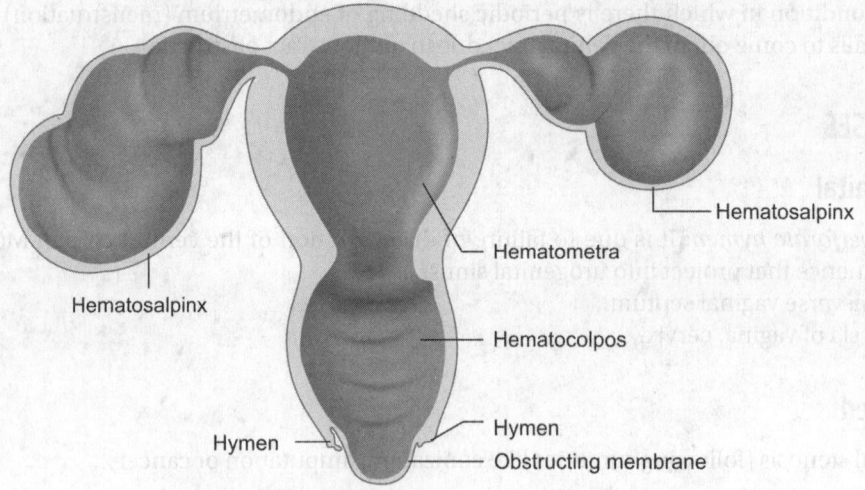

Fig. 3.1: Hematocolpos and hematometra due to imperforate hymen.

Q. Define menorrhagia. Causes of menorrhagia.

■ DEFINITION

Menorrhagia (heavy periods) is greater than 80 mL of blood loss per cycle and/or duration of menses more than 7 days, occurring at regular and normal cycle intervals. It is one of the most common gynecological complaints.

A normal menstrual cycle is 21–35 days in duration, with bleeding lasting an average of 5 days and flow measuring 25–80 mL (usually 30–50 mL).

Chapter 3: Menstrual Disorders

In actual practice, measuring menstrual blood loss is difficult. So, the diagnosis is usually based upon the patient's history.

■ CAUSES (TABLE 3.1)

- *Organic*: Pelvic, systemic, endocrinal, hematological.
- *Functional*: Dysfunctional uterine bleeding (DUB) due to disturbed HPO axis.
- *Iatrogenic*: Use of anticoagulants, steroids, improper use of hormones.

Pelvic (Due to Increased Surface Area or Hyperplasia of the Endometrium)

- Fibroids
- Polyps
- Adenomyosis, endometriosis
- Intrauterine contraceptive device (IUCD) in utero
- Early phase of tuberculous endometritis, pelvic inflammatory disease
- Granulosa cell tumor of ovary
- *Pregnancy complications*: Miscarriage or ectopic pregnancy should always be ruled out in reproductive age group
- *Cancer*: Rarely, uterine cancer, ovarian cancer and cervical cancer can cause excessive menstrual bleeding.

Systemic

- Liver failure
- Renal failure

Endocrinal

- Hypothyroidism
- Hyperthyroidism.

Hematological

Inherited bleeding disorders such as von Willebrand disease, idiopathic thrombocytopenic purpura (ITP).

Table 3.1: Important causes of menorrhagia in different age groups.		
Puberty	*Reproductive age*	*Perimenopausal*
HPO axis immaturity	Always first rule out pregnancy-related complications (like incomplete abortion) in this age group	DUB, infrequent ovulation
Dysfunctional uterine bleeding (DUB)	Fibroids, polyps, adenomyosis, endometriosis	Endocrine problems
Coagulation defects [idiopathic thrombocytopenic purpura (ITP), von Willebrand disease]	DUB	Fibroids, polyps, adenomyosis, endometriosis
Endocrine abnormalities	Endocrine abnormalities	Endometrial hyperplasia, carcinomas

Q. Pathophysiology of DUB.

Q. Investigations in case of DUB.

Q. Management of DUB.

Q. Medical management of DUB.

DEFINITION

Dysfunctional uterine bleeding is abnormal uterine bleeding that occurs in the **absence of any clinically detectable organic, systemic and iatrogenic cause (pelvic pathology like fibroids, etc., and pregnancy excluded).** It is considered a diagnosis of exclusion.

This condition is usually associated with anovulatory menstrual cycles but also can present in patients with oligoovulation (dysfunction of HPO axis: endocrine origin).

INCIDENCE

Dysfunctional uterine bleeding is more prevalent in extremes of reproductive period: puberty and perimenopause. It is a common diagnosis, making up 5–10% of cases in the OPD.

About 20% of affected individuals are in the adolescent age group, and 50% of affected individuals are aged 40–50 years.

PATHOPHYSIOLOGY

Types

- Ovulatory (10%)
- Anovulatory (90%).

Ovulatory

Polymenorrhea: Rare; condition occurs following childbirth, abortion or during adolescence and premenopausal period. Short follicular phase.

Oligomenorrhea: Very rare during adolescence and premenopausal period. Prolonged follicular phase.

Menorrhagia: Uncommon.

Two varieties:
1. ***Irregular shedding of endometrium (Halban's disease):*** Persistent corpus luteum → persistent progesterone.
   The desquamation is continued for a variable period with simultaneous failure of regeneration. Histology reveals mixture of secretory and proliferative endometrium done on day 5 or 6 of cycle.
2. ***Irregular ripening of endometrium:*** Inadequate function of corpus luteum/luteal phase defect → progesterone deficiency.
   Premenstrual spotting occurs prior to start of proper flow.
   Serum progesterone levels are less than 5 ng/mL and histology shows patchy area of secretory changes amidst proliferative endometrium.

Anovular Menorrhagia

Dysfunctional uterine bleeding (menorrhagia) due to anovulation in premenopausal women is called as **metropathia hemorrhagica or Schroeder's disease.**

Anovulatory cycles are associated with a variety of bleeding manifestations. Estrogen withdrawal bleeding and estrogen breakthrough bleeding are the most common patterns encountered in clinical practice.

As anovulatory cycles have no corpus luteal formation, progesterone is not produced. So the endometrium continues to proliferate under the influence of unopposed estrogen leading to a phase of amenorrhea for about 6–8 weeks.

Eventually, either the estrogen levels fall or the endometrium outgrows its blood supply and this out-of-phase endometrium is shed in an irregular manner that would be prolonged and heavy. Also there is no vasoconstrictor effect of prostaglandin F2 (PGF2) alpha resulting in heavy bleeding.

There is myohyperplasia with symmetrical enlargement of uterus to size of about 8–10 weeks.

The endometrium looks thick, congested, and polypoidal.

Microscopy

- Hyperplasia of all endometrial components
- Cystic glandular hypertrophy
- **Swiss cheese pattern**
- Empty glands lined by columnar epithelium
- Absence of secretory changes.

■ MANAGEMENT

History

- Most patients are adolescents or are older than 40 years.
- The history of excessive bleeding is confirmed by asking about the number of pads soaked/day and passage of clots and duration of bleeding. Keeping a menstrual calendar is helpful.
- Rule out the presence of signs or symptoms indicative of bleeding disorders such as: history of easy bruising, bleeding gums, epistaxis, and excessive bleeding episodes during childbirth, surgery, or dental procedures.
- Rule out iatrogenic causes of bleeding like IUCD, steroidal hormone intake.
- Patients who report irregular menses since menarche may have polycystic ovary syndrome (PCOS).
- Patients with adrenal enzyme defects, hyperprolactinemia, thyroid disease, or other metabolic disorders also might present with an ovulatory bleeding.
- Typically, the usual premenstrual syndrome (PMS) that accompany ovulatory cycles will be absent.

Examination

- The physical examination can elicit several anatomic and organic causes of abnormal uterine bleeding.

- Suspect DUB when a patient presents with unpredictable bleeding despite a normal pelvic examination.
- A complete physical examination should begin with assessment of hemodynamic stability and proceed with evaluation of the following:
  - Obesity [body mass index (BMI)], height and weight.
  - Signs of androgen excess (acne, hirsutism).
  - Thyroid enlargement or manifestations of hyperthyroidism or hypothyroidism.
  - Galactorrhea (may suggest hyperprolactinemia).
  - Ecchymosis, purpura (signs of bleeding disorder).
  - Signs of anemia or chronic blood loss.
  - A careful gynecologic examination (PS and PV), including Papanicolaou test (Pap smear) is warranted except in cases of puberty menorrhagia (virgins). Rule out the presence of uterine fibroids or polyps, any adnexal mass, forniceal, and cervical movement tenderness.

Investigations

- Laboratory studies for patients with DUB include:
  - Exclude pregnancy first by doing urine pregnancy test (UPT) or beta-human chorionic gonadotropin (beta-hCG). The most common cause of abnormal uterine bleeding during the reproductive years is abnormal pregnancy. Rule out threatened abortion, incomplete abortion, and ectopic pregnancy.
  - Complete blood count (CBC) with platelets.
  - Thyroid stimulating hormone (TSH) and prolactin.
  - Pap smear/LBC
  - Liver functions.
  - Coagulation studies [bleeding time (BT), clotting time (CT), prothrombin time (PT), activated partial thromboplastin time (aPTT)] in cases of *puberty menorrhagia*.
- **Endometrial sampling** (the aim is to rule out hyperplasia and endometrial cancer):
  - *Perimenopausal age group:*
    - **Histopathological diagnosis [dilatation and curettage (D&C)/endometrial biopsy/hysteroscopy and biopsy] should always be made first** to rule out endometrial hyperplasia/cancer before proceeding with any treatment.
    - **Hysteroscopy and biopsy are preferred** to blind D&C.
  - *Puberty age group:*
    - Dilatation and curettage is used as the last resort **only when all the medical methods fail** to control bleeding.
    - It is both diagnostic and therapeutic.
  - *Reproductive age group:*
    - In cases of DUB, three cycles of hormonal manipulation is given (OC pills or cyclical progesterone).
    - If the menorrhagia persists then histopathological diagnosis (D&C/endometrial biopsy/hysteroscopy and biopsy) should be made.

Ultrasonography (TVS Preferred) and Color Doppler

- Ultrasound can be used to examine the status of the endometrium and endometrial thickness (ET). Endometrial hyperplasia, endometrial carcinoma, endometrial polyps (**feeding vessel sign on color Doppler**), and uterine fibroids can be identified.

Chapter 3: Menstrual Disorders

- Saline-infusion sonohysterography is also very useful in evaluating for intracavitary (submucosal) fibroids and endometrial polyps. MRI (not routinely done) better than USG for diagnosis of adenomyosis and fibroid mapping
  - *Hysteroscopy*: It is preferred over D&C. It helps in better evaluation of the lesion and also helps in taking the biopsy. **Hysteroscopy is also therapeutic in cases of polyps and submucous fibroids.**
  - *Laparoscopy*: Needed only if adnexal pathology/endometriosis/PID is suspected.

Treatment

General and specific (medical and surgical).

General

To correct anemia with hematinics, diet, and blood transfusion in severe cases.

Medical

It is considered first-line treatment for DUB. Various drugs used are:

Hormones	Nonsteroidal anti-inflammatory drugs (NSAIDs)	Antifibrinolytics
Combined oral contraceptive (COC)	Mefenamic acid	Tranexamic acid (500–1000 mg) BID or TID
Progestins [norethisterone, medroxyprogesterone acetate (MPA), dydrogesterone]		Epsilon-aminocaproic acid (EACA)
Conjugated equine estrogen (CEE)		
Androgens, danazol		
Levonorgestrel-releasing intrauterine device (LNG-IUD; Mirena)		
Gonadotropin-releasing hormone (GnRH) analogs		
Desmopressin		

Progesterones

- Medroxyprogesterone acetate (MPA) 10 mg or norethisterone 5 mg three to four times a day for 4–7 days can be used to control the acute bleeding.
- Cyclical progesterone can be used from day 5 to day 25 or from day 20 to 25 of the cycle.
- Progestins activate 17-hydroxysteroid dehydrogenase in endometrial cells, converting estradiol to the less active estrone.
- Synthetic progestins have an antimitotic effect, allowing the endometrium to become atrophic if administered continuously. These drugs are very effective in cases of endometrial hyperplasia.
- **Treatment with a progestin for 10–12 days/month will allow for controlled, predictable menses and will also protect the patient against the development of endometrial hyperplasia.**
- MPA is the drug of choice for patients with anovulatory DUB.
- Depot MPA works by causing progesterone induced amenorrhea.

Combined Oral Contraceptive (COC)

- Contraceptive pills containing estrogen and progestin have been advocated in patients with DUB.
- It is preferred in women who desire contraception.
- It is also used to treat acute episodes of hemorrhagic uterine bleeding. They are also very effective in long-term management of DUB.
- Low dose and very low dose OC pills are preferred now.

Estrogen

- The role of only estrogen is limited.
- Estrogen alone in high doses is indicated only in certain clinical situations.
- Prolonged uterine bleeding would mean that the epithelial lining of the cavity has become denuded over time. In this setting, a progestin is unlikely to control bleeding. Estrogen alone will induce return to normal endometrial growth rapidly.
- It is effective in controlling acute, profuse bleeding. It exerts a vasospastic action on capillary bleeding by affecting the level of fibrinogen, factor IV, and factor X in blood, as well as platelet aggregation and capillary permeability.
- It also induces formation of progesterone receptors, making subsequent treatment with progestins more effective.
- Intravenous estrogen (not available in India) or conjugated equine estrogens (CEE) tablets can be used.

Mirena/Levonorgestrel Releasing Intrauterine Device (LNG-IUD)

- It releases 20 µg LNG per day and causes a state of **progesterone induced amenorrhea**, induces endometrial atrophy. Up to 97% reduction in blood loss is achieved.
- It can be used for up to 5 years and is hysterectomy can be avoided.

Danazol

Very rarely used because of androgenic side effects.

Gestrinone

2.5 mg orally twice a week for 3 months is also effective.

Gonadotropin-Releasing Hormone (GnRH) Analogs

- Work by reducing concentration of GnRH receptors in the pituitary via receptor down regulation and induction of postreceptor effects, which **suppress gonadotropin release.**
- This form of medical castration is very effective in inducing amenorrhea.
- Because prolonged therapy with this form of medical castration is associated with osteoporosis and other postmenopausal side effects, its use is often limited in duration.
- Because of the expense of these drugs, they usually are not used as a first-line approach but can be used to achieve short-term relief from a bleeding problem, particularly in patients with renal failure or blood dyscrasia.

Desmopressin Acetate (DDAVP)

It has been used to treat abnormal uterine bleeding in patients with coagulation defects. Transiently elevates factor VIII and von Willebrand factor. Available in tablet form/IV route/intra nasal spray (0.3 µg/kg)

Ormeloxifene (SERM)

Also known as Centchroman is a non hormonal, oral contraceptive.

Dose: 30–60 mg twice weekly for 3 months

Surgical

Most cases of DUB can be treated medically. Surgical measures are reserved for situations when medical therapy has failed or is contraindicated.
1. D&C
2. Endometrial ablation
3. Hysterectomy
   - D&C is an appropriate diagnostic step in a patient who fails to respond to hormonal management.
   - The addition of hysteroscopy will aid in the treatment of endometrial polyps or the performance of directed uterine biopsies.
   - Therapeutic D&C alone for DUB has not been shown to be very efficacious.
   - Laparoscopic, abdominal or vaginal hysterectomy might be necessary in patients who have failed or declined medical management and who experience a disruption in their quality of life from persistent, unscheduled bleeding.
   - **Also in cases of hyperplasia with atypia, hysterectomy is preferred if the family is complete.**
   - **Ovaries should be preserved during hysterectomy**.
   - Endometrial ablation is an alternative for those who wish to avoid hysterectomy or who are not candidates for major surgery.

Uterus Conserving Surgeries for DUB

(Endometrial Ablation/Resection) The various surgeries are:
1. Transcervical resection of endometrium (TCRE) in which the basal endometrium is removed using diathermy loop.
2. Roller ball endometrial ablation.
3. Laser [neodymium-doped yttrium aluminum garnet (Nd:YAG)] endometrial ablation.
4. Microwave of 9.2 GHz used for endometrial ablation (MEA).
5. Uterine thermal balloon in which hot saline (85°C for 10–15 minutes) is circulated within the balloon after it is placed inside the uterus.
6. Hydrothermablator in which heated saline is circulated within uterine cavity. In a D&C, only superficial endometrium is removed which grows back, but in above minimally invasive surgeries **the basal endometrium is destroyed** so that it does not regenerate back.

Prerequisites

- Patient's family should be complete.
- *Histopathology*: There should be no evidence of malignancy.

Advantages

- Day-care procedure.
- Major surgery such as hysterectomy is avoided.

Results

- Forty percent patients will become amenorrheic.
- Forty percent will have hypomenorrhea.
- Only 20% will require hysterectomy.

■ RECENT ADVANCES

FIGO classification system (PALM-COEIN) for causes of abnormal uterine bleeding in nongravid women of reproductive age: There is general inconsistency in the nomenclature used to describe abnormal uterine bleeding (AUB). It seems clear that the development of consistent and universally accepted nomenclature is a step toward rectifying this unsatisfactory circumstance. Another requirement is the development of a classification system, on several levels, for the causes of AUB, which can be used by clinicians, investigators, and even patients to facilitate communication, clinical care, and research.

The PALM-COEIN (P = polyp; A = adenomyosis; L = leiomyoma; M = malignancy and hyperplasia; C = coagulopathy; O = ovulatory dysfunction; E = endometrial; I = iatrogenic; and N = not yet classified) classification system for AUB, has been approved by the International Federation of Gynecology and Obstetrics (FIGO) Executive Board as a FIGO classification system.

Q. Dysmenorrhea.

■ DEFINITION

Dysmenorrhea is defined as painful menstruation so as to incapacitate day to day activities.

■ TYPES

- *Primary (spasmodic)*: In absence of any pelvic pathology.
- *Secondary (congestive)*: In presence of pelvic pathology.

Primary Dysmenorrhea

Primary dysmenorrhea is mostly confined to adolescent, more common among affluent society, generally with a positive family history.

The pain always occurs in ovulatory cycles and is usually cured after pregnancy and vaginal delivery.

The various theories for primary dysmenorrhea are:
- Uterine myometrial hyperactivity, junctional zone (JZ: subendometrial layer of myometrium) hyperplasia, dysperistalsis and hyperactivity of JZ.
- Overactivity of sympathetic nerves → hypertonicity of circular fibers of isthmus.
- PGFα → is more in ovulatory cycles which cause ischemia of myometrium.
- Vasopressin, endothelins, leukotrienes, and platelet activating factor are all increased which cause uterine hyperactivity, hyperperistalsis, dysrhythmic contractions, ischemia, and pain.
- Psychosomatic factors, anxiety lower pain threshold.

Clinical Features

- The pain begins few hours or just before the menses.
- The pain last for few hours to 24 hours, rarely beyond 48 hours.
- Spasmodic in nature, lower abdomen and may radiate to back and medial aspect of thigh.
- May be associated with nausea, vomiting, diarrhea, tachycardia, pallor, cold sweats.
- Fainting, syncope in severe cases.
- Clinical examination does not reveal any abnormalities.
- Ultrasonography helps in ruling out any pelvic pathology.

Treatment

Assurance, counseling, encourage normal activities.

Drugs

- NSAIDs: Given for 1–3 days, for 3–6 cycles.
- Mefenamic acid 250–500 mg three times a day (tds).
- Ibuprofen (400 mg) tds or naproxen [250 mg; four times a day (qds)].
- Indomethacin (25 mg) tds.
- Newer selective cyclooxygenase-2 (COX-2) inhibitors may also be used.
- Glyceryl trinitrate (GTN) transdermal patches are also used.
- Oral contraceptive pills (suppresses ovulation and hence used) 3–6 cycles.
- The patients wanting contraception, those with associated menorrhagia and patients unresponsive to NSAIDs or in whom NSAIDs are contraindicated are good candidates for OC pills.
- Dydrogesterone (from day 5–25) has also been tried.
- Transcutaneous electrical nerve stimulation (TENS) has also been used to relieve the pain.

Surgery

Surgery is **very rarely required.** Laparoscopy may be very rarely needed to rule out pelvic causes especially endometriosis.

- Laparoscopic uterine nerve ablation (LUNA) has not been found to be very beneficial.
- Laparoscopic presacral neurectomy (LPSN) to cut down sensory pathways (T11–T12) from uterus.
- Cervical dilatation very rarely done. May lead to incompetence in future.

Secondary Dysmenorrhea

Etiology

- Endometriosis
- Pelvic inflammatory disease (PID)
- Ovarian cysts and tumors
- Cervical stenosis
- Adenomyosis
- Fibroids
- Uterine polyps
- Intrauterine adhesions

- Congenital malformations (e.g., bicornuate uterus)
- Intrauterine contraceptive device (IUCD) in utero
- Transverse vaginal septum
- Pelvic congestion syndrome
- Allen-Masters syndrome.

Clinical Features

The patient is usually in her thirties.
- The pain usually appears **3–5 days prior to the period and relives with start of bleeding**.
- The pain is dull, situated in back and front. The onset and duration of pain depends on the pathology producing the pain.
- There is no systemic discomfort unlike primary dysmenorrhea.
- There may be other symptoms related to the underlying pelvic pathology.
- Clinical examination would reveal the pathology.
- The underlying pathology may be detected by USG, laparoscopy or hysteroscopy.

Treatment

Treatment is aimed at underlying cause (e.g., myomectomy, polypectomy, adhesiolysis, chocolate cystectomy, hysterectomy, etc.) and depends on the patients' age and parity.

Q. Define primary amenorrhea. Differentiate between MRKH syndrome and CAIS.

■ DEFINITION

Primary amenorrhea is defined as:
- **In absence** of secondary sexual characters, no menses till the age of **13 years**; or
- **In presence** of secondary sexual characters, no menses till the age of **15 years**.

■ CAUSES

- *Most common cause of primary amenorrhea is ovarian dysgenesis/Turner syndrome.*
- Müllerian agenesis (Mayer-Rokitansky-Küstner-Hauser or MRKH syndrome) is the second main cause and androgen insensitivity syndrome or testicular feminizing syndrome (AIS/TFS) is the third main cause of primary amenorrhea.
- *Each and every case of primary amenorrhea karyotyping should be done.*
- In the *entire gynecology, these are only two conditions in which there is primary amenorrhea and absent uterus*:

	Müllerian agenesis (RMKH)	Complete androgen insensitivity syndrome (CAIS)
Karyotype	XX	XY
Gonads	Ovaries	Testes (inguinal)
Axillary/pubic hair	Present	Absent/sparse
Associated anomalies	Renal and skeletal/vertebral defects and deafness may be present	Absent
Reproduction	Possible with surrogacy as ovaries function normally (they can have their own biological child)	Not possible but gonadectomy, vaginoplasty, and estrogen replacement therapy (ERT) are required

Chapter 3: Menstrual Disorders

Breasts are well-developed in both the above cases. In CAIS breast development is due to peripheral aromatization of testosterone to estrogen.

Key Points to Remember about CAIS

- They do not have ambiguous genitalia at birth. The external genitalia look like females.
- Testes secrete both testosterone and anti-Müllerian hormone/Müllerian inhibiting factor (AMH/MIF), but testosterone functions are absent (as receptors are insensitive).
- Since the testes have a risk of developing gonadoblastoma/seminoma, orchidectomy should be done.
- Vaginoplasty should be done for sexual activity and ERT given for bone protection and maintenance of secondary sexual characters.
- Patients of CAIS should be continued to be reared as females.

CHAPTER 4

Fibroids

Q. Etiology and clinical features of fibroids.

Q. Signs and symptoms and management of fibroids.

■ INTRODUCTION

Fibroids are benign smooth muscle tumors arising from the myometrium.

They are the **most common benign tumors of uterus, and they are also the most common pelvic tumors in females.**

■ INCIDENCE

Incidence increases with the age of patient. It is estimated that at the age of 30 years around 20% of women will have fibroids. Prevalence is highest between 35–45 years of age. By the age of 45 years it is estimated that every third or fourth women would have a fibroid.

■ ETIOLOGY

- It is **predominantly an estrogen-dependent tumor:**
  - Associated with early menarche, late menopause.
  - Associated anovulation and polycystic ovary syndrome (PCOS).
  - Grows in size during pregnancy, and following menopause there is cessation of growth.
- Nulliparity (a uterus which does not bear a baby consoles itself by having a fibroid). Multiparity is protective.
- Deletions in chromosome 7 and t(12; 14) are associated with fibroids.
- More common in colored races or black women.
- *Infertility:* Fibroids can cause infertility and infertile women are more prone to develop fibroids.
- *Obesity:* Epidermal growth factor (EGF), insulin-like growth factor (IGF-1) and transforming growth factor (TGF) stimulate the growth of fibroid either directly or via estrogen.
- **Smoking is protective for fibroids.**

CLINICAL FEATURES
- The patients are usually nulliparous or have primary infertility or having a long duration of secondary infertility.
- Prevalence is highest between 35 and 45 years of age.

Symptoms
- **Majority (75%) of the fibroids remain asymptomatic.**
- They are discovered accidently during ultrasonography (USG)/laparoscopy/laparotomy or during pelvic examination.
- **Symptoms depend on the location and size of the fibroid.**

Menstrual Abnormalities
They are mainly associated with submucous and intramural fibroids.

Menorrhagia
Menorrhagia is the classic and most common symptom. It is due to:
- Increased surface area of endometrium.
- Endometrial hyperplasia due to hyperestrogenism and anovulation.
- Interference with normal uterine contractility.
- Congestion of subjacent endometrial venous plexus and pelvic congestion.
- Relative deficiency of thromboxane A2 (TXA2).

Metrorrhagia
Metrorrhagia may be due to ulceration of submucous fibroid.

Dysmenorrhea
Congestive or secondary dysmenorrhea is due to pelvic congestion or associated endometriosis.

Infertility
It is due to:
- Submucous or intramural fibroid distorts the cavity and thereby makes the uterus unsuitable for implantation.
- Congestion of endometrial plexus and ulceration of endometrium over submucous fibroid may also prevent implantation.
- Also, elongation of the cavity and prevention of rhythmic uterine contraction may impair sperm transport.
- Cornual fibroid may block the fallopian tube.
- Menorrhagia and dyspareunia may also contribute to infertility.

Lump in Abdomen
- Subserous fibroids or large intramural fibroids are most likely to cause this.
- The patient may feel lump or heaviness in lower abdomen without any other symptoms.

Pressure Symptoms

- It can press the bladder causing frequency, dysuria or retention. It can press the rectum causing constipation.
- Broad ligament fibroid can press the ureter causing **hydroureter and hydronephrosis.**

Pregnancy Complications

Effects of Fibroids on Pregnancy

- Recurrent abortions
- Impacted posterior fibroid can lead to retroverted gravid uterus and urinary retention
- Malpresentations
- Preterm labor
- Intrauterine growth restriction (IUGR)
- Prolonged labor or obstructed labor
- Cervical dystocia (due to cervical or broad ligament fibroid)
- Abruption
- Atonic postpartum hemorrhage (PPH)
- Increased risk of obstetric hysterectomy.

Effects of Pregnancy on Fibroids

- Red degeneration
- Increase in size (due to increase in vascularity, edema and hypertrophy and hyperplasia of fibromuscular tissue)
- Torsion of pedunculated subserosal fibroid
- Infection and polypoidal changes (more in puerperium).

Pain in Abdomen

Fibroids are usually painless. Pain is due to some complications (like degeneration, torsion) or associated pathology like endometriosis.

Signs

- Pallor (due to menorrhagia).
- **Abdominal examination:** If the uterus size is less than 12 weeks, it is not palpable on abdominal examination.

Palpation

If uterus is enlarged to 12-14 weeks or more, the following features are noted:
- Feel is **firm to hard**, may be cystic in cases of cystic degeneration.
- Well defined margin, lower pole cannot be reached suggesting of pelvic origin.
- **Generally bosselated, nodular surface,** may be uniformly enlarged in case of single fibroid.
- Mobility is restricted from above downwards but can be moved from side to side.
- Swelling is dull on percussion.

PV Examination

- Bimanual examination reveals irregularly enlarged uterus.

- The mass or swelling **is not felt separately from the uterus.**
- **The cervix moves with the movement of the mass felt per abdomen** and movement of the mass moves the cervix.

INVESTIGATIONS

To confirm the diagnosis:
- **Preoperative evaluation:** Blood group, complete blood count (CBC), blood sugars, electrocardiography (ECG), chest X-ray, etc.
- **Ultrasonography is the imaging modality of choice** for detection and evaluation of uterine fibroids.
    - Uterus is enlarged and can be distorted.
    - Fibroids most often appear as **concentric, solid, hypoechoic masses.** As these solid masses absorb sound waves they cause a variable amount of acoustic shadowing.
    - Fibroids may vary in their degree of echogenicity; they can be heterogeneous or hyperechoic, depending on the amount of fibrous tissue and/or calcification. Fibroids may have anechoic components resulting from necrosis.
    - The echogenic endometrial stripe may be displaced by a fibroid. Calcifications appear hyperechoic, with sharp acoustic shadowing.
    - Also, hydroureter and hydronephrosis can be detected by USG.
    - Doppler ultrasound shows vascularity of the uterus and fibroids. Besides it can differentiate between the fibroid and localized adenomyosis. **The blood flow surrounds a fibroid, but diffuses through adenomyosis.**
    - Ultrasonography has a sensitivity of 60%, a specificity of 99%, and an accuracy of 87%.
    - **3D USG** is also available nowadays and can locate the fibroids accurately.
- **Saline infusion sonography** is very helpful to **detect submucous fibroid or polyp.**
- **Magnetic resonance imaging (MRI)** is more accurate for fibroid mapping but is expensive and not routinely used.
- **Computed tomography (CT)** scanning has a limited role in the diagnosis of uterine fibroids. On CT scans, fibroids are usually indistinguishable from healthy myometrium unless they are calcified or necrotic. Calcifications may be more visible on CT scans conventional radiographs.
- **Hysteroscopy** not only recognizes a submucous fibroid, but also allows its excision under direct vision.
- Dilation and curettage (D&C) is required to rule out endometrial cancer in a woman complaining of menstrual disorders, irregular bleeding and postmenopausal bleeding. Histopathology of endometrium gives clue to its etiology and rules out endometrial cancer.
- **Laparoscopy:** Can be diagnostic as well as therapeutic.

Myomectomy or hysterectomy can be done through laparoscopic route. Associated pelvic inflammatory disease (PID) and endometriosis can be detected. Also the tubal patency can be established in infertile patient.

DIFFERENTIAL DIAGNOSIS

- Pregnancy
- Full bladder
- Adenomyosis

- ❖ Ovarian tumor
- ❖ Myohyperplasia [in cases of dysfunctional uterine bleeding (DUB)]
- ❖ Tubo-ovarian mass.

TREATMENT

- ❖ General and specific **(Flowchart 4.1)**.
- ❖ **All fibroids do not require treatment but all symptomatic fibroids require treatment.**

General

To correct anemia: Iron supplements and even blood transfusion may be needed in cases of severe anemia.

Specific

Medical and surgical.

Medical Management

- ❖ **To control menorrhagia and dysmenorrhea:** Nonsteroidal anti-inflammatory drugs (NSAIDs), low dose oral contraceptive (OC) pills, progesterone.

Flowchart 4.1: Management protocol of uterine fibroids.

- To decrease the size and vascularity of fibroids:
- Drugs which decrease the size of fibroids (never for permanent treatment, as the fibroid grows back to its usual size after the action of drug is over; they are **mainly used preoperatively**):
  - Gonadotropin-releasing hormone (GnRH) analogs (most commonly used)
  - Danazol
  - Progesterone [depot medroxyprogesterone acetate (DMPA)/Mirena/progesterone-only pill (POP)/low-dose OC pills]
  - Mifepristone (RU-486): Available in 10 mg and 25 mg. Once a day
  - Gestrinone
  - Anastrozole (aromatase inhibitor)
  - Asoprisnil and ulipristal acetate both are selective progesterone receptor modulators (SPRMs). They reversibly block the progesterone receptors and act as potent, orally active antiprogestational agents. Ulipristal acetate has shown efficacy with a significant reduction in uterine bleeding, fibroid volume and improved quality of life, without the side effects associated with other medications such as GnRH agonists. Dose of ulipristal acetate is 5 mg-10 mg once a day oral tablet, taken for 3 months ahead of surgery.
- GnRH analogs are used preoperatively:
  - Decrease the vascularity and blood loss during surgery.
  - To induce amenorrhea to build up hemoglobin in cases of anemia.
  - May facilitate laparoscopic or hysteroscopic surgery.
  - May help to convert an abdominal surgery to a vaginal surgery.

Surgical Management

It is the mainstay of treatment.

Myomectomy: Laparotomy, laparoscopy, hysteroscopy, vaginal.

Hysterectomy: Laparotomy, laparoscopic, vaginal.

- The type of surgery depends on the patient's age, parity, desire for pregnancy, symptoms and number of fibroids.
- The route of surgery is decided by location of fibroid, size of the fibroid and the uterus and the surgeon expertise.
- Fibroids causing infertility, or recurrent abortions or symptomatic fibroid in a young patient myomectomy is the surgery of choice.
- For submucous fibroids hysteroscopic myomectomy is the gold standard.
- For subserous and intramural fibroids laparoscopic surgery is preferred today over laparotomy.
- Old patients or family is complete, hysterectomy is preferred.

Indications of Surgery in Asymptomatic Fibroid

- Size >12 weeks of pregnancy.
- Diagnosis not certain.
- Fibroid grows during follow-up.
- Subserosal pedunculated fibroid (because of risk of torsion).
- Situated in the lower part of the uterus and likely to complicate deliveries in future.
- Fibroids compressing ureter and causing hydroureter or hydronephrosis.
- Unexplained infertility with distortion of uterine cavity.
- Unexplained recurrent abortions.

Uterine Artery Embolization (UAE)

In this procedure, the femoral artery is cannulated, and artificial clot of polyvinyl alcohol is used to block the uterine artery and its branches supplying the fibroids. It decreases the blood loss during surgery. The same technique can also be used as a therapy for symptomatic patients who refuse or want to avoid surgery. After embolization there is 60–65% decrease in size of fibroids over a period of 6–9 months, and so the patient's symptoms may decrease or disappear. If the patient is still symptomatic after 1 year, then surgery should be considered.

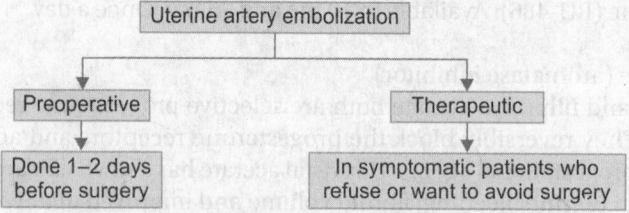

RECENT ADVANCES

High-intensity focused ultrasound (HIFU or FUS) is a highly precise medical procedure using high-intensity focused ultrasound waves to heat and destroy fibroids rapidly through ablation.

Clinical HIFU procedures are typically image-guided (MRI or USG) to precisely target the fibroids before applying of ultrasound energy.

When MRI is used for guidance, the technique is called magnetic resonance-guided focused ultrasound (**MRgHIFU or MRgFUS**). MRI is used to identify fibroids before they are destroyed by the ultrasound waves.

When USG is used to localize the fibroids, the technique is called **ultrasound-guided focused ultrasound (USgFUS)**.

Q. Degenerations in fibroids.

Q. Red degeneration.

DEGENERATIONS/SECONDARY CHANGES IN FIBROIDS

Fibroids can undergo various types of degenerations/secondary changes.

Hyaline Degeneration

It is the most common type (65%).
- It can occur in fibroids of all sizes. It is more common in fibroids having more connective tissues. The central part of the fibroid (being the least vascular) is the common site. The fibroid feels soft and elastic.
- On cut section there are irregular homogenous areas with **loss of whorl-like appearance**.
- Microscopy reveals hyaline changes in muscle and fibrous tissue.

Cystic Degeneration

More common in interstitial fibroids and usually occurs following menopause. It is formed by liquefaction of areas within hyaline changes.

Fatty Degeneration

Found after menopause. There is deposition of fat globules in the muscle cells.

Calcareous Degeneration

- In calcareous degeneration, phosphates and carbonates of lime are deposited in the periphery along the course of the vessels. The best examples of calcareous myomas are those in old patients with long-standing myomas. They have been found as **"womb-stones"** in graveyards.
- Calcareous tumors are easily identified by radiography.

Red Degeneration (Also Known as Carneous Degeneration)

- Occurs because fibroid overgrows its blood supply (**micronecrothrombosis**).
- Most commonly occurs in **second trimester of pregnancy** followed by in the puerperium.
- **Cut section:** Raw beefy appearance, fishy odor.
- Patient presents with acute abdomen, vomiting, fever, and leukocytosis.

Differential Diagnosis

- Acute appendicitis
- Pyelonephritis
- Abruption.

Management

Always conservative management (never surgery):
- Hospitalization
- Bed rest
- Analgesics
- Intravenous (IV) fluids
- Intravenous antibiotics (SOS).

Atrophy

- As a result of diminished vascularity after menopause, there is a shrinkage in the size of the tumor, which becomes firmer and more fibrotic. A similar change occurs in myomas after pregnancy enlargement.
- Temporary shrinkage by 50% occurs following GnRH therapy, but regrows after stoppage of therapy.

Sarcomatous Change

- Sarcomatous change in a myoma is extremely rare, and the incidence is 0.1–0.5% of all myomas.
- Intramural and submucous tumors have a higher potential for sarcomatous change than subserosal tumor.
- It is rare for malignant change to develop in a woman under the age of 40. It is commonly seen in a postmenopausal woman when the tumor is noticed to grow suddenly, causing pain and postmenopausal bleeding.

- To the naked eye, a sarcomatous myoma is yellowish grey in color and hemorrhagic. The consistency is soft and friable, and not firm like a simple myoma. Another important sign is the nonencapsulation of the tumor.
- Sarcoma is highly malignant and spreads via the bloodstream.

Infection

- Infection (Streptococcal and *Bacteroides*) is common in submucous and myomatous polyps if they project into the cervical canal or into the vagina.
- An infected polyp causes blood-stained purulent discharge. This generally happens following delivery or abortion.

Q. FIGO classification for fibroids.

A classification system for submucosal fibroids that reported the relationship of the fibroid to the mucosal surface of the uterus was introduced by Wamsteker et al. and was later adopted by the European Society of Hysteroscopy. FIGO adopted and extended this classification system to all fibroids in the uterus by describing the relationship of fibroids to both the serosal and mucosal uterine surfaces.

The FIGO classification system retains the original submucosal relationship of types 0–2, but extends staging to an additional six categories. Type 3 fibroids abut the endometrium but are completely intramural. Type 4 describes a completely intramural fibroid; types 5 and 6 are defined by the relationship to the serosal layer; type 7 describes fibroids that are pedunculated on the sub-serosal surface; and type 8 refers to fibroids found in ectopic locations such as the cervix. Additionally, FIGO staging allows a range of stages if the fibroid traverses multiple layers; for instance, a fibroid with less than half of its volume in the uterine cavity and extending to the sub-serosal layer could be labeled type 2–5.

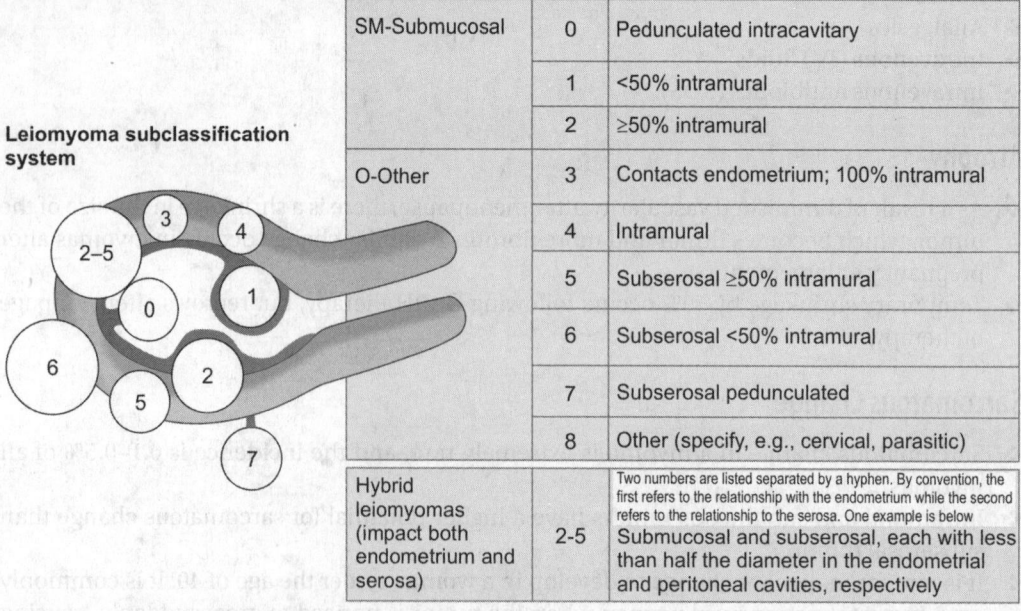

Leiomyoma subclassification system

SM-Submucosal	0	Pedunculated intracavitary
	1	<50% intramural
	2	≥50% intramural
O-Other	3	Contacts endometrium; 100% intramural
	4	Intramural
	5	Subserosal ≥50% intramural
	6	Subserosal <50% intramural
	7	Subserosal pedunculated
	8	Other (specify, e.g., cervical, parasitic)
Hybrid leiomyomas (impact both endometrium and serosa)	2-5	Two numbers are listed separated by a hyphen. By convention, the first refers to the relationship with the endometrium while the second refers to the relationship to the serosa. One example is below Submucosal and subserosal, each with less than half the diameter in the endometrial and peritoneal cavities, respectively

CHAPTER 5

Prolapse

Q. Supports of the uterus.

■ INTRODUCTION

- ❖ Normal position of uterus is anteverted and anteflexed.
- ❖ The external os is at the level of ischial spine.
- ❖ The uterus is held in this position by **three tier support systems—upper, middle and inferior (Figs. 5.1 and 5.2).**

■ 3 TIER SUPPORT SYSTEM

Upper Tier

- ❖ Endopelvic fascia covering the uterus
- ❖ **Round ligaments:** They are remnants of the gubernaculum, extend from the uterine horns to the labia majora via the inguinal canal. They function to maintain the anteverted position of the uterus
- ❖ **Broad ligaments:** Double layer of peritoneum attaching the sides of the uterus to the pelvis. It acts as a mesentery for the uterus
- ❖ **Broad ligament and round ligament** are considered as false supports of the uterus.

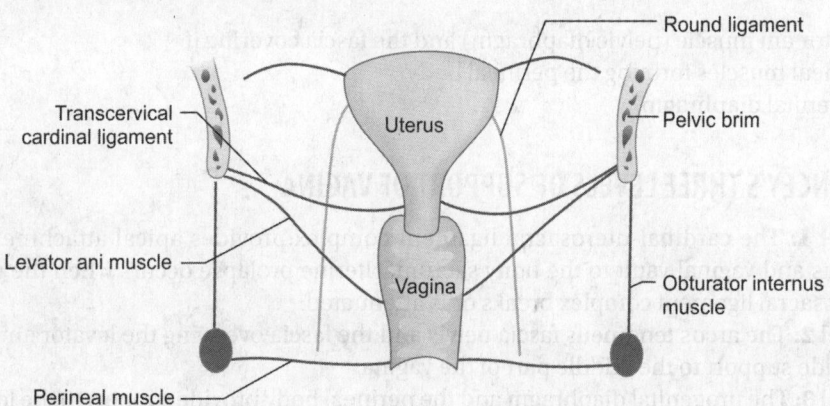

Fig. 5.1: Supports of the uterus.

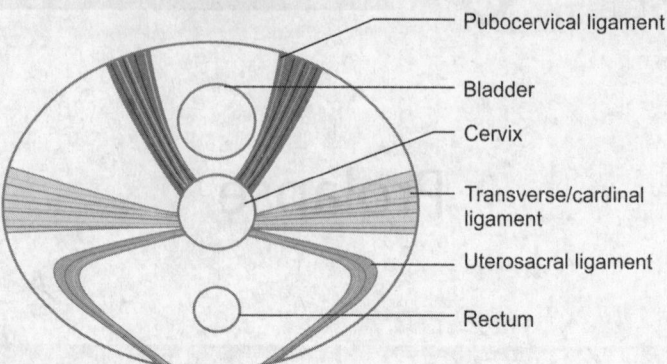

Fig. 5.2: Ligamentous supports of uterus.

Middle Tier

- Strongest support
- **Pericervical ring:** Collar of fibroelastic connective tissue encircling the supravaginal cervix
- The ligaments (pubocervical, cardinal and uterosacral) are attached anteriorly, laterally, and posteriorly to the ring, respectively
- **Endopelvic fascia/ligaments/pelvic cellular tissues**
- The endopelvic fascia is condensed at places to form ligaments:
  - **Pubocervical ligament:** From pubic symphysis to anterior part of cervix and pericervical ring
  - **Cardinal/Mackenrodt's/transverse cervical ligament:** It is located at the base of the broad ligament, it extends laterally from the cervix and the pericervical ring to the lateral pelvic walls (condensation of parietal fascia covering the obturator internus). It contains the uterine vessels (artery and vein)
  - **Uterosacral ligaments:** From the periosteum of 2nd, 3rd, and 4th sacral vertebrae to the posterolateral part of cervix and the pericervical ring.
- **This hammock like arrangement of condensed pelvic cellular tissue is the cardinal support of uterus.**

Inferior Tier

- Levator ani muscle (pelvic diaphragm) and the fascia covering it
- Perineal muscles forming the perineal body
- Urogenital diaphragm.

■ DELANCEY'S THREE LEVELS OF SUPPORT OF VAGINA

- **Level 1:** The cardinal-uterosacral ligament complex provides apical attachment of the uterus and vaginal vault to the bony sacrum. Uterine prolapse occurs when the cardinal-uterosacral ligament complex breaks or is attenuated.
- **Level 2:** The arcus tendineus fascia pelvis and the fascia overlying the levator ani muscles provide support to the middle part of the vagina.
- **Level 3:** The urogenital diaphragm and the perineal body provide support to the lower part of the vagina.

Q. Etiology of prolapse.

INTRODUCTION

Prolapse is defined as the displacement of an organ from its normal anatomical position. Genital prolapse occurs due to weakness of the supports.

ETIOLOGY

- **Predisposing factors:** This could be acquired or congenital
- Aggravating factors.

Predisposing Factors

Acquired

- Vaginal delivery with consequent injury to the supports is the single most important factor.
- Prolapse is unusual in cases delivered by cesarean section.
- The injury caused by:
  - Overstretching of cardinal and uterosacral ligaments
  - Overstretching of perineum
  - Overstretching and breaks in endopelvic fascia. This could be due to:
    - Premature bearing down efforts prior to full dilatation
    - Forceful traction with forceps or vacuum or application prior to full dilatation
    - Prolonged 2nd stage of labor
    - Precipitate labor
    - Undue fundal pressure
    - Delivery of large baby
    - Repeated frequent childbirths
    - Poorly timed episiotomy
    - Improperly conducted delivery
- Imperfect repair of perineal injuries.
- *Neuromuscular damage of levator ani:* **Internal rotation causes maximum damage** of levator ani muscle.
- *Subinvolution of supporting structures:* Ill-nourished asthenic women, with early resumption of activities which greatly increase the intra-abdominal pressure.

Congenital

Congenital weakness of supports can cause nulliparous prolapse or prolapse following easy vaginal delivery:
- Connective tissue disorders (Ehlers-Danlos syndrome, Marfan syndrome)
- Neurological anomalies (spina bifida occulta).

Aggravating Factors

- Postmenopausal atrophy **(decrease in estrogen decreases collagen strength)**
- Chronic cough/constipation (increase in intra-abdominal pressure)
- Malnourishment

- Large ovarian tumor, fibroid (can cause pressure on uterus)
- Obesity.

Q. Types of prolapse and degrees of prolapse.

■ TYPES OF GENITAL PROLAPSE

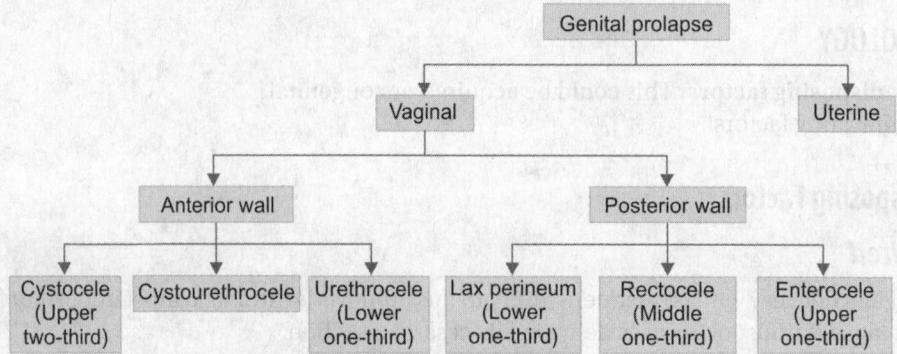

Cystocele is the most common type of vaginal prolapse.

Vaginouterine prolapse (more common)	Uterine/uterovaginal prolapse (less common)
Traction variety	Pulsion variety
• Vagina prolapses first and then, due to traction, pulls cervix and uterus • Supravaginal elongation is present • Uterocervical length (UCL) is increased	• Uterus prolapses first and then drags vagina later • Supravaginal elongation not seen • UCL is not increased

Vault prolapse can occur following:
- Vaginal hysterectomy.
- Abdominal hysterectomy.
- Laparoscopic hysterectomy.

■ DEGREES OF PROLAPSE

- **First degree:** Descent of cervix into the vagina (external os is at the level of ischial spine in normal anatomical position)
- **Second degree:** Descent of cervix up to the introitus
- **Third degree:** Descent of cervix outside the introitus
- **Fourth degree (procidentia):** Whole uterus (including the fundus) is outside the introitus.

■ STAGES OF PROLAPSE

The five stages of prolapse (POPQ = Pelvic Organ Prolapse Quantitative) Scoring:
- **Stage 0:** No prolapse
- **Stage I:** The most distal portion of the prolapse is more than 1 cm above the level of the hymen
- **Stage II:** The most distal portion of the prolapse extends from 1 cm above to 1 cm below the hymen

- **Stage III:** The most distal portion of the prolapse is more than 1 cm below the hymen but protrudes no further than 2 cm less than the total length of the vagina
- **Stage IV:** Complete eversion of the vagina.

Q. Clinical features/signs and symptoms of genital prolapse.

INTRODUCTION

Prolapse is defined as the displacement of an organ from its normal anatomical position. Genital prolapse occurs due to weakness of the supports.

SYMPTOMS

- Variable
- There may not be any symptoms even with severe degree of prolapse or the following symptoms may be present:

Patient Profile

Generally **postmenopausal** or premenopausal multiparous women with complaints of:
- Something coming out through per vagina or fullness within the vagina
- Backache or lower pelvic dragging pain during walking, working
- The above two symptoms are usually **relieved on lying down**.

Vaginal Symptoms

- Sensation of a bulge or protrusion
- Seeing or feeling a bulge
- Pressure
- Heaviness
- Excessive whitish discharge (due to venous congestion)
- Blood-stained discharge due to decubitus ulcer in dependent part.

Urinary Symptoms (in Presence of Cystocele)

- **Urgency or frequency** (may be due to cystitis or due to incomplete evacuation)
- Weak or prolonged urinary stream
- Feeling of incomplete emptying
- **Manual reduction** of prolapse needed to start or complete voiding
- Stress urinary incontinence (SUI), due to bladder neck descent
- Rarely retention of urine
- Painful micturition (due to infection).

Bowel Symptoms (in Presence of Rectocele)

- Feeling of incomplete emptying
- Pushing of posterior vaginal wall needed to start or complete defecation
- Straining during defecation

- Digital evacuation needed to complete defecation
- Incontinence of flatus, or liquid or solid stool.

Sexual Symptoms

Dyspareunia or difficulty in coitus.

■ CLINICAL EXAMINATION

Composite Examination

- Inspection and palpation: Vaginal, rectal, rectovaginal examination may be needed.
- Findings will depend on type of prolapse.

General Examination

- Nutritional status
- Body mass index (BMI)
- Signs of myopathy or neuropathy
- Chronic airway disease
- Abdominal mass
- Abdominal tone (help in planning type of conservative surgery).

Local Examination

Pelvic organ prolapse (POP) is evaluated in dorsal position and standing position if needed.
The patient is asked to strain/Valsalva maneuver, which would demonstrate prolapse not seen at rest.
Prolapse of uterus may be associated with prolapse of adjacent organ—bladder and rectum.

Cystocele

- Bulge of varying degree of anterior vaginal wall, increase on straining may be seen or may be seen on separation of labia and depressing the posterior vaginal wall
- Mucosa over the bulge: Transverse rugosities
- Impulse on coughing, diffuse margins, and reducible.

Cystourethrocele

- The bulging will include the lower one-third of the anterior wall
- There may be associated SUI—leakage of urine on coughing.

Lax Perineum

- Gaping introitus with old scar of perineal tear may be seen.
- Lower part of posterior vaginal wall is visible with or without straining.

Rectocele and Enterocele

- Bulging in posterior vaginal wall with transverse sulcus between the two
- The midvaginal one is rectocele

❖ The enterocele bulge is in the upper third, close to the cervix and cannot be reached by finger in rectum.

Uterine Prolapse

❖ In 2nd or 3rd degree prolapse or procidentia: Inspection reveals a mass protruding out of introitus, the leading part of which is external os
❖ In 1st degree on per speculum (PS), there would be descent of cervix below ischial spines on straining
❖ To diagnose 4th degree prolapse palpation is essential. Thumb placed anteriorly and fingers posteriorly above the mass outside the introitus will appose (**pinch test**)
❖ Degree of prolapse or POP Quantification (POP-Q) system should be done.
❖ Evidence of decubitus ulcer or pigmentation may be present
❖ Bimanual examination: Shallow fornices, with normal length of vaginal cervix and normal size of uterine body
❖ Uterocervical length (UCL) with uterine sound will reveal **increase in length** of uterine cavity which signifies **supravaginal elongation** of cervix seen in vaginouterine variety
❖ Levator ani muscle tone to be assessed
❖ Pubovaginalis is palpated in lower third of vagina for its tone (patient is asked to squeeze the anus)
❖ Rectal examination helps to detect deficient perineum.

Q. Decubitus ulcer.

■ INTRODUCTION

❖ **Decubitus ulcer is a tropic ulcer.**
❖ It is always found at the dependent part of prolapsed mass lying outside the introitus.
❖ So it will be present **only in 3rd and 4th degree prolapse** and never in 1st and 2nd degree.
❖ It is due to **friction, congestion, and circulatory changes** in the dependent part of the prolapse.
❖ The diminished circulation is due to constriction of prolapsed mass by vaginal opening and narrowing of uterine vessels by stretching effect.
❖ Ulcer must be treated before operation otherwise:
  ▹ Difficulty in incision
  ▹ Postoperative healing slowed
  ▹ Increased bleeding
  ▹ Postoperative infection.

Initial surface keratinization
↓
Cracks
↓
Infection
↓
Sloughing
↓
Ulceration and complete denudation of surface epithelium

■ MANAGEMENT

❖ Cervical cytology to rule out malignancy
❖ Reduction of the prolapse in to the vagina
❖ Daily packing with roller bandage or tampon soaked in **glycerin and acriflavine** heals the ulcer in a week or two.
  ▹ Glycerin: Hygroscopic agent, decrease edema and acriflavine = yellow colored dye that helps in epithelization.
❖ Estrogen cream can also be used in postmenopausal women.

Q. Key points of various surgeries for prolapse.
Q. Surgeries for young/nulliparous patient with prolapse.
Q. Treatment options for old/postmenopausal lady with prolapse.

INTRODUCTION

Prolapse is defined as the displacement of an organ from its normal anatomical position.

SURGICAL TREATMENT FOR PROLAPSE

Age, parity, type and degree of prolapse are the factors that decide the type of surgery.

Young patients desirous of further childbearing/menstrual function	For old patients, family complete, postmenopausal women
Vaginal route: • Fothergill's operation • Shirodkar's uterosacral ligament advancement Anterior colporrhaphy Posterior colporrhaphy	• Vaginal hysterectomy with or without anterior and posterior colporrhaphy • LeFort's repair (complete colpocleisis) • Goodell-Powel surgery (partial colpocleisis) Anterior colporrhaphy Posterior colporrhaphy
Abdominal route: Sling surgery (preferred choice) • Purandare • Shirodkar • Khanna • Virkud (composite sling)	

Anterior Colporrhaphy ("A" Repair)

Indications

Cystocele, urethrocele.

Principles

❖ Separation of anterior vaginal, wall from bladder
❖ Separation and mobilization of bladder from cervix.
❖ Plication of the pubovesicocervical (uterovesical fascia), thus elevating the bladder base and obliterating the cystocele.
❖ Excising the redundant portion of vaginal wall thus narrowing the vagina.

Posterior Colporrhaphy (Colpoperineorrhaphy; "P" Repair)

Indications

Rectocele, old torn perineum, relaxed vaginal outlet as a part of all vaginal operations of prolapse.

Principles

❖ Removal of triangular piece of posterior vaginal wall
❖ Rectocele corrected by suturing pararectal fascia

Chapter 5: Prolapse

- Approximation of levator ani by deep suturing **(Young's stitch)**
- Suturing the vaginal edges longitudinally thus narrowing the vaginal opening.

Manchester (Fothergill) Operation

Devised by Archibald Donald and William Fothergill.

Indications

- Young patient with second (sometimes even third) degree prolapse with supravaginal elongation of cervix and who wants to preserve menstrual function.
- Initially, the operation was thought to preserve the fertility status of the patient. But as it is associated with a lot of complications (mentioned below), **it is not a preferred option in nulliparous patients.**
- **Main step is amputation of cervix.**

Principles

- Anterior colporrhaphy is done
- Cervix is dilated. It helps in passage of sutures, ensures adequate drainage and prevents cervical stenosis. Curettage can be done
- **Amputation of cervix**
- Plication of Mackenrodt's ligaments in front of the cervix. This facilitates their shortening and raising the cervix
- Posterior lip of the amputated cervix is covered by vaginal flap using a **Sturmdorff suture**
- Colpoperineorrhaphy is done.

Complications

- Primary hemorrhage or secondary hemorrhage
- Repeated second trimester abortions due to **cervical incompetence**
- Preterm labor/premature rupture of membranes (PROM)
- Cervical stenosis
- Cervical dystocia
- Infertility due to cervical factor.

Shirodkar's Modification of Fothergill's Operation/Shirodkar's Uterosacral Ligaments Advancement

Principles

- The vaginal wall is dissected upward all around the cervix.
- The uterosacrals are dissected, mobilized and brought forward and sutured in front of the cervix.
- **Cervical amputation is NOT done**
- Posterior repair is done
- The modified Fothergill's operation has the advantage that **childbearing function is preserved.**
- This operation is not advisable if the uterosacrals are atrophic.

Sling Operations

Following sling operations **fertility is not impaired** and hence considered **best or most suitable for nulliparous young patients.**

When the supporting tissues have become atrophic or torn, slings of Mersilene tape or mesh are used. These slings produce minimal tissue reaction and remain unabsorbed giving lifelong support.

Types of Sling Operations

- **Shirodkar's sling:** Tape is anchored to sacral promontory and posterior aspect of isthmus—static, closed loop, posterior sling.
- **Purandare's cervicopexy:** Tape is anchored to anterior abdominal wall and anterior aspect of isthmus—dynamic, closed loop, anterior sling.
- **Khanna's sling:** Tape is anchored to anterior superior iliac spines and anterior aspect of isthmus—static, open, neutral sling.
- **Virkud's composite sling:** Tape is anchored to sacral promontory as well as anterior abdominal wall and posterior aspect of isthmus; left uterosacral ligament is also plicated—static sling + dynamic, open, anterior + posterior sling.

1. Purandare's Sling Operation

- Pfannenstiel incision
- Two strong linen stay sutures are transfixed to the isthmus anteriorly.
- Middle portion of a 30 cm Mersilene tape is transfixed to the isthmus anteriorly with the stay sutures.
- The left end tape is then passed between left broad ligament, through left internal inguinal ring, piercing the transversalis fascia and turned medially at linea semilunaris between the rectus muscle and sheath where it is sutured with linen/vicryl/prolene **to rectus sheath.**
- The same is repeated on the other side.
- **Good abdominal muscle tone is prerequisite for this surgery.** If the anterior abdominal tone is poor, this surgery should not be done.

Advantages:
- Technically very easy to perform
- Provides dynamic support to uterus.

Disadvantages:
- Postsurgery the uterus becomes **retroverted** and the Pouch of Douglas (POD) becomes deep and hence **enterocele is a long-term complication** of this surgery. It can be prevented by Moskowitz/Halban's surgery in which POD is obliterated.
- As the tape is anchored to the isthmus anteriorly, it may be damaged at subsequent cesarean section (LSCS)
- Bladder may be advanced on uterus and may make exposure of lower uterine segment difficult
- As it is a closed loop sling; in case it becomes tight, there is a risk of bowel loops being trapped between uterus and anterior abdominal wall.

2. Khanna's Sling Operation

The Mersilene tape is attached to the isthmus anteriorly and it is anchored to the periosteum of the anterior superior iliac spines.

Advantages:
- Technically easy to perform
- Does not antevert or retrovert the uterus
- No risk of bowel obstruction.

Disadvantages:
- Tape is very superficial and can be very easily felt by the patient and the tape constantly rubs against dress worn tightly at the hip
- If skin wound gets infected, periostitis results which is painful and there is a risk of the tape getting detached.

3. Shirodkar's Abdominal Sling Operation

- Any cystocele present must be repaired before this operation
- The disc between the fifth lumbar and the first sacral vertebra is exposed. Two strong linen stay sutures are passed through the disc (anterior longitudinal ligament) with the ends kept long
- The left psoas muscle is exposed, a loop of Mersilene strip is passed through the muscle belly and ends firmly sewn together to form a loop to avoid obstruction to the rectosigmoid
- A sufficiently long strip of Mersilene tape is taken and its middle portion is sutured to the back of the cervix at the level of the uterosacrals
- On the left side, the tape has to pass below the mesentery of sigmoid colon, through the loop to reach sacral promontory
- The psoas loop on the right side is not essential
- The two ends of the tape are anchored to the disc (anterior longitudinal ligament) with the linen stay sutures.

Advantages:
- Anatomically the **most correct operation** as it maintains the uterus in its correct anatomical position. It provides a strong static bony support
- There is no tendency to enterocele formation.

Disadvantages/Complications:
- Technically very difficult to perform
- Injury to sigmoid colon, mesentery, and ureters
- Hemorrhage from presacral or mesenteric vessels
- Intestinal obstruction
- Injury to genitofemoral nerve (present in psoas muscle).

4. Virkud's Composite Sling Operation

As the complications of Shirodkar sling are mainly on the left side, in this surgery, on right side the tape is attached to sacral promontory and on left side the tape is attached to rectus sheath **(left-sided Purandare + right-sided Shirodkar)**.
- Pfannenstiel incision
- One end of the Mersilene tape (30 cm long) is fixed to the sacral promontory posteriorly with two strong linen stay sutures
- It is then passed subperitoneally on the right side of pelvic wall; then through right broad ligament and fixed to posterior surface of isthmus of cervix with linen stay sutures
- The tape is then passed between left broad ligament, through left internal inguinal ring, piercing the transversalis fascia and turned medially at linea semilunaris between the rectus muscle and sheath where it is sutured with linen to rectus sheath

- ❖ The left uterosacral ligament is then plicated with linen in order to correct the dextrorotation of uterus (this also helps in anteverting the uterus).

Advantages:
- ❖ Technically the operation is easy to perform
- ❖ Provides double support: Bony (sacral promontory) + dynamic (rectus sheath)
- ❖ Uterus remains anteverted
- ❖ No tendency to enterocele formation
- ❖ No risk of injury to sigmoid mesentery/colon or the genitofemoral nerve
- ❖ No risk of bowel obstruction (open sling)
- ❖ No difficulty in subsequent LSCS: As tape is posterior.

Vaginal Hysterectomy

- ❖ With or without anterior and posterior colporrhaphy (pelvic floor repair) is the **best and definitive surgery.**
- ❖ Suitable for old patients, family complete, postmenopausal women **who are medically fit** for surgery.

Principles
- ❖ Bladder separated and mobilized
- ❖ Anterior pouch is opened
- ❖ Posterior pouch is opened
- ❖ Bilateral uterosacrals and transverse cervical ligaments are clamped, cut and transfixed
- ❖ Uterine vessels, clamped, cut and ligated
- ❖ Uterus is delivered through anterior and posterior pouch
- ❖ Uppermost pedicles of ovarian ligament, tube and round ligament are clamped, cut and ligated, uterus removed
- ❖ Anterior colporrhaphy done
- ❖ Peritoneum closed by purse string suture
- ❖ The vaginal vault is then closed and **vault suspension is done**
- ❖ Posterior colpoperineorrhaphy done.

Le Forte's Operation (Complete Colpocleisis)

- ❖ It is done in very elderly **postmenopausal** women who are **unfit for vaginal hysterectomy** (e.g., with medical complications such as heart failure, past history of myocardial infarction, severe hypertension, etc.)
- ❖ This procedure can be performed under **local anesthesia and sedation**
- ❖ **Prior to the procedure, Pap smear should be done to rule out cervical dysplasia** and pelvic ultrasonography (USG) to rule out pelvic pathology.
- ❖ Sexual function **not** preserved.

Principle
Rectangular pieces of anterior and posterior vaginal walls are excised and edges are sutured to produce colpocleisis.

Goodell and Powell Surgery (Partial Colpocleisis)

- ❖ Modification of Le Forte's operation

Chapter 5: Prolapse

- Same indication as Le Forte's operation (patient medically not fit for vaginal hysterectomy).
- Sexual function is preserved.

Principle

Triangular pieces of anterior and posterior vaginal walls are excised and edges are sutured to produce partial colpocleisis.

MEDICAL TREATMENT

Ring Pessary

- It is never curative, **only palliative** (relieves the symptoms).
- **Additional benefit:** Improvement in urinary symptoms.

Indications of Ring Pessary

- Early pregnancy (up to 18 weeks)
- Puerperium
- Patients absolutely unfit for surgery
- Patient refuses surgery
- While waiting for surgery.

Q. Vault prolapse (short note).

Q. Post-hysterectomy vault prolapse (PHVP).

INTRODUCTION

Vaginal vault prolapse is a **long-term complication** following vaginal hysterectomy (less likely with abdominal/laparoscopic hysterectomy) with negative impact on women's quality of life due to associated urinary, anorectal and sexual dysfunction.

Definition

Vaginal vault prolapse has been defined by the International Continence Society as descent of the vaginal cuff below a point that is 2 cm less than the total vaginal length above the plane of the hymen. It occurs when the upper vagina bulges into or outside the vagina.

Coexistent pelvic floor defects which may be a cystocele, rectocele or enterocele are present in 72% of patients with vault prolapse.

Causes

Prolapse of the vaginal vault after hysterectomy may occur when the structures that support the top of the vagina and uterus are not reattached at the time of the initial procedure or due to weakening of these supports over time.

Prevention

The following can be done at the time of hysterectomy to prevent PHVP:

- **Moschcowitz operation:** The goal is to fix and suture the strong connective tissue that normally supports the uterus to the top of the vagina and at the same time, the pouch of Douglas is reduced with a purse-string type suture.
- **McCall culdoplasty** at the time of vaginal hysterectomy is effective in preventing subsequent PHVP. McCall culdoplasty involves approximating the uterosacral ligaments using continuous sutures, so as to obliterate the peritoneum of the posterior cul-de-sac as high as possible.
- **Vault suspension:** Suturing the cardinal and uterosacral ligaments to the vaginal cuff at the time of hysterectomy is effective in preventing PHVP following both abdominal and vaginal hysterectomies.
- **Sacrospinous fixation (SSF)** at the time of vaginal hysterectomy should be considered when the vault descends to the introitus during closure.

Conservative Management

- **Pelvic floor muscle training** is an effective treatment option for women with stage I–II vaginal prolapse, including post-hysterectomy vault prolapse.
- **Vaginal pessaries** are an alternative treatment option for women with stage II–IV PHVP.

Surgical Management

- **Sacrospinous fixation (SSF):** Vault is attached to sacrospinous ligament.
  The technique comprises dissection into the paravaginal space and the ischial spine is identified.
  Two nonabsorbable sutures are placed through the sacrospinous ligament, one and a half to two finger breadths medial to the ischial spine. One end of each suture is attached to the under surface of the posterior vaginal wall at the apical area
- **Abdominal or laparoscopic sacrocolpopexy:** Vault anchored to sacrum with use of mesh Interposition of a synthetic mesh or tissue graft between the vaginal vault and Sacrum
- **Colpocleisis:** Involves surgical obliteration of the lumen of the vagina.
  The prolapse is reduced by placing progressive sutures anteroposteriorly, till the prolapsed tissues are above the level of the levator plate.
  It is suitable for the frail elderly woman who is not sexually active and for whom conservative methods like the pessary is not ideal. It has the advantage that it can also be carried out under local anesthesia and involves a shorter operation time.

CHAPTER 6

Polycystic Ovarian Syndrome and Endometriosis

Q. Polycystic ovarian syndrome (PCOS).
Q. Clinical features of PCOS.
Q. Management of PCOS.

INTRODUCTION

- Polycystic ovarian syndrome (PCOS) is the **most common endocrinopathy** in women of reproductive age.
- It was first reported by **Stein and Leventhal in 1935** as a syndrome manifested by amenorrhea, hirsutism and obesity associated with enlarged polycystic ovaries.
- It is, however, a misnomer as there are no cysts in the ovary (there are multiple small follicles which look like cysts).

DEFINITION

It is a heterogeneous syndrome complex characterized by **chronic anovulation** and **hyperandrogenism**, frequently associated with **insulin resistance**, resulting in menstrual irregularity, infertility and hirsutism.

INCIDENCE

It is most important and extremely common disorder affecting 4–12% of women of reproductive age. It is **one of the leading causes of infertility**.

DIAGNOSTIC CRITERIA

- **Rotterdam 2003** criteria for diagnosis of polycystic ovarian syndrome or polycystic ovarian disease (PCOS/PCOD)—**at least two out of three** should be present:
  - Oligo- or anovulation
  - **Hyperandrogenism:** Biochemical or clinical
  - Twelve or more than 12 follicles 2–9 mm in size present within one or both ovaries on ultrasonography (USG) (necklace of pearl pattern) and/or ovarian volume more than 10 mL.

- Obesity is **not required** to make the diagnosis and even the ratio of FSH/LH = 1/2 or 1/3 not essential to make the diagnosis of PCOS.

PATHOPHYSIOLOGY (FIG. 6.1)

Complex and not yet well understood.
Hyperandrogenism and chronic anovulation with hyperinsulinemia.
- **Hyperthecosis**—increased testosterone from the ovaries due to stimulation of theca cells by persistently elevated *luteinizing hormone* (LH)
- **Defective aromatization** within the ovaries (hyperandrogenic microenvironment within the ovaries) which prevents follicular maturation
- Normal aromatization in periphery (unopposed estrogenic action) and **no progesterone due to anovulation**
- Insulin resistance (IR) is considered to be the hallmark in pathophysiology of PCOS.
- **IR through P450c17 enzyme dysfunction causes excessive androgen production from ovary and adrenals.**

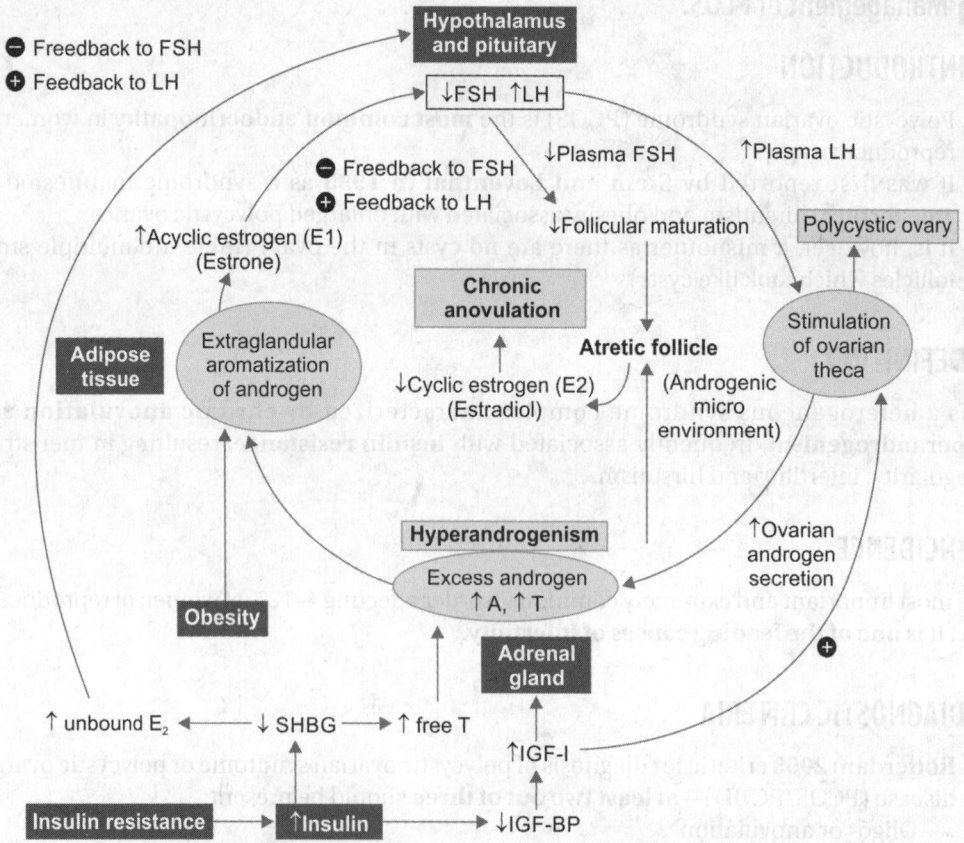

Fig. 6.1: Pathophysiology of polycystic ovarian syndrome (PCOS).

(FSH: follicle stimulating hormone; LH: luteinizing hormone; E1: estrone; E2: estradiol; T: testosterone; A: androstenedione; SHBG: sex hormone binding globulin; IGF-1: insulin-like growth factor 1; IGF-BP: insulin-like growth factor-binding protein)

Chapter 6: Polycystic Ovarian Syndrome and Endometriosis

It also decreases sex hormone-binding globulin (SHBG) and thereby increases free testosterone and estrogen levels.

CLINICAL FEATURES

The clinical features with frequency are listed in the table below:

Signs/symptoms	Frequency (%)
Oligomenorrhea	50–90
Amenorrhea	25–50
Infertility	55–75
Obesity	50–60
Hirsutism	60–90
Acne	25–30
Acanthosis nigricans	
Male pattern alopecia	
First trimester abortions	
Menorrhagia following prolonged amenorrhea	

PCOS patients have android obesity: Waist to hip ratio more than 0.85.

Acanthosis Nigricans

- Diffuse, velvety thickening and hyperpigmentation of the skin
- It is generally present at the nape of the neck, axillae, area beneath the breasts, intertriginous areas, and exposed areas
- Marker of insulin resistance
  - HAIR–AN syndrome
    [Hyperandrogenism (HA), insulin resistance (IR) and acanthosis nigricans (AN)]
- **Long-term complications** associated with PCOS:
  - Diabetes mellitus (because of IR)
  - Endometrial hyperplasia
  - Endometrial carcinoma (both due to unopposed estrogen stimulation).
- **Metabolic syndrome or syndrome X:** Insulin resistance (IR), obesity, hypertension, ↑triglycerides, and ↑ fasting blood sugar (↑FBS) associated with coronary artery disease.

INVESTIGATIONS

Serum Values

- Serum follicle stimulating hormone (FSH) and *luteinizing hormone* (LH) **(done on day 2 or day 3 of menstrual cycle)**
- **Serum FSH/LH = 1:2 OR 1:3**. Raised LH and decreased or normal FSH (serum FSH/LH: 2:1 = Normal ratio)
- **Serum testosterone is elevated** but generally less than 150 ng/dL (normal: 20–80 ng/dL)
- Androstenedione elevated

- SHBG: Reduced
- Free or unbound estradiol: Increased
- Estrone is increased
- Dehydroepiandrosterone (DHEAS) is normal or elevated
- Serum fasting insulin: Increased (>25 micro IU/mL)
- Serum FBS or serum fasting insulin <4.5 indicates insulin resistance
- Serum AMH (can be done on any day of the cycle) levels are elevated
- Serum thyroid stimulating hormone (TSH) and PROLACTIN levels must also routinely done
- Lipid profile is also to be done [(increase in total cholesterol and low-density lipoproteins (LDL) and decrease in high-density lipoproteins (HDL)].

Ultrasonography (USG)

Transvaginal ultrasonography (TVS) is preferred (100% detection rate).

Necklace of Pearls Pattern

- Twelve or more than 12 follicles 2–9 mm in size present within one or both ovaries and/or ovarian volume >10 mL
- Increase in echogenicity and volume of stroma and increase in stromal blood flow velocity
- USG shows a necklace-of-pearl pattern in 60–80% cases only. **Ovaries can be normal on USG** in a case of PCOS
- Increase in endometrial thickness due to unopposed estrogen stimulation.

Laparoscopy (not routinely done for diagnosis purpose, but as a part of infertility workup)

Laparoscopy (can be diagnostic and therapeutic also)
- Oyster ovaries: Bilaterally **enlarged** (2–5 times of normal size), white, smooth sclerotic ovaries with thickened capsule.
- No evidence of corpus luteum or stigma of ovulation.

■ TREATMENT

- Individualization of patients
- Treatment depends on patients need and symptoms
- Patient counseled about the disease
- **Lifestyle modification and weight loss:** Weight loss in obese patients is very important. Weight loss of 5–10% can restore ovulation and fertility in majority of patients and also improves menstrual irregularity and hirsutism
- **Multidisciplinary approach** for weight loss (Gynecologist, Endocrinologist, Dietician, exercise program).

Treatment Options as per Symptoms

- **Irregular periods/amenorrhea:** Regularization of menses with oral contraceptive (OC) pills/cyclical progesterone
- **Hirsutism/acne:** Suppression of androgens with OC pills/antiandrogens/mechanical methods

- **Infertility:** Ovulation induction with drugs/laparoscopic electrocoagulation of ovarian surface (LEOS)/assisted reproductive technology (ART)
- **Obesity:** Diet/exercise/insulin sensitizers
- **Hyperinsulinemia:** Insulin sensitizers/weight loss.

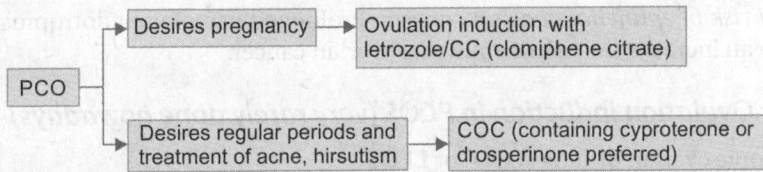

Insulin sensitizers (**metformin, myoinositol**) should be added to the treatment **if there is insulin resistance (IR)**.

Infertility/Desirous of Child

Ovulation has to be induced as infertility is due to anovulation.

Ovulation Induction Agents

1. Clomiphene Citrate (CC) (was the 1st Drug of Choice for Anovulatory Infertility)

It is a racemic mixture of enclomiphene and zuclomiphene. Enclomiphene is a more potent isomer responsible for its ovulation-inducing action.

- Dose: 50–250 mg/day for 5 days: From day 2 to day 6 or day 5 to day 9. However, the US Food and Drug Administration (FDA) approved maximum dose for CC is 100 mg
- CC blocks 'E' receptors → increase FSH from pituitary → growth of follicles
- With CC success rate for ovulation is 80% and success for pregnancy is 40%.

In cases of elevated DHEAS, dexamethasone 0.5 mg/day at bedtime combined with CC is found to be useful.

2. Letrozole, Anastrozole, Tamoxifen

Letrozole (2.5–5 mg for 5 days)/anastrozole/tamoxifen: Aromatase inhibitor blocks conversion of testosterone to estrogen, leading to increased FSH from pituitary.

As per ESHRE/ASRM 2018 guidelines now letrozole is the 1st line DOC for PCOS patients with anovulatory infertility.

3. Gonadotropins

HMG (human menopausal gonadotropin) (from the urine of the menopausal women) and recombinant FSH.

- With gonadotropins, success rate for ovulation is 80–99% and pregnancy rate is 40–70%
- Follicular study through TVS is done along with ovulation induction to monitor the growth of follicles and when the **dominant follicle is 18–20 mm**, ovulation trigger is given to rupture the follicle
- For ovulation trigger, most common drug used is **injection human chorionic gonadotropin (hCG) 5,000–10,000 IU IM** (derived from the urine of pregnant women or by recombinant technology). Recombinant LH is can also be used but is very expensive
- Ovulation occurs **36 hours after injecting hCG**.

Side Effects of Ovulation Induction

- *Multiple pregnancies:* 3–8% with CC, 15–30% with gonadotropins
- *Ovarian hyperstimulation syndrome (OHSS):* Most dangerous complication, more common with gonadotropins and very unlikely with CC
- *Increased risk of epithelial ovarian cancers:* Prolonged use of gonadotropins/CC (>6–12 months) can increase the risk of epithelial ovarian cancer.

Surgery for Ovulation Induction in PCOS (very rarely done nowadays)

- Laparoscopic ovarian drilling (LOD) or LEOS
- In this surgery, monopolar current is passed within the ovary to destroy the ovarian theca
- This surgery is done **only for infertile patients of PCOS who are resistant to ovulation with gonadotropin** or when very high doses of gonadotropins are required for ovulation
- *Advantages:* No risk of OHSS and multiple pregnancy
- *Disadvantages:* Surgical procedure, risk of premature ovarian failure if excessive ovarian tissue is damaged, and adhesion formation postsurgery.

Success rate for ovulation is 70–90% and pregnancy rate is 40–70%.

ART/IVF

When all the above treatment fails then in vitro fertilization (IVF) is used as the last resort for infertile patients.

Insulin Sensitizers

- MC used drug till now was metformin
- Metformin (starting from 500 mg once and can be increased up to 1,000 mg twice a day or 850 mg TDS) will help the patient to lose weight and will either cause spontaneous ovulation or *increase the success of ovulation induction drugs*. It reduces fasting insulin, testosterone and body mass index (BMI)
- **MC side effects:** Nausea or vomiting and bloating (GI upset)
- **Most dangerous side effect:** Lactic acidosis
- Metformin was thought to be teratogenic, but recent consensus is that metformin **can be continued throughout pregnancy and it decreases the risk of spontaneous abortion and development of [gestational diabetes mellitus (DM) (GDM)]**
- Newer insulin sensitizer **myoinositol** is now available. It is better tolerated than metformin and preferred nowadays.

Desires Regular Periods and Treatment of Acne, Hirsutism

Best treatment is oral contraceptive (**OC**) **PILLS as it regularizes the cycle and can also suppress acne and hirsutism.**
    OC pills containing cyproterone or drospirenone are preferred.
    OCs significantly decrease free testosterone levels. Progestin suppresses LH and estrogen increases SHBG.

Antiandrogens for Hirsutism

- Spironolactone 25–100 mg twice a day.
- Flutamide

- ❖ Finasteride
- ❖ Cyproterone acetate.
  Mechanical methods like plucking or shaving or electrolysis or laser can also be used.
  Eflornithine hydrochloride 13.9% cream for local use.

Q. Define endometriosis. Give clinical features and management of endometriosis.

Q. Laparoscopy in endometriosis.

■ DEFINITION

It was first described by Von Rokitansky. Endometriosis is defined as the presence of normal functional endometrial mucosa (glands and stroma) abnormally implanted in locations other than the uterine cavity (ectopic functional endometrium).

■ MOST COMMON SITES IN ORDER OF FREQUENCY

- ❖ Ovaries (ovarian endometriosis = endometrioma = chocolate cyst of the ovaries)
- ❖ Pouch of Douglas (POD)
- ❖ Uterosacral ligaments.

■ THEORIES FOR DEVELOPMENT OF ENDOMETRIOSIS

- ❖ **Sampson's theory of retrograde menstruation:** The most accepted theory
- ❖ **Ivanoff and Meyer:** Celomic metaplasia
- ❖ Hematogenous spread
- ❖ Lymphatic spread (Halban's theory)
- ❖ Direct implantation.

■ CLINICAL FEATURES

Symptoms

About one-third of women with endometriosis remain asymptomatic.

When they do occur, symptoms, such as the following, typically reflect the area of involvement:

- ❖ **Dysmenorrhea (50%):** Progressively increasing **secondary dysmenorrhea** (due to PGF2 and thromboxane)
- ❖ Menorrhagia and premenstrual spotting (50–60%)
- ❖ **Pelvic pain** or backache due to adhesions, scarring or impingement of nerves
- ❖ Lower abdominal or back pain
- ❖ **Deep dyspareunia:** Mostly seen in endometriosis of rectovaginal septum or Pouch of Douglas and with fixed retroverted uterus
- ❖ **Infertility:** Around 40–60% patients have infertility due to multiple factors like tubal adhesions, or anatomical distortion ovarian dysfunction, dyspareunia, defective implantation and increased sperm phagocytosis
- ❖ **Dyschezia (pain on defecation):** Often with cycles of diarrhea and constipation, rectal bleeding in cases of involvement of colon and rectum
- ❖ Pain on micturition and/or urinary frequency, **cyclical hematuria if bladder is involved**.

Clinical Examination

Abdominal

Examination may be normal. Very rarely, enlarged chocolate cyst or a tubo-ovarian mass may be felt in the lower abdomen arising from the pelvis. The mass is tender with restricted mobility.

Pelvic Examination

It may be normal or may reveal the following:
- **Fixed retroverted uterus**
- Pelvic tenderness
- **Nodules in the POD**
- Nodularity of the uterosacral ligaments
- Unilateral or bilateral adnexal mass
- Speculum examination may reveal bluish nodules in posterior fornix.

INVESTIGATIONS

Laparoscopy is the investigation of choice.
Laparoscopy findings are (**Fig. 6.2**):
- Chocolate cysts
- Powder burn spots
- Matchstick burnt spots
- Blueberry lesion
- Red/purple raspberry lesion
- White lesion
- Red/flame lesion
- Subovarian adhesions
- Subtle peritoneal defects associated with endometriosis are called Allen-Master syndrome.

USG, CT Scan, MRI may detect ovarian chocolate cysts but can also be normal.

Ca125 is a nonspecific marker, may be **moderate elevations** in levels (up to 35 IU/mL is normal).

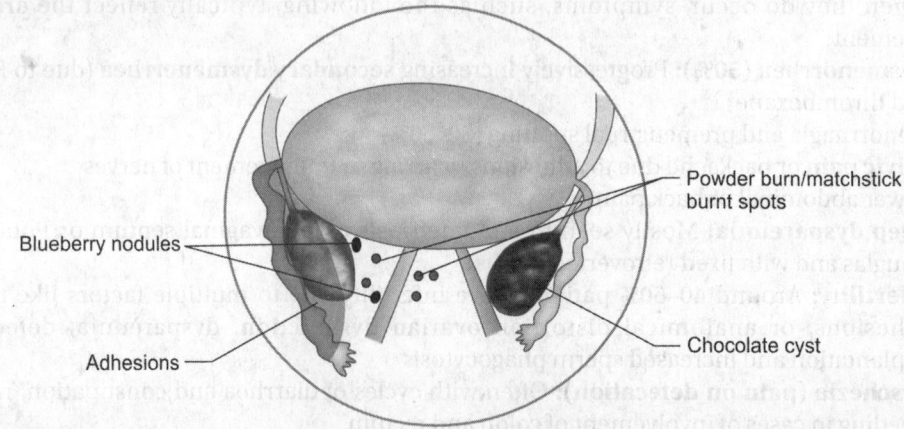

Fig. 6.2: Laparoscopy in endometriosis.

TREATMENT

The treatment depends on the patient's age, size and extent of lesion and desire for fertility.
- ❖ Medical
- ❖ Surgical
- ❖ Combined.

Generally surgery is done first followed by medical management or **sandwich therapy** is done in which medical → surgical → medical treatment is done.

Medical Management

The aim of medical management is **to induce amenorrhea** in the patient thereby causing atrophy of the implants. The treatment is considered suppressive rather than curative as recurrence is high on stopping the treatment.

The medical management provides symptomatic relief from pain, dysmenorrhea, and also decrease the size of lesions:
- ❖ **Pseudopregnancy regimen:** OC pills, DMPA, POP (progestogen-only pill) and Mirena.
- ❖ **Pseudomenopause regimen:** Danazol (Hardly ever used today because of androgenic side effects).
- ❖ **Medical castration: Gonadotropin-releasing hormone (GnRH) analogs (most common drug used for medical management).** Treatment is usually restricted to monthly injections for 6 months. Loss of trabecular bone density caused by GnRH is restored by 2 years after cessation of therapy. Other prominent adverse effects include hot flashes and vaginal dryness.

Hormones used in endometriosis		
Drugs	Dose	Mechanism
Combined estrogen progestogen (oral pill)	1–2 tablets 6–9 months	Pseudopregnancy
Progestogens *Oral* Medroxyprogesterone acetate	10 mg thrice daily × 6–9 months 10–20 mg daily × 6–9 months	Pseudopregnancy
Dydrogesterone Norethisterone	10–30 mg daily × 6–9 months	
IM Medroxyprogesterone	150 mg 3 months interval × 2	Pseudopregnancy
IUCD Levonorgestrel-releasing IUCD		Pseudopregnancy
Danazol	400–800 mg orally in 4 divided doses × 6–9 months	Pseudomenopause
Gestrinone	1.25 or 2.5 mg twice a week × 6–9 months	Pseudomenopause
GnRH analogs	Leuprolide 3.75 mg IM monthly × 6 months Nafarelin 200 µg intranasally daily × 6 months Goserelin 3.6 mg depot IM monthly × 6 months	Medical oophorectomy

Recent Advances

Dienogest is an orally-active semisynthetic, steroidal progestogen. It also has antiandrogenic activity.

It binds to the progesterone receptor with high specificity, and produces a potent progestogenic effect.

It has been investigated extensively for long-term treatment of endometriosis (**up to 65 weeks**). **Dienogest 2 mg daily** effectively alleviates the painful symptoms of endometriosis, reduces endometriotic lesions, and improves indices of quality of life.

When given continuously, dienogest causes decidualization of endometrial tissue followed by atrophy of the endometriotic lesions.

- In 2018, the Food and Drug Administration (FDA) approved the first **oral** gonadotropin-releasing hormone **(GnRH) antagonist**, called **Elagolix**, to help with moderate to severe pain from endometriosis.
- **Letrozole** (aromatase inhibitor) and **cabergoline** (appears to inhibit angiogenesis) have shown to be effective in the treatment of endometriosis-related pain.

Surgery

Age, desire for future childbearing, and deterioration of quality of life are the main considerations when deciding on the extent of surgery.

Surgical care can be broadly classified as conservative when reproductive potential is retained, semiconservative when reproductive ability is eliminated but ovarian function is retained, and radical when the uterus and ovaries are removed.

Conservative Surgery

Surgical efforts **(laparoscopy preferred over laparotomy)** are aimed at **removal of the endometrial implants and correction of anatomic distortions.** Implants can be ablated using either laser energy or electrosurgical techniques.

Patients with infertility: **Laparoscopic ovarian cystectomy, adhesiolysis, and electrocoagulation of endometriotic implants** with bipolar current.

Chocolate Cyst/Endometrioma

- Treatment options include drainage/aspiration or cystectomy
- After drainage the cyst wall epithelium is removed or destroyed with coagulation
- This decreases the risk of recurrence but can lead to loss of ovarian reserve
- Pregnancy rates are about 60% in moderate cases and 35% in severe cases. Maximum rates are observed in first 6 months postsurgery.

In severe cases In vitro fertilization-embryo transfer (IvF-eT) is required.

For Pain Relief

- **Presacral neurectomy** can be done to relieve severe dysmenorrhea. The nerve bundles are transected at the level of the third sacral vertebra, and the distal ends are ligated.
- Nodularity of the uterosacral ligaments may contribute to low backache and dyspareunia. The transmission of neural pathways is via the Lee-Frankenhäuser plexus. **Laparoscopic uterine nerve ablation (LUNa)** can be performed to interrupt these pain fibers.

Radical Surgery

If the family is complete and the patient has severe pain or menstrual complaints: Hysterectomy with bilateral salpingo-oophorectomy with resection of all endometriotic implants.

CHAPTER 7

Hysterolaparoscopy

Q. Indications of laparoscopy. Add a note on advantages of laparoscopy.
Q. Contraindications and complications of laparoscopy.

■ INTRODUCTION

- Laparoscopy is a technique of visualization of peritoneal cavity by means of fiber optic endoscope introduced through abdominal wall.
- Laparoscopic surgery (key hole surgery), also called minimally invasive surgery (MIS), is a modern surgical technique in which operations in the abdomen and pelvis are performed through small incisions (usually 0.5–1.5 cm). This is in contrast to the larger incisions needed in laparotomy.
- Prior pneumoperitoneum is achieved with the help of CO_2 gas.

The intra-abdominal pressure should be between 10–15 mm Hg.

■ INDICATIONS

- Diagnostic
- Therapeutic.

Diagnostic

Infertility: Tubal factor evaluation, chromopertubation (**Fig. 7.1**), tubal adhesions, fibroids, endometriosis (**Fig. 7.2**), etc.
- Chronic pelvic pain.
- *Pelvic mass:* Fibroids, ovarian tumors.
- Müllerian anomalies.
- Uterine perforation.
- Patients with primary amenorrhea.
- *Acute pelvic lesions:* Ectopic pregnancy, acute salpingitis, etc.

Therapeutic

- *Tubes:* Tubal ligation, adhesiolysis, tuboplasty, tubal ligation reversal.

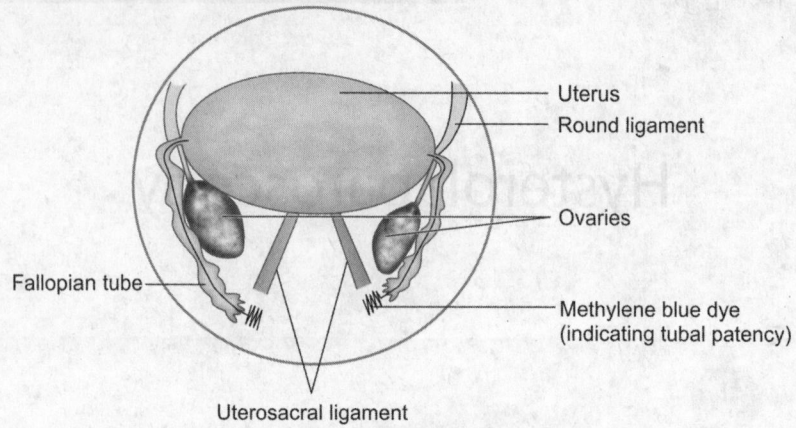

Fig. 7.1: Laparoscopy and chromopertubation.

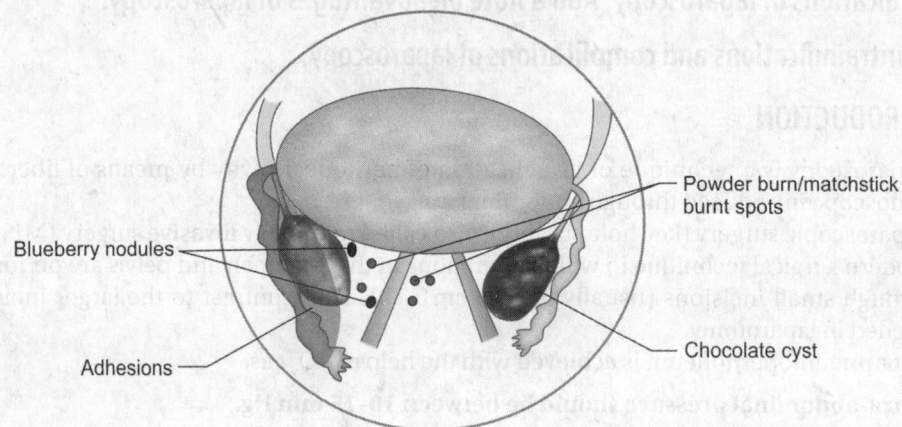

Fig. 7.2: Laparoscopy in endometriosis.

- *Uterus:* Myomectomy, hysterectomy [laparoscopic-assisted vaginal hysterectomy (LAVH), total laparoscopic hysterectomy (TLH)].
- *Ovary:* Cystectomy, oophorectomy, cyst aspiration.
- *Ectopic pregnancy:* Salpingectomy, salpingostomy.
- Laparoscopic electrocoagulation of the ovarian surface (LEOS) for polycystic ovary syndrome (PCOS).
- *Endometriosis:* Excision/aspiration of chocolate cyst and coagulation/ablation of endometriotic implants
- Urinary incontinence.
- Sacrocolpopexy for vault prolapse
- Oncosurgeries.

Advantages of Laparoscopic Surgery

There are several advantages of laparoscopic surgery over laparotomy:
- Rapid postoperative recovery
- Less morbidity
- Shorter hospital stay and back to normal life sooner.

- Excellent visualization of tissues (better and magnified images with HD cameras and availability of 3D technology)
- Very small abdominal scars (cosmetic value) and avoidance of large incisions and quick healing as the scar is small.
- Reduce likelihood of infection: As exposure of internal organs gets reduced for external contaminants, hence the risk of infections reduced.
- Require less sutures to close it. This reduces the likelihood of complications from the wound
- Less tissue cutting less adhesion formations
- Reduced blood loss
- Less postoperative pain—lesser use of analgesics
- Lesser risk of incisional hernia
- Overall increase patient satisfaction.

CONTRAINDICATIONS OF LAPAROSCOPY

- Severe cardiopulmonary disease
- Patient hemodynamically unstable
- Generalized peritonitis
- Significant hemoperitoneum
- Intestinal obstruction
- Extensive peritoneal adhesion
- Large pelvic tumor
- Large hiatal hernia
- Advanced malignancy
- Anticoagulation therapy
- Pregnancy (considered relative contraindication, as nowadays laparoscopy is done during pregnancy when indicated).

COMPLICATIONS

Due to Laparoscopy

- Extraperitoneal insufflation—surgical emphysema.
- Omental emphysema.
- Trauma/injury to:
  - Blood vessels: Mesenteric, omental, aorta, inferior epigastric vessels
  - Bowel
  - Bladder
  - Ureter
  - The trauma may be mechanical or thermal by electrical or laser energy.
- Electrosurgical complications causing thermal injury.
- Gas embolism (CO_2) causing hypotension, cardiac arrhythmia.

ANESTHETIC COMPLICATIONS

- Hypoventilation—due to pneumoperitoneum and Trendelenburg position.
- Hypercarbia and metabolic acidosis.

- Basal lung atelectasis.
- Aspiration, cardiac arrest.

Complications Common to any Surgical Procedure
- Hemorrhage
- Infection
- Wound dehiscence and incisional hernia.

Q. Indications of hysteroscopy.

INTRODUCTION

Hysteroscopy is a procedure to visualize the uterine cavity by means of fiberoptic endoscope introduced through cervix.

Indications
- Diagnostic
- Therapeutic.

Diagnostic

Various indications for diagnostic hysteroscopy are as follows:
- **Abnormal uterine bleeding/menorrhagia/postmenopausal bleeding:** Hysteroscopy has nearly replaced standard dilatation and curettage for the management of abnormal uterine bleeding (AUB), as it allows for direct visualization and diagnosis of intrauterine abnormalities (like polyps, submucous fibroids; **Figs. 7.3 to 7.5**).
- **Infertility:** Hysteroscopy increases accuracy in diagnosing the cause of intrauterine filling defects detected on hysterosalpingography (HSG). Intracavitary lesions (fibroids, septum, and adhesions) are implicated as causes of infertility. In unexplained infertility, hysteroscopy may be performed simultaneously with laparoscopy to evaluate the uterine cavity.

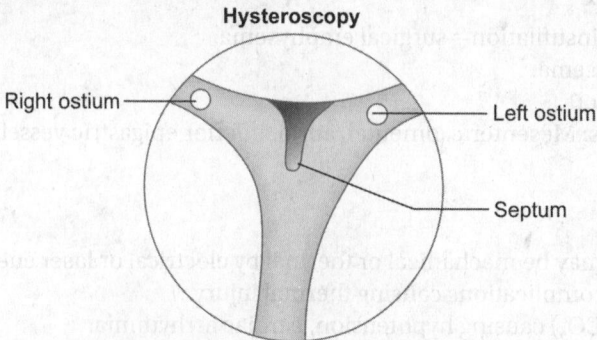

Fig. 7.3: Hysteroscopy in septate uterus.

- **Recurrent spontaneous abortions:** Intracavitary lesions (fibroids, septum, and adhesions) are implicated as causes of infertility and recurrent abortions.
- Misplaced intrauterine contraceptive device (IUCD).

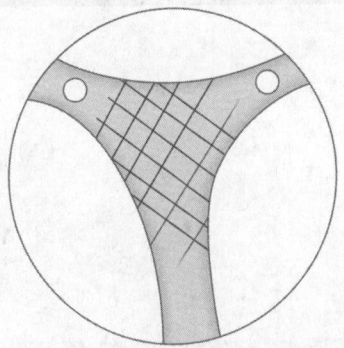
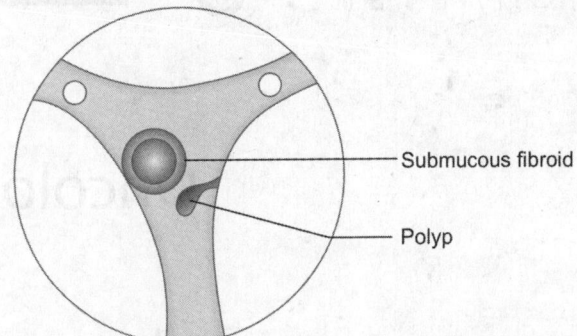

Fig. 7.4: Intrauterine adhesions (Asherman's syndrome).

Fig. 7.5: Hysteroscopy detecting submucous fibroid and polyp.

Therapeutic/Operative Hysteroscopy

For all intracavitatory pathologies hysteroscopy is the gold standard for treatment. The indications for therapeutic hysteroscopy are:

- **Polyps and fibroids**: Endometrial polyps and submucous fibroids are well known to cause vaginal bleeding and can be removed with hysteroscopy (polypectomy, myomectomy).
- **Transcervical resection of the endometrium (TCRE) and endometrial ablation** can be done in cases of dysfunctional uterine bleeding (DUB).
- **Intrauterine adhesions (IUAs):** Asherman's syndrome was first identified in 1948 as uterine synechiae. These IUAs are often associated with amenorrhea or infertility. Hysteroscopy is the gold standard to diagnose and treat these adhesions. Benefits include visually directed lysis.
- **Lateral wall metroplasty** can be done in cases of T-shaped uterus and **septal resection** in cases of septum.
- Removal of IUCD which is in the cavity when threads are missing.
- Endometrial biopsy of suspected endometrium under direct vision.
- **Cornual catheterization** in cases of cornual blocks of Fallopian tubes.
- **Sterilization:** Essure coil insertion.

CHAPTER 8

Oncology

Q. Risk factors for cervical intraepithelial neoplasia (CIN) and its management.
Q. Management of CIN III.

INTRODUCTION

Cervical intraepithelial neoplasia (CIN) is a premalignant lesion that is diagnosed by histology as CIN I, CIN II, or CIN III. If left untreated, CIN II or CIN III can progress to cervical cancer.

RISK FACTORS FOR CA CERVIX AND CIN

- Young age at first intercourse (<16 years)
- Multiple sexual partners
- Cigarette smoking
- Race
- Early age at first pregnancy
- High parity
- Low socioeconomic status
- **Human papillomavirus (HPV) infection, herpes simplex virus (HSV)**
- Human immunodeficiency virus (HIV)
- Immunosuppression.

Over 90% cases with CIN and invasive cancer are positive with HPV deoxyribonucleic acid (DNA).

Human Papillomavirus and CIN

- HPV produces CIN in 90% cases

HPV type	Oncogenic potential	Comment
6, 11	Low	Anogenital warts
31, 33, 35, 51, 52	Intermediate	CIN I, II, III
16, 18, 45, 56	High	• CIN II, III • Invasive CA

Chapter 8: Oncology

- HPV-16 is the most common HPV seen in invasive CA and CIN II/III and is found in 50% cases
- HPV-16 is not very specific and is also the most common HPV type in women with normal cytology
- **HPV-18 is more specific than HPV-16** for invasive tumors.

Life cycle of unstable cervical epithelium			
Cervical epithelium	CIN I	CIN II	CIN III/CIS
Regression to normal (%)	60	40	30
Persistence (%)	30	35	50
Progression to CIN 3/CIS (%)	10	20	–
Progression to invasion (%)	<1	5	20

DIAGNOSIS

Exfoliative Cytology (Pap Smear)

It is the gold standard for screening.
- The Papanicolaou test is a method of cervical screening used to detect potentially precancerous and cancerous processes in the transformation zone. The test was invented by and named after the prominent Greek doctor Georgios Papnikolaou.
- **Pap test reduces the incidence of cervical cancer by 60-90% and the death rate by 90%.**
- The cells are examined under a microscope to look for abnormalities. The test aims to detect potentially precancerous changes (called CIN or cervical dysplasia).
- Traditional Pap tests can be hard to read because cells can be dried out, covered with mucus or blood, or clump together on the slide.

ACOG Guidelines for Cervical Cancer Screening

- Women aged 21-29 years should have a Pap test alone **every 3 years**. HPV testing is not recommended.
- Women aged 30-65 years should have a Pap test and an HPV test (co-testing) every 5 years (preferred). It is also acceptable to have a Pap test alone every 3 years.
- Patient should stop having cervical cancer screening **after age 65 years** if:
  - The woman does not have a history of moderate or severe abnormal cervical cells or cervical cancer.
  - The woman had either three negative Pap test results in a row or two negative co-test results in a row within the past 10 years, with the most recent test performed within the past 5 years.

Liquid-based Cytology

It is superior to Pap smear and has a better sensitivity and specificity.
- The sample is collected in a similar way to the Pap smear but instead of smearing the sample onto a microscope slide (as in Pap smear), the head of the spatula, where the cells are lodged, is broken off into a small glass vial containing preservative fluid, or rinsed directly into the preservative fluid.

- The sample is then spun and treated to remove any obscuring material like blood, mucus or pus.
- A thin layer of the cells is deposited onto a slide. The slide is examined under a microscope.

HPV DNA Test

- The HPV test is a screening test for cervical cancer. The test detects the presence of HPV, the virus that causes cervical cancer. Certain types of HPV—including types 16 and 18—increase cervical cancer risk.
- The sample is taken at the same time as Pap smear.
- Visual inspection with acetic acid (VIA): Acetic acid is applied on cervix and if there is acetowhite area, colposcopy and biopsy is recommended.

Colposcopy and Cervical Biopsy

An abnormal cytology report warrants further evaluation with colposcopy and cervical biopsy.

- Colposcope is an instrument which gives an illuminated and magnified (6–16 fold) view of the cervix and the tissues of the vagina.
- The main goal of colposcopy is to prevent cervical cancer by detecting precancerous lesions early and treating them.
- 3% acetic acid is applied on the cervix and biopsy is to be taken from **acetowhite areas** (due to coagulation of nucleic acid).
- The abnormal findings include:
  - Leukoplakia/acetowhite areas
  - Punctuation (dilated capillaries seen end on)
  - Mosaic pattern
  - Neovascularization/atypical blood vessels and branching (green filter is used).

If colposcopy is not available then Schiller's test directed biopsy can be taken.

Confirmation of diagnosis is by biopsy.

Diagnostic Cone Biopsy

Indications are:
- If there is a mismatch between cytology and histology (If Pap smear is abnormal but cervical biopsy is normal)
- If entire transformation zone (TZ) is not visualized on colposcopy (unsatisfactory colposcopy)
- If endocervical curettage is positive.

■ TREATMENT

Definitive treatment will depend on:
- CIN I/II/III or CIS
- Patients age
- Parity desire for reproduction
- Facilities available for follow-up (colposcopy and cytology).

The principal treatments for CIN available are:
1. Local ablation (**no tissue available for histopathology**):
    - Cryotherapy
    - Cold coagulation
    - Electrodiathermy
    - Laser vaporization.
2. Excisional methods (**tissue is available for histopathology**):
    - Large loop excision of the transformation zone, or loop electrosurgical excision procedure (LLETZ, or LEEP)
    - Cold knife or laser conization.
3. **Simple hysterectomy** (Abdominal/vaginal/laparoscopic): **Never radical**
    Indications of simple hysterectomy are:
    - If the family is complete
    - If the patient is not ready for regular follow-ups or
    - Has associated problems such as prolapse or fibroids
    - Cancerphobia.

Management according to CIN grading:
- **CIN I:** Wait and watch and regular follow-up. If it is not possible it can be treated like CIN III
- **CIN II:** Follow-up or cryosurgery
- **CIN III and CIS:** If patient wants to **conserve the uterus/desirous of further child bearing**, complete destruction of the lesion by any of the following techniques after the following criteria are fulfilled:
    - The entire lesion is visualized within the TZ
    - Exclusion of microinvasion
    - No endocervical glandular involvement.

The techniques of destruction of the lesion are:
1. Cryotherapy: Crystallizing intracellular water at −90°C
   Nitrous oxide or CO_2 is used
   Depth of destruction = 5 mm
2. Cold coagulation: Temperature of 100–120°C
3. Electrodiathermy: Unipolar needle electrode is used
   Depth of destruction = 8–10 mm
4. CO_2 laser vaporization
   Depth of destruction = 7 mm
5. Cold knife or laser conization: However **therapeutic conization is reserved for stage IA1 microinvasive cervical cancer in young patients to preserve the uterus.**
   Complications of the procedure are:
    - Hemorrhage
    - Infections
    - Cervical stenosis
    - Cervical incompetence.
6. **Loop electroexcision procedure/large loop excision of transformation zone (LEEP/LLETZ)**
    - **Most commonly done and considered the best conservative treatment for CIN III**
    - Two to three cm loop of thin stainless steel wire used to excise the TZ
    - Blended current (cutting and coagulation)
    - Depth of destruction = 10 mm

FOLLOW-UP

- Post treatment cytology at 6 months till negative and then repeated at 12 months
- Thereafter repeated yearly for 5 years and
- Then 3 yearly.

- Simple and quick procedure under local anesthesia
- Tissue removed and send for histopathology
- Minimal complications.

PREVENTION

- To delay sexual exposure
- To avoid multiple sexual partners
- To avoid smoking
- Barrier contraception
- Local vaginal and penile hygiene
- **HPV vaccination:**
  - Highly effective intervention to prevent CIN and CA cervix.
  - **Bivalent (against HPV types 16, 18) and quadrivalent (against HPV types 6, 11, 16, 18) vaccines are now available in India and recommended for females 9–45 years of age.**

Q. Risk factors, pathogenesis and diagnosis of cervical cancer.

Q. Clinical features and management of cervical cancer.

INTRODUCTION

Carcinoma cervix is the second most common cancer affecting women in India today, breast cancer being the most common. One women dies of cervical cancer every eight minutes in India. The most common variety of Ca cervix is squamous cell carcinoma (85–90%).

RISK FACTORS FOR CARCINOMA CERVIX/CIN

- Young age at first intercourse (<16 years)
- Multiple sexual partners
- Cigarette smoking
- Race
- High parity
- Low socioeconomic status
- Human papillomavirus (HPV) infection
- HIV
- Immunosuppression.

The cervix is composed of the columnar epithelium, which lines the endocervical canal, and squamous epithelium, which covers the exocervix. The point at which they meet is called as squamocolumnar junction (SCJ).

- ❖ The SCJ is a dynamic point that changes in response to puberty, pregnancy, menopause, and hormonal stimulation. In neonates, SCJ is located on the exocervix. At menarche, the production of estrogen causes the vaginal epithelium to fill with glycogen. Lactobacilli act on the glycogen and lower the pH, stimulating the subcolumnar reserve cells to undergo metaplasia.
- ❖ Metaplasia advances from the original SCJ inward, toward the internal os and over the columnar villi. This process establishes an area called the transformation zone (TZ). The TZ extends from the original SCJ to the physiologically active SCJ.

PATHOGENESIS OF CIN AND INVASIVE CARCINOMA

The initial event in cervical dysplasia and carcinogenesis is likely to be infection with HPV. The mechanism by which HPV affects cellular growth and differentiation to interactions of **viral E6 and E7 proteins with p53 and Rb resulting in gene activation (Fig. 8.1).**

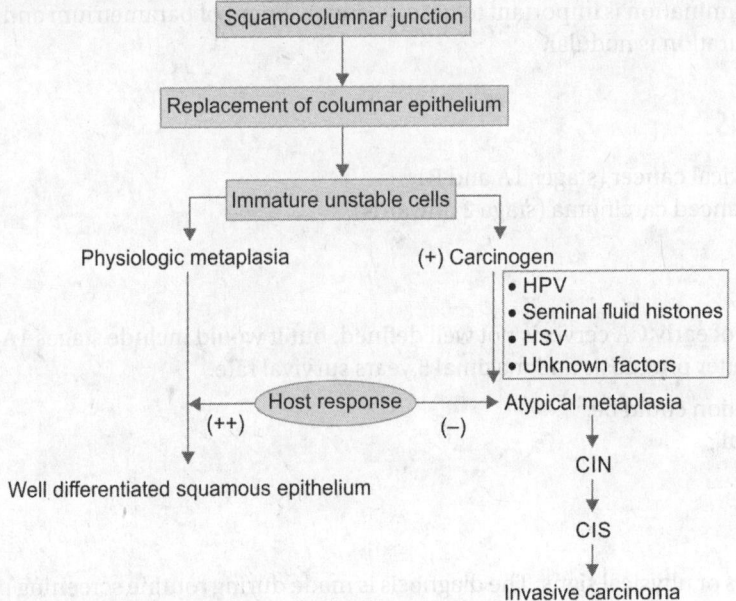

Fig. 8.1: Pathogenesis of CIN and invasive carcinoma.

CLINICAL FEATURES

Symptoms

- ❖ **Patient profile:** Patients are usually multiparous and in premenopausal age group (30–45 years) or even postmenopausal age
- ❖ In early stages there may be no symptoms
- ❖ Clinically, the first symptom of cervical cancer is **abnormal vaginal bleeding**, intermittent or continuous
- ❖ Usually its **postcoital bleeding**
- ❖ Postmenopausal bleeding
- ❖ Vaginal discomfort

- Malodorous vaginal discharge
- Pelvic pain
- **Dysuria, frequency, hematuria** due to bladder involvement
- It can invade the rectum directly, leading to constipation, fistula
- Ureteral obstruction, with or without **hydroureter or hydronephrosis leading to uremia**
- The triad of leg edema, pain, and hydronephrosis suggests pelvic wall involvement
- Cachexia, anemia, and uremia.

On Examination

- Physical examination (PS): Growth could be **ulcerative or fungating** which **bleeds on touch**
- Bimanual examination, the indurated growth is felt and extent to vagina and sides can be felt
- Induration of the bladder base may be felt through anterior fornix
- Rectal examination is important to note the involvement of parametrium and lateral pelvic wall. Induration is nodular.

DIAGNOSIS

- Early cervical cancer (stages 1A and B)
- Late/advanced carcinoma (stage 2 onwards).

Early

The concept of early CA cervix is not well defined, but it would include stages 1A and B which have got a better prognosis and maximal 5 years survival rate.

The presentation could be:
- Preclinical
- Clinical.

Preclinical

No symptoms or physical signs. The diagnosis is made during routine screening procedures or incidental on histopathology.

Exfoliative Cytology (Pap Smear)

- It is the gold standard for screening.
- The Papanicolaou test is a method of cervical screening used to detect potentially precancerous and cancerous processes in the transformation zone. The test was invented by and named after the prominent Greek doctor Georgios Papnikolaou
- The cells are examined under a microscope to look for abnormalities
- Abnormal smears should be subjected to colposcopic-guided cervical biopsy
- In the absence of colposcopy, **Schiller's test** directed biopsy can be done.

Liquid-based Cytology

- Superior to Pap smear and has a better sensitivity and specificity

Chapter 8: Oncology

- The sample is collected in a similar way to the Pap smear and the head of the spatula, where the cells are lodged, is broken off into a small glass vial containing preservative fluid, or rinsed directly into the preservative fluid
- The sample is then spun and treated to remove any obscuring material like blood, mucus or pus
- A thin layer of the cells is deposited onto a slide.

HPV DNA Test

- The HPV test is a screening test for cervical cancer. The test detects the presence of HPV, the virus that causes cervical cancer. Certain types of HPV—including types 16 and 18—increase cervical cancer risk.
- The sample is taken at the same time as Pap smear.

Colposcopy and Cervical Biopsy

- An abnormal cytology report warrants further evaluation with colposcopy and cervical biopsy.
  - 3% acetic acid is applied on the cervix and biopsy is to be taken from acetowhite areas (due to coagulation of nucleic acid)
  - The abnormal findings include:
    - Leukoplakia/acetowhite areas
    - Punctuation (dilated capillaries seen end on)
    - Mosaic pattern
    - Neovascularization/atypical blood vessels and branching.
- If colposcopy is not available, then Schiller's test directed biopsy can be taken.
- **Confirmation of diagnosis is by biopsy.**
- Depending on the depth of invasion the diagnosis of stage 0 (carcinoma in situ) or stage 1A (up to 5 mm invasion below the basement membrane) or 1B (>5 mm invasion) is made.

Diagnostic Cone Biopsy

It should be done in following cases:
- If there is a mismatch between cytology and histology (if Pap smear is abnormal but cervical biopsy is normal)
- If entire TZ is not visualized on colposcopy (unsatisfactory colposcopy)
- If endocervical curettage is positive.

Early Stage Clinical and Advanced/Late Carcinoma

Cervix may be abnormal in appearance, with red granular gross erosion, ulcer, or nodular growth. These abnormalities can extend to the vagina.

Punch biopsy (and histopathology) taken from the growth or ulcer on cervix is mandatory and confirmatory.

Once the diagnosis is established:
- Complete blood count (CBC)
- Renal function test (RFT) and
- Liver function test (LFT) (to look for abnormalities from possible metastatic disease)
- **Cystoscopy and proctoscopy** should be performed in patients with a bulky primary tumor to help rule out local invasion of the bladder and the colon

- Barium enema studies can be used to evaluate extrinsic rectal compression from the cervical mass
- A routine chest radiograph is obtained to help rule out pulmonary metastasis
- A computed tomography (CT) scan of the abdomen and pelvis is performed to look for metastasis in the liver, lymph nodes, or other organs and to help rule out hydronephrosis or hydroureter
- MRI or positron-emission tomography (PET) scanning is an alternative to CT scanning.

Staging Procedure

Physical examination	- Palpate lymph nodes - Examine vagina - Bimanual rectovaginal examination (under anesthesia recommended)
Radiologic studies	- Intravenous pyelogram - Barium enema - Chest X-ray - Skeletal X-ray
	- Biopsy - Conization - Hysteroscopy - Colposcopy - Endocervical curettage - Cystoscopy - Proctoscopy
Optional studies	- Computerized axial tomography - Lymphangiography - Ultrasonography - Magnetic resonance imaging - Radionuclide scanning - Laparoscopy

MANAGEMENT OF CANCER OF CERVIX (STAGEWISE)

Stage IA1

- Young patient/family not complete (to retain uterus) = **therapeutic conization**
- Old patient/family complete = **simple extrafascial hysterectomy.**

Stage IA2, IB, and IIA

Radical/Wertheim's hysterectomy	Concurrent chemoradiation (CTRT)
Only for stages: IA2, IB, IIA	I–IV IIb–IV

RT includes combined external beam radiation with brachytherapy.

Cisplatin is given before RT as a radiosensitizer hence the preferred terminology is concurrent chemoradiation.
- **All stages (I–IV) are radiosensitive**
- Stages of carcinoma cervix that are operable (radical/Wertheim's hysterectomy) are IA2, IB, and IIA

Chapter 8: Oncology

- Stages iiB–iV are not operable and have to be treated with cardiotoxicity of radiotherapy (CTRT) only
- IA2, IB, IIA are radiosensitive and surgically operable, but **surgery is preferred over CTRT** for these stages for the following reasons:
  - Preservation of ovarian function
  - Preservation of vagina for coital function
  - Psychological benefit to the patient.
- **Carcinoma cervix almost never spreads to ovary and so when radical hysterectomy is done, oophorectomy is not required.**

Indications of postoperative Radiotherapy: A randomized trial showed that patients with **parametrial involvement, positive pelvic nodes, or positive surgical margins** benefit from a postoperative combination of cisplatin containing chemotherapy and pelvic irradiation.

Postoperative radiation therapy is also recommended in patients who have at least two intermediate risk factors (including tumor size greater than 2 cm, deep stromal invasion, or lymphovascular space invasion).

Comparison between the two modalities of treatment for carcinoma cervix

Points of comparison	Surgery	Radiation
Survival	85%	85%
Serious complications	Urologic fistulas 1–2%	Intestinal and urinary strictures and fistulas 1.4–5.3%
Vagina	Initially shortened but may lengthen with regular intercourse	Fibrosis and possible stenosis, particularly in postmenopausal patients
Ovaries	Can be conserved	Destroyed
Chronic effects	Bladder atony in 3%	Radiation fibrosis of bowel and bladder in 6–8%
Surgical mortality	1%	1% (from pulmonary embolism during intracavitatory therapy)

Point A and Point B are in relation to radiotherapy for carcinoma cervix

	Point A	Point B
Location	2 cm above and 2 cm lateral to external os	2 cm above and 5 cm lateral to external os
Structure present	Paracervical/parametrial lymph node	Obturator lymph node
Dose of radiation	7000–8000 cGy	6000 cGy

■ RECENT ADVANCES

Radical trachelectomy: This involves removal of cervix, parametrium, vaginal cuff and pelvic lymphadenectomy. The uterus is preserved for further fertility.

The eligibility criteria include:
- Desire to preserve fertility/young patients
- International Federation of Gynecology and Obstetrics (FIGO) stage 1A2 and 1B1
- Lesion size of 2 cm or smaller
- No lymph node metastasis.

However, it is not yet considered the standard of care, Wertheim's hysterectomy is the standard care for stages 1A2 and 1B1.

Q. FIGO staging of cervical cancer.

CLINICAL STAGING OF CANCER CERVIX (FIGO)

Preinvasive carcinoma	
Stage 0	Carcinoma in situ, intraepithelial carcinoma (cases of stage 0 should not be included in any therapeutic statistics)
Invasive carcinoma	
Stage I	Carcinoma strictly confined to the cervix (extensions to the corpus should be disregarded)
Stage Ia	Preclinical carcinomas of the cervix, i.e. those diagnosed only by microscopy Stage 1a1: Lesion with <3 mm invasion Stage 1a2: Lesions detected microscopically and can be measured The upper limit of the measurement should show a depth of invasion of >3–5 mm taken from the base of the epithelium, either surface or glandular, from which it originates, and a second distinction, the horizontal spread, must not exceed 7 mm. Larger lesions should be staged as Ib
Stage 1b	Lesion invasive >5 mm Stage 1b1: Lesions less than or equal to 4 cm Stage 1b2: Lesions larger than 4 cm
Stage II	The carcinoma extends beyond the cervix but has not extended onto the wall The carcinoma involves the vagina, but not the lower one-third Stage IIa: No obvious parametrial involvement Stage IIb: Obvious parametrial involvement
Stage III	The carcinoma has extended onto the pelvic wall. On rectal examination, there is no CA free space between the tumor and the pelvic wall. The tumor involves the lower one-third of the vagina. All cases with hydronephrosis or nonfunctioning kidney Stage IIIa: No extension to the pelvic wall Stage IIIb: Extension onto the pelvic wall and/or hydronephrosis or nonfunctioning kidney
Stage IV	The carcinoma has extended beyond the true pelvis or has clinically involved the mucosa of the bladder or rectum. A bullous edema, as such, does not permit a case to be allotted to stage IV Stage IVa: Spread of the growth to adjacent organs Stage IVb: Spread to distant organs

FIGO (2009) STAGING FOR CARCINOMA CERVIX

IA1	Confined to the cervix, diagnosed only by microscopy with invasion of <3 mm in depth and lateral spread 7 mm
IA2	Confined to cervix, diagnosed with microscopy with invasion of >3 mm and <5 mm with lateral spread of 7 mm
IB1	Clinically visible lesion or greater than A2, <4 cm in greatest dimension
IB2	Clinically visible lesion, >4 cm in greatest dimension
IIA1	Involvement of the upper two-thirds of the vagina, without parametrial invasion, <4 cm in greatest dimension
IIA2	>4 cm in greatest dimension
IIB	With parametrial involvement
IIIA/B	Unchanged
IVA/B	Unchanged

Chapter 8: Oncology

■ RECENT ADVANCES: FIGO (2018) STAGING OF CARCINOMA CERVIX

Stage	Description
I	The carcinoma is strictly confined to the cervix (extension to the uterine corpus should be disregarded)
IA	Invasive carcinoma that can be diagnosed only by microscopy, with maximum depth of invasion <5 mm[a]
IA1	Measured stromal invasion <3 mm in depth
IA2	Measured stromal invasion ≥3 mm and <5 mm in depth
IB	Invasive carcinoma with measured deepest invasion ≥5 mm (greater than Stage IA), lesion limited to the cervix uteri[b]
IB1	Invasive carcinoma ≥5 mm depth of stromal invasion, and <2 cm in greatest dimension
IB2	Invasive carcinoma ≥2 cm and <4 cm in greatest dimension
IB3	Invasive carcinoma ≥4 cm in greatest dimension
II	The carcinoma invades beyond the uterus, but has not extended onto the lower third of the vagina or to the pelvic wall
IIA	Involvement limited to the upper two-thirds of the vagina without parametrial involvement
IIA1	Invasive carcinoma <4 cm in greatest dimension
IIA2	Invasive carcinoma ≥4 cm in greatest dimension
IIB	With parametrial involvement but not up to the pelvic wall
III	The carcinoma involves the lower third of the vagina and/or extends to the pelvic wall and/or causes hydronephrosis or nonfunctioning kidney and/or involves pelvic and/or para-aortic lymph nodes[c]
IIIA	The carcinoma involves the lower third of the vagina, with no extension to the pelvic wall
IIIB	Extension to the pelvic wall and/or hydronephrosis or nonfunctioning kidney (unless known to be due to another cause)
IIIC	Involvement of pelvic and/or para-aortic lymph nodes, irrespective of tumor size and extent (with r and p notations)[c]
IIIC1	Pelvic lymph node metastasis only
IIIC2	Para-aortic lymph node metastasis
IV	The carcinoma has extended beyond the true pelvis or has involved (biopsy proven) the mucosa of the bladder or rectum (a bullous edema, as such, does not permit a case to be allotted to Stage IV)
IVA	Spread to adjacent pelvic organs
IVB	Spread to distant organs

When in doubt, the lower staging should be assigned.
[a]Imaging and pathology can be used, where available, to supplement clinical findings with respect to tumor size and extent, in all stages.
[b]The involvement of vascular/lymphatic spaces does not change the staging. The lateral extent of the lesion is no longer considered.
[c]Adding notation of r (imaging) and p (pathology) to indicate the findings that are used to allocate the case to Stage IIIC. Example: If imaging indicates pelvic lymph node metastasis, the stage allocation would be Stage IIIC1r, and if confirmed by pathologic findings, it would be Stage IIIC1p. The type of imaging modality or pathology technique used should always be documented.
Source: Bhatla et al.[17]

Q. Causes of postmenopausal bleeding.

■ INTRODUCTION

Postmenopausal bleeding (PMB) is vaginal bleeding that happens at least 12 months after the periods have stopped due to menopause.

It should never be neglected and the patient should always be evaluated further.

CAUSES

Uterus/Endometrium

- Atrophic endometrium/senile endometritis
- Use of hormone replacement therapy (HRT)
- Endometrial hyperplasia; simple, complex, and atypical
- Endometrial cancer. The probability of a woman presenting with PMB having endometrial cancer is 10%. However, 75–90% of women with endometrial cancer present with PMB
- Endometrial polyps
- Uterine sarcoma
- Fibroids (very rare, suspect sarcomatous degeneration).

Cervix

- Cancer
- Erosion
- Cervicitis
- Polyps.

Vagina

- Vaginal atrophy
- Cancer of vagina.

Ovary

Ovarian cancer, especially estrogen secreting (granulosa and theca cell) ovarian tumors.

Vulva

Vulval cancer.

Fallopian tube

Cancer (very rare)
- Nongynecological causes including trauma or a bleeding disorder
- Bleeding from the urinary tract or rectum may be confused with postmenopausal bleeding.

Q. Risk factors, clinical features and management of endometrial carcinoma.

INTRODUCTION

It the most common genital malignancy in **developed countries**. However, in India and in developing countries carcinoma cervix is the most common.

Adenocarcinoma is the most common variety of carcinoma endometrium.

Chapter 8: Oncology

■ RISK FACTORS/ETIOLOGY

Estrogen-dependent cancer.
- **Persistent unopposed stimulation of endometrium with estrogen is the single most important factor** for the development of carcinoma endometrium.
  - PCOS (anovulation, hyperestrogenism)
  - Granulosa cell tumor of ovary (secretes estrogen)
  - Unopposed estrogen therapy in HRT (in HRT both estrogen and progesterone to be given in patients with intact uterus)
  - Early menarche and late menopause (more exposure to estrogen. Risk is increased if menopause has not occurred by 52 years).
- Age: 75% patients are postmenopausal with **median age 60 years**
- 10% of patients with postmenopausal bleeding have carcinoma endometrium
- Nulliparity
- **Obesity, hypertension, and diabetes mellitus** associated with carcinoma endometrium = **corpus carcinoma syndrome**. Obesity leads to high level of free estradiol
- Tamoxifen therapy: It is used for breast cancer treatment, it has weak estrogenic action on endometrium
- Lynch 2 syndrome: Hereditary nonpolyposis colon cancer with increased risk of endometrial, breast, and ovarian cancer
- Atypical endometrial hyperplasia can progress to carcinoma in about 29% cases.

Type of hyperplasia	Progression to carcinoma (%)
Simple	1
Complex	3
Simple with atypia	8
Complex with atypia	29

- COC, POP, DMPA, MIRENA and PREGNANCY all are protective for CA endometrium
- COCS lower the risk of endometrial cancer by about 50%; the effect lasts for up to 15 years.

■ PATHOLOGY

The uterus may be enlarged due to myohyperplasia, pyometra.

Localized
- Sessile or pedunculated
- Usual site fundus
- Myometrial involvement late.

Diffuse
Spreads through endometrium to invade myometrium may reach serosa.

■ MICROSCOPY

- Adenocarcinoma is the MC variety of carcinoma endometrium (80%)

- Papillary serous
- Clear cell
- Adenosquamous
- Mucinous
- Adenoacanthoma
- Squamous cell
- Mixed
- **Papillary serous variety and clear cell variety have worst prognosis**
- Among the two, **clear cell variety has poorer prognosis.**

SPREAD

- Direct: Myometrium, serosa, peritoneal cavity and cervix, tubes, and ovaries
- Lymphatic: Pelvic, para-aortic and rarely inguinal femoral nodes and ovary and tubes and vagina
- Pelvic lymph node involved in 4% cases in stage 1, grade 1 and 2 whereas it is 35–40% in stage 2
- Hematogenous: Lungs, liver, bones and brain.

CLINICAL FEATURES

Symptoms

- **Postmenopausal bleeding:** Approximately 75% of women with endometrial cancer are postmenopausal. The most common symptom is postmenopausal bleeding. Bleeding may vary from slight to heavy and may be continuous or irregular.
- **Perimenopausal/premenopausal polymenorrhagia:**
  - 25% of endometrial cancers are in patients who are perimenopausal or premenopausal
  - Heavy frequent menstrual periods or intermenstrual bleeding.
- Offensive watery discharge (pyometra)
- Pain: **Simpson's pain** = colicky pain in patients of CA endometrium.

On Examination

- Pallor may be present.
- **Per speculum (PS):** Cervix is healthy looking, blood or purulent discharge may be seen coming from os.
- **Per vaginum (PV):** The uterus may be atrophic or normal or enlarged, mobile unless in late stages where it becomes fixed.
- Regional lymph nodes and breast to be examined.

INVESTIGATIONS AND DIAGNOSIS

The diagnosis of carcinoma endometrium has to be **by histopathological examination of endometrium (fractional curettage, D&C, endometrial biopsy).**

- **Fractional curettage is the investigation of choice for patients with postmenopausal bleeding.**
  - Be gentle to prevent perforation

Chapter 8: Oncology

- If pyometra, give antibiotics and delay the procedure by one week to avoid perforation and systemic infection
  - Endocervical curettage
  - UCL with sound
  - Dilatation of os
  - Uterine curettage
  - Specimens of cervical curettage and endometrium to be send separately for histopathology.
- D&C
- Endometrial biopsy using a curette or pipelle can be done as an outpatient procedure
- Hysteroscopically directed biopsy
- Pap smear is not reliable test but can also detect 50–60% of endometrial carcinomas. Endometrial cancerous cells present in the posterior vaginal fornix can be detected by Pap smear.
- TVS: Findings suggestive are:
  - Thickened endometrium **(even >5 mm in postmenopausal lady is significant)**
  - Hyperechoic endometrium with irregular outline
  - Increased vascularity on color Doppler
  - Intrauterine fluid.
- Special studies, such as CT scans of the abdomen and pelvis or magnetic resonance imaging (MRIs) are not routinely performed
- Preoperative evaluation includes:
  - CBC
  - FBS
  - PLBS
  - RFT
  - LFT
  - HIV, HBsAg, HCV
  - Chest X-ray
  - ECG.

■ TREATMENT

- Mainstay of treatment is surgery and postoperative radiotherapy.
- Carcinoma endometrium is **surgically staged** and hence all patients **will first require staging laparotomy.**

Stage 1

Surgery (total abdominal hysterectomy with bilateral salpingo-oophorectomy with lymph node sampling), followed by radiotherapy.

Postoperative radiotherapy:
- Vaginal cuff radiation 6,000–7,000 cGy for stage 1B
- Pelvis external beam radiation 4,500–5,000 cGy plus vaginal cuff boost for stage 1C.

Stage 2

- Modified radical hysterectomy, bilateral salpingo-oophorectomy with lymph node dissection, followed by radiotherapy
- Pelvis external beam radiation 4,500–5,000 cGy plus vaginal cuff boost for stage 2.

Stages 3 and 4
- Debulking surgery followed by radiotherapy
  - Pelvis external beam radiation 4,500–5,000 cGy plus vaginal cuff boost for stage 3 and whole abdominal radiation for stage 4.

Only patients with stage 1A, grade 1 and 2 do not require postoperative radiotherapy.

A 2012 review found that for early stage primary endometrioid adenocarcinoma of the endometrium, laparoscopy and laparotomy are associated with similar rates of disease-free and overall survival and that laparoscopy is associated with reduced operative morbidity and shorter hospital stays.

- Chemotherapy and hormonal therapy is used in advanced or recurrent cases or in metastatic lesion
- Cytotoxic agents which can be used singly or in combination are:
  - Cisplatin
  - Carboplatin
  - Cyclophosphamide
  - Paclitaxel
  - Adriamycin.

Hormone treatment for endometrial cancer can include:
- Progestins—which are the main hormone treatment used
- Tamoxifen
- Gonadotropin-releasing hormone (GnRH) analogs
- Aromatase inhibitors.

If a tumor is well-differentiated and known to have progesterone and estrogen receptors, progestins may be used in treatment. About 25% of metastatic endometrioid cancers show a response to progestins.

The main hormone treatment for endometrial cancer uses progesterone. The two most commonly used progestins are medroxyprogesterone acetate which can be given as an injection or as a pill and megestrol acetate. These drugs work by slowing the growth of endometrial cancer cells.

Q. FIGO staging carcinoma endometrium.

FIGO GRADING OF ENDOMETRIAL CARCINOMA

Histopathologic degree of differentiation:
- G1: ≤5% nonsquamous or nonmorular growth pattern
- G2: 6–50% nonsquamous or nonmorular growth pattern
- G3: >50% nonsquamous or nonmorular growth pattern.

SURGICAL STAGING FOR ENDOMETRIAL CANCER

Stage	Finding
Ia G1 2 3	No myometrial invasion
Ib G1 2 3	<½ myometrial invasion
Ic G1 2 3	>½ myometrial invasion
IIa G 1 2 3	Extension to endocervical glands

Chapter 8: Oncology

IIb G1 2 3	Cervical stromal invasion
IIIa G 1 2 3	Positive uterine serosa, adnexa, and/or peritoneal cytology
IIIb G 1 2 3	Vaginal metastasis
IIIc G 1 2 3	Metastasis to pelvic and/or paraaortic lymph nodes
IVa G 1 2 3	Tumor invasion of bladder and/or bowel mucosa
IVb	Distant metastasis including intraabdominal and/or inguinal lymph nodes.

■ RECENT ADVANCES

FIGO (2009)	Staging for Carcinoma Endometrium
IA	Tumor confined to the uterus, no or <½ myometrial invasion
IB	Tumor confined to the uterus, >½ myometrial invasion
II	Cervical stromal invasion, but not beyond uterus
IIIA	Tumor invades serosa or adnexa
IIIB	Vaginal and/or parametrial involvement
IIIC1	Pelvic node involvement
IIIC2	Paraaortic involvement
IVA	Unchanged
IVB	Unchanged.

Q. Clinical features of epithelial ovarian carcinoma.

Q. How will you manage a case of epithelial ovarian malignancy?

■ INTRODUCTION

❖ Ovarian malignancy constitutes about 15–20% of all genital malignancies
❖ 20% of all ovarian neoplasms are malignant
❖ 85–90% of all primary ovarian malignancies are epithelial in origin
❖ Germ cell tumors constitute 6–10% of all ovarian malignancies and sex cord stromal tumors accounts for 5–7% of all primary ovarian malignancies.

■ CLINICAL FEATURES OF EPITHELIAL OVARIAN MALIGNANCY

Patient Profile

❖ Epithelial cancer mainly occurs in postmenopausal age group
❖ The peak incidence is at **55–60 years of age**
❖ Increase association with nulliparity and family history.

Symptoms

Most women with epithelial ovarian cancer have **no symptoms** for very long periods of time. When symptoms develop they are very **vague and nonspecific**.

❖ Bloating; abdominal distention, discomfort
❖ Dyspepsia, flatulence
❖ Early satiety, loss of appetite
❖ Indigestion and acid reflux

- Pressure effects on the bladder and rectum (increase frequency to urinate, constipation)
- Abdominal swelling, dull pain and discomfort in lower abdomen
- Shortness of breath, respiratory distress (in advanced cases, due to ascites or pleural effusion)
- Tiredness
- Sudden weight loss
- Dyspareunia
- Irregular menses or postmenopausal bleeding (very rarely).

Signs

General Examination

- Pallor
- Cachexia
- Jaundice
- Left supraclavicular lymph gland (Virchow's node) may be enlarged
- Lower limb and vulval edema.

Per Abdomen

- Hepatomegaly: Firm and nodular
- Mass in hypogastrium, may be bilateral with the following characteristics:
  - Solid or heterogenous
  - Restricted mobility
  - Irregular surface
  - Lower pole not reached
  - Dull on percussion
- Ascites.

PV

- The uterus is felt separately from the mass
- **Solid, irregular, fixed, pelvic mass is highly suggestive of ovarian malignancy**
- **Nodules may be felt through the posterior fornix.**

INVESTIGATIONS

- Serum CA-125: It is not diagnostic and is for prognosis. However, it is useful to differentiate benign and malignant pelvic mass. For postmenopausal patient with adnexal mass, a high CA-125 levels (>95 IU/mL), there is a 96% positive predictive value for malignancy
- **Human Epididymis protein 4 (HE4) is a new and specific biomarker for ovarian cancer.**

Combination of these 2 markers provides higher accuracy for detecting epithelial ovarian cancer.

- **The diagnosis of ovarian cancer requires exploratory laparotomy.**
- **Preoperative evaluation includes:**
  - CBC
  - FBS
  - PLBS

Chapter 8: Oncology

- RFT
- LFT
- HIV, HBsAg, HCV
- ECG
- Chest X-ray
- Intravenous pyelogram (IVP)
- Ultrasonography (USG) pelvis and abdomen, limited value, but would detect ascites, involvement of omentum and the other ovary
- CT Scan and MRI: Limited role but will give an idea of extent of disease, lymph nodes, ascites and liver involvement
- **To rule out primary gastric and colon malignancy with ovarian metastasis:**
  - Upper and lower endoscopy
  - Barium enema
  - Upper GI series
  - Mammography if any breast mass
  - Cervical cytology (Pap smear)
  - Endometrial biopsy, endocervical curettage to exclude uterine or endocervical cancer
- Fine-needle aspiration (FNA) or percutaneous biopsy of an adnexal mass **is not routinely recommended.** In most cases, this approach may only serve to delay diagnosis and treatment of ovarian cancer. Instead, if a clinical suggestion of ovarian cancer is present, the patient should undergo a laparotomy for diagnosis and staging.

■ TREATMENT

Surgery is the initial treatment of choice provided patients are medically fit. Patients who are not fit for surgery may be given chemotherapy and considered for surgery later. The aim of surgery is to confirm the diagnosis, define the extent of disease, and resect all visible tumor. The role of cytoreduction was demonstrated by Griffiths in 1975.

Cytoreductive Surgery

- This should be performed by a gynecologic oncologist at the time of initial laparotomy. **The volume of residual disease at the completion of surgery represents one of the most powerful prognostic factors.**
- **Residual disease of less than 1 cm is evidence of optimal cytoreduction**, although the best possible effort should be made to remove all obvious disease.
- **For all stages 1–4: The main treatment consists of staging laparotomy, primary cytoreductive surgery followed by chemotherapy.**
- Basic steps involved in surgical staging: Midline or paramedian incision.
  - Send free fluid for cytology
  - If no free fluid, perform peritoneal washings and send it for cytology
  - Inspect and palpate all the intraabdominal organs
  - Any suspicious area on peritoneal surfaces should be biopsied
  - Sample the diaphragm either by biopsy or scraping
  - Perform the infracolic omentectomy
  - Evaluate the pelvic and para-aortic lymph nodes. Enlarged nodes should be resected. If no metastasis are present, pelvic lymphadenectomy should be performed.

Primary Cytoreductive Surgery

❖ The ovarian tumor should be removed intact (if possible) and a frozen histologic section should be obtained.
❖ The following steps are performed:
  ➢ Total abdominal hysterectomy
  ➢ Bilateral salpingo-oophorectomy
  ➢ Infracolic omentectomy
  ➢ Lymph node dissection and
  ➢ Removal of all the metastatic deposits (as much as possible). All visible tumor should be removed. This may require extensive surgery, including bowel resection, excision of peritoneal implants, liver resection and splenectomy.

Conservative Surgery (Unilateral Salpingo-oophorectomy)

❖ **Not recommended routinely except in young patients**, desirous of reproduction provided
❖ The tumor is stage 1A, well differentiated and opposite biopsy normal on frozen section
❖ The patient to be regularly followed up with TVS pelvis and CA-125 and definitive surgery done in future after family is complete.

Chemotherapy

❖ Postsurgery chemotherapy improves survival
❖ **Given in all cases except Stage 1A, grade 1: no adjuvant chemotherapy required.**
❖ Given for 6 cycles at 3–4 weeks interval
❖ Platinum compounds (cisplatin, carboplatin) are most effective
❖ Taxane derivatives (paclitaxel, docetaxel) also very effective
❖ **Currently chemotherapy with carboplatin and paclitaxel is preferred in most patients as it is found to have better survival rate and better tolerated.**

Immunotherapy

Cytokines, interferon alpha and gamma, and interleukin 2 are being used as second line therapy along with chemotherapy. Use of monoclonal antibodies is under trial.

Interval Cytoreduction (after NACT)

In patients with advance stages (stages 3 and 4) and not fit for surgery (severe ascites and pleural effusion) or inadequate primary cytoreductive surgery.

Patients receive three cycles of neoadjuvant chemotherapy (NACT). Carboplatin and paclitaxel followed by interval cytoreductive surgery which is followed by three more cycles of NACT.

■ PREVENTION

Factors Reducing the Risk of Ovarian Cancer

❖ Use of oral contraceptive pills (OCP)/depot medroxyprogesterone acetate (DMPA) (since they cause anovulation)

- ❖ Breastfeeding
- ❖ Multiparity
- ❖ Pregnancy.

Management Options in High-risk Women: BRCA1/2 Carriers

- ❖ Six monthly TVS
- ❖ OCPs (when not interested in fertility)
- ❖ Prophylactic oophorectomy (as soon as family is completed)
- ❖ Annual mammography.

Q. Etiology and staging of vulval cancer.

- ❖ Vulval cancer is rare, and accounts for 3–5% of genital malignancies
- ❖ Squamous cell carcinoma accounts for most vulvar cancers (90%) followed by melanoma (8–10%)

Etiology

The exact etiology is unclear, but the following factors play a role:

- ❖ **Increasing age:** The risk of developing vulval cancer increases with age. Most cases develop in women age 65 or over, although very occasionally women under 50 can be affected.
- ❖ **Vulval intraepithelial neoplasia (VIN):** VIN is a precancerous condition, malignancy transformation is a gradual process that usually takes well over 10 years. It can be subdivided into two categories: **HPV dependent usual type (uVIN) and HPV independent differentiated type (dVIN).**
- ❖ **Human papillomavirus (HPV) infection:** Infection with high-risk oncogenic HPV, type 16, 18, 31, 33, 45. HPV is present in at least 4 out of 10 women with vulval cancer
- ❖ Associated vulval epithelial disorders such as lichen sclerosus
- ❖ More common amongst whites
- ❖ Smoking
- ❖ Immunodeficiency (HIV, AIDS) and other STIs
- ❖ Increased association with obesity, hypertension, diabetes
- ❖ Other primary malignancies (like carcinoma cervix) have been observed in 20% cases of vulval cancers

Staging

- ❖ Vulvar cancer staging is by the International Federation of Gynecology and Obstetrics (FIGO)
- ❖ Treatment and prognosis are related to the surgical stage.

Stage I

Tumors confined to the vulva or perineum, no nodal metastasis.
- ❖ **IA:** Tumor ≤2 cm with stromal invasion ≤1 mm
- ❖ **IB:** Tumor >2 cm or stromal invasion >1 mm

Stage II

Tumor of any size with extension to adjacent perineal structures (lower 1/3 urethra, 1/3 lower vagina, anus), no nodal metastasis

Stage III

Tumor of any size with or without extension to adjacent perineal structures (lower urethra, lower vagina, anus), with inguinofemoral nodal metastasis
- **IIIA:** 1 node metastasis (≥5 mm) or 1 to 2 node metastasis(es) (<5 mm)
- **IIIB:** ≥2 node metastases (≥5 mm) or ≥3 node metastases (<5 mm)
- **IIIC:** Node metastases with extracapsular spread

Stage IV

Tumor invades other regional or distal structures.
- **IVA:** Tumor invades any of the following: Upper urethra and/or vaginal mucosa, bladder mucosa, rectal mucosa, or fixed to the pelvic bone, or fixed or ulcerated inguinofemoral nodes
- **IVB:** Any distant metastasis, including pelvic nodes

CHAPTER 9

Contraception

Q. Lactational amenorrhea as birth control.

■ INTRODUCTION

The period of lactational amenorrhea can act as method of contraception, though **not a very reliable method as** patient can conceive in this period.

■ MECHANISM OF ACTION

Excessive secretion of prolactin, which controls lactation, **inhibits the ovarian function**.

Prolactin inhibits luteinizing hormone (LH) but has no effect on follicle-stimulating hormone (FSH). However, it partially inhibits ovarian response to both of these gonadotropins. As a result, while the prolactin level remains high, the ovary produces little estrogen and no progesterone. Hence, it **suppresses ovulation** and hence, ovulation and menstruation are affected.

■ FAILURE RATE

It is effective **maximum up to 6 months postpartum** and not reliable beyond that if there is exclusive breastfeeding, the failure rate of lactational amenorrhea method (LAM) (for 6 months only) is less than 2% when correctly and consistently used, but it is more otherwise. If any time during these 6 months the menses resumes, then it is not effective as contraception.

■ ADVANTAGES

The breastfeeding practices required for LAM have other health benefits for mother and baby:
- It provides the healthiest food to the baby.
- It protects from life-threatening diarrhea.
- It protects the baby from diseases such as measles and pneumonia by passing on the mother's immunities.
- It helps to develop a close relationship between mother and baby.
- It protects the mother from diseases such as subinvolution, fibroadenosis, and fibroadenoma of the uterus.
- Breastfeeding reduces risks of breast cancer and epithelial ovarian cancer.

Q. Condoms.

INTRODUCTION

Male condoms are contraceptive sheaths meant to cover the penis during coitus. Condoms are barrier method of contraception. They are also known as French letters.

The condom is the **oldest and most widely used birth control device in the world**. Its invention is attributed to a physician named **Dr Condom**, who recommended it to Charles II.

CHARACTERISTICS

Condoms are mostly made of **fine latex rubber**. They are circular cylinders, 15–20 cm in length, 3–3.5 cm in diameter and 0.003–0.007 cm in thickness; they are closed at one end and open at the other with an integral rim.

Nonlatex forms of male condoms are now commercially made of **polyurethane**. Polyurethane condoms have a longer shelf life and can be used with oil-based lubricants, which can damage latex condoms.

It is the most harmless method of contraception.

MECHANISM OF ACTION

Barrier method, they prevent the union of egg and the sperm.

FAILURE RATE

They have got a **very high failure rate**. Total condom failure rates (breakage and slippage rate combined) range from **4% to 13%**.

ADVANTAGES AND NONCONTRACEPTIVE BENEFITS

- Cheap, easily available.
- No side effects.
- No medical supervision required [as in cases of intrauterine contraceptive device (IUCD) and oral contraceptive (OC) pills].
- When used properly, the condoms give very good **protection against sexually transmitted diseases (STDs).**
- These include not only traditional syphilis and gonorrhea but also trichomoniasis, moniliasis, nongonococcal urethritis, and infection with *Chlamydia* and herpes virus. The condom seems to give best protection against sexually transmitted AIDS. Condoms also give protection against sexually transmitted hepatitis B virus. Protection against STD benefits male and female partners.
- When used for more than 5 years, condom, reduce the chance of developing severe cervical dysplasia and cervical cancer as compared to the use of oral pills or to nonuse of contraceptives.
- Condom catheter in males.
- To cover the transvaginal sonography (TVS) probe.
- After vaginoplasty, molds are used to prevent fibrosis, which are covered with condoms.

Chapter 9: Contraception

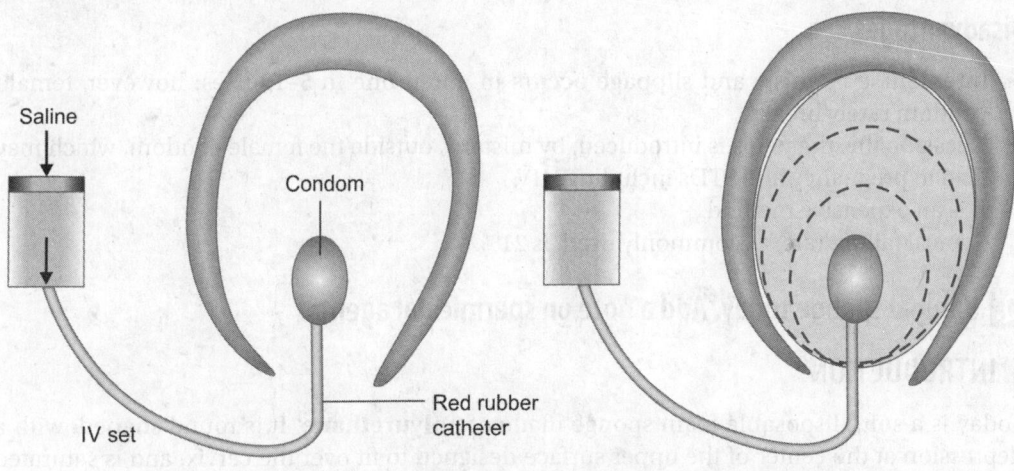

Fig. 9.1: Shivkar's pack.

- **Shivkar's pack (condom tamponade)** for atonic postpartum hemorrhage (PPH) **(Fig. 9.1)**.
- In cases of antisperm antibodies are present in cervical mucus.

■ DISADVANTAGES

- **High failure rates**
- **Coitus dependent and male dependent**
- May slightly decrease the sexual pleasure
- Storage and disposal problems affect village people reduce the use of condoms.

■ DISPOSAL OF CONDOMS

They should be wrapped in a piece of paper and thrown in dustbins or buried underneath the soil but should never be left in commodes or flushing-type latrine pans.

Female Condom

- A female condom, by the trade names of "Femidom" or "Reality," is a new disposable barrier contraceptive for women. It consists of soft, loose-fitting polyurethane sac about 15 cm long and 7 cm in diameter **(Fig. 9.2)**.
- Sexual intercourse takes place within the cavity of the device.
- It is a women-controlled method and can even be used without the partner's cooperation. It prevents STDs including HIV/AIDS.

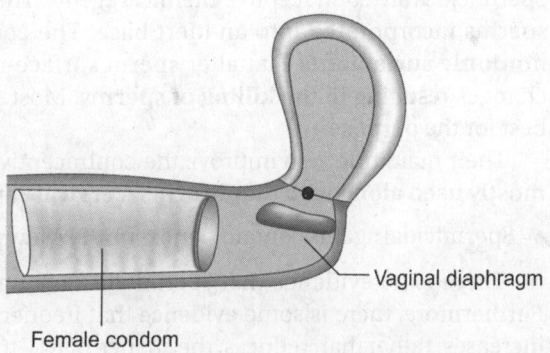

Fig. 9.2: Female condom and diaphragm.

Disadvantages

- ❖ Intercourse is noisy, and slippage occurs in about one in 5-10 uses; however, female condom rarely breaks.
- ❖ Occasionally, the penis is introduced, by mistake, outside the female condom, which may lead to pregnancy and STDs including HIV.
- ❖ It is an expensive method.

Typical failure rate, as commonly used, is 21%.

Q. Vaginal sponge today. Add a note on spermicidal agents.

■ INTRODUCTION

Today is a soft, disposable foam sponge made of **polyurethane**. It is round shaped, with a depression at the center of the upper surface designed to fit over the cervix, and is saturated with **nonoxynol-9, the most powerful spermicide**. It has an attached nylon loop that helps in its removal.

■ MECHANISM OF ACTION

It **releases spermicidal agent** which kills the sperms. It is moistened with water, squeezed gently to remove excess water and inserted high up in the vagina to cover the cervix. It **acts for 24 hours**, and intercourse may be repeated as often as desired during this period. Like the cervical cap, it can be introduced long before the sex act. It is **not a barrier method**.

■ FAILURE RATE

The failure rate varies **between 9 and 27 per 100 users** in the first year.

It must be removed and thrown away after 8-24 hours **but not before 6 hours** of the last act. The real danger of the sponge is the **development of toxic shock syndrome (TSS)**, although it happens very rarely.

■ SPERMICIDES

Spermicides are contraceptive chemical agents. They comprise a chemical capable of destroying sperms incorporated into an inert base. The commonly used spermicidal agents contain **nonionic surfactants** that alter sperm surface membrane permeability, causing osmotic changes resulting in the **killing of sperms**. Most spermicides contain nonoxynol-9, which is best for the purpose.

Their main role is to improve the contraceptive effect of other barrier methods. **They are mostly used along with diaphragms, cervical caps, and condoms**.

Spermicidal agents contain nonoxynol-9. A few products contain octoxynol-9 and menfegol.

There is no evidence that spermicides offer any protection against HIV and other STIs. Furthermore, there is some evidence that frequent use of nonoxynol-9 (twice a day or more) increases, rather than reduces, the chance of HIV transmission, perhaps by irritating the vaginal and cervical mucosa.

Typical average failure rate, as commonly used, is 21%.

Chapter 9: Contraception

Q. Generations of IUD. Mechanism of action of IUD and failure rates.

INTRODUCTION

The intrauterine device (IUD) is the **second most commonly** used family planning method, after voluntary female sterilization (in India).

The IUD is one of the best methods of contraception during lactation.

Generations of IUD:
- **First:** Inert devices, e.g., Lippes loop
- **Second:** All the copper-containing devices, e.g., multiload Cu 250, 375, Cu T 200, 220C, Cu T 380A, etc.
- **Third:** Hormonal devices, e.g., Progestasert and Mirena.

MECHANISM OF ACTION

The precise mechanism of action of the IUD is still unknown.
- New studies prove that the IUDs act mostly by preventing sperms from fertilizing ova. The primary mechanisms of action of **copper-releasing IUD are by impeding sperm transport and inhibiting their capacity to fertilize ova**.
- All unmedicated and copper devices **produce an inflammatory or foreign body reaction, which in turn causes cellular and biochemical changes in the endometrium.** Prostaglandin level increase and the fibrinolytic mechanism needed for hemostasis are affected. Numerous polymorphs, giant cells, mononuclear cells, plasma cells, and macrophages appear in the endometrium as well as in the uterine and tubal fluids. These cells engulf or consume sperms and ova by the process of phagocytosis and thus prevent fertilization. Besides, normal cyclical changes in the endometrium may be delayed or deranged by the inflammatory reaction and liberation of prostaglandins, **making it inhospitable for implantation of the blastocyst.**
- When inserted postcoitally, IUDs **can prevent implantation of the fertilized ovum.**
- Copper causes more intense inflammatory reaction and interferes with enzymes in the uterus, the amount of DNA in endometrial cells, glycogen metabolism, and estrogen uptake by the uterine mucosa.
- Sperm motility, capacitation, and survival are also affected by the biochemical changes in the cervical mucus produced by copper.
- IUDs containing progesterone prevent sperm passing through the cervical mucus and maintain high progesterone level, and inconsequence, relatively low estrogen levels locally. They, thereby, **keep the endometrium in a state in which implantation is hindered**.

FAILURE RATE

Pearl Index of IUD

IUDs can be divided into three groups according to the pregnancy rate, indicating their contraceptive efficacy:
1. Group I (pregnancy rates greater than 2.0 per 100 women-year): Lippes loop, Cu 7 T 200
2. Group II (pregnancy rates less than 2.0 but more than 1 per 100 women-year): Nova T, ML Cu 250, and Cu T 220C

3. Group III [pregnancy rates less than 1 (mostly less than 0.5) per 100 women-year]: Cu T 380A, Cu T 380S, ML Cu 375, and levonorgestrel (LNG) 20.

Q. Mirena/LNG IUD/LNG 20/Levonova/LNG IUS.

INTRODUCTION

- Mirena is a hormone-containing third generation IUCD.
- Mirena contains a total of **52 mg LNG**. LNG is released into the uterine cavity at a rate of approximately **20 µg/day**.
- These devices act mainly by local progestogenic effects and act for up to **5 years**.

FAILURE RATE

Pearl index after 5 years is **0.09/100 women-year** (**most effective reversible contraception available today**).

MECHANISM OF ACTION

- Mirena **releases progesterone** in the uterine cavity and also has a **foreign body reaction in the uterus, it alters the endometrium and thus, makes it unsuitable for implantation**.
- It also makes the **cervical mucus thick** and hence prevents the sperms from entering the uterus.
- It may also affect the sperm capacitation.
- Mirena eventually leads to **progesterone-induced amenorrhea**.

ADVANTAGES AND NONCONTRACEPTIVE BENEFITS

Health benefits of Mirena include:
- **Reduction of blood loss**, which benefits patients with anemia and dysfunctional uterine bleeding
- Reduction of pain and dysmenorrhea in **endometriosis and adenomyosis**
- Beneficial effect on fibroids
- The advantage that IUDs introduced 6 weeks after delivery do not influence lactation or affect infant growth and development
- It can be used in **prevention and treatment of endometrial hyperplasia**
- Decreases the risk of endometrial cancer
- Decreases the risk of pelvic inflammatory disease (PID) and hence **protects against ectopic pregnancy**.

DISADVANTAGES

- Irregular bleeding and oligomenorrhea, which happen quite commonly in the first 3–4 months
- Amenorrhea, which affects up to 20–50% cases by 1 year. But this is not at all harmful as it is a progesterone-induced amenorrhea
- Difficulty of introduction, needing local anesthesia in many cases.

Q. Contraindications for use of IUD. Complications of IUD.

INTRODUCTION

The IUD is the **second most commonly** used family planning method, after voluntary female sterilization (in India).

Contraindications for IUD use are absolute and relative.

Absolute contraindications include:
- Immediate postseptic abortion
- Pregnancy
- Pelvic tuberculosis
- Vaginal bleeding suspicious/unexplained
- Current PID
- Puerperal sepsis
- Malignant trophoblastic disease
- Current STDs
- Cervical cancer
- Uterine fibroids with distortion of uterine cavity
- Endometrial cancer
- Uterine anomalies like bicornuate, septate uterus.

Nulliparity, heart disease, fibroids with no cavity distortion and past history of PID are **relative contraindications**.

COMPLICATIONS OF IUD

- **Menorrhagia and dysmenorrhea:** Increased bleeding is the greatest disadvantage of IUDs and, along with **pain**, accounts for their removal in 2-10 per 100 users in the first year.
- **Misplaced IUD:** If the device is detected inside the peritoneal cavity, it should be removed as early as possible. Copper devices produce irritative reactions, inflammations, and a lot of adhesions. Copper devices in the peritoneal cavity usually need laparotomy for their removal, as they produce a good amount of adhesions, although it is possible to remove them by laparoscopy. Perforation occurs rarely, not more than **1.2 per 1000 insertions.**
  - The device may migrate into the peritoneal cavity or become embedded in the uterine musculature. Most perforations occur at the time when faulty insertion technique is followed.
  - The copper T devices are known to produce omental masses and adhesions, and progesterone devices can cause intraperitoneal bleeding and should always be removed urgently with laparoscopy (preferred) or laparotomy.
- **Infections:** Doxycycline 200 mg or, better still, azithromycin 500 mg, administered orally 1 hour before insertion, reduces chance of infection.
  - The presence of actinomyces has been found to increase with duration of use, especially after use of inert-tailed devices.
  - The infection in IUD users can be prevented by: (a) proper selection of patients, excluding those cases who have active infection or are likely to have infection from the husband or other partners, (b) prophylactic antibiotic course, and (c) proper disinfection and the practice of aseptic techniques.

- ❖ **Pregnancy:** As soon as pregnancy is confirmed, the IUD should be removed (if it can be done easily) to **reduce the risk of pelvic infection and miscarriage which is the most frequent complication of pregnancy with an IUD in place.**
  - ➢ If the IUD cannot be removed easily, it can also be left *in situ.*
  - ➢ There is **no risk at all of any congenital malformations** if IUD is left *in situ.*
- ❖ **Ectopic pregnancy:** Several studies, including a WHO multicenter study, have found that actually **IUD users are 50% less likely to have ectopic pregnancy than women using no contraception.** The chance of ectopic pregnancy in IUD users is rare and varies from 0.25 to 1.5 per 1000 women-year. However, when pregnancy occurs, the chance of ectopic pregnancy is higher (about 30%) than in general population (about 0.5–0.8%) of all pregnancies.
- ❖ **Spontaneous expulsion (5%):** Usually, in the first few months, more commonly during periods; more likely to occur in postabortal and puerperal insertions.

Immediate (postinsertion) complications include:
- ❖ **Cramp like pain:** Transient can last for few hours. Relieved by analgesics and antispasmodics
- ❖ **Syncopal attack (rare)**
- ❖ **Partial or complete perforation:** Due to faulty technique and more likely in lactational period (soft uterus).

Q. Types of OC pills. Mechanism of action of oral contraceptive pills. What are the noncontraceptive benefits of OC pills?

■ INTRODUCTION

OC pills contain both estrogen **(ethinyl estradiol)** and progesterone (e.g., levonorgestrel/desogestrel/drospirenone/cyproterone).

They are highly effective method of birth control.

■ TYPES

OC pills are of two types: Monophasic pills and multiphasic pills.

Monophasic Pills

These pills contain estrogen and progestogen in the same amount in each pill. They are divided into four subgroups:
1. Standard dose containing ethinyl estradiol (EE) 50 µg/pill
2. Low-dose pills containing EE 30 µg/pill
3. Very low-dose containing EE 20 µg/pill
4. Ultra low-dose pills containing EE 10–15 µg/pill.

Each pill contains a progestogen such as levonorgestrel or other newer varieties such as desogestrel, cyproterone, gestodene, norgestimate, norethisterone, and drospirenone.

Multiphasic Pills

These phasic formulations employ low doses and variable amounts of estrogen and progestogen in two (biphasic) or three (triphasic) periods within the menstrual cycle. The dose of progestogen is low at the beginning and higher at the end, while the estrogen remains either constant or rises slightly in mid-cycle. The total doses of steroids in a whole cycle are less in these pills. Very rarely used today.

MECHANISM OF ACTION

- **Inhibition of ovulation:** The combined pills inhibit ovulation by suppressing hypothalamic-releasing factors, which in turn leads to inappropriate secretion of FSH and LH. As a result, no LH surge occurs and **ovulation is suppressed**.
- **Alteration of endometrium:** OCs alter maturation of the endometrium, rendering it unsuitable for implantation of the fertilized ovum.
- **Changes in cervical mucus:** Cervical mucus becomes scanty, viscous, and cellular with low spinnbarkeit and no ferning; these changes impair sperm transport and penetration.

PEARL INDEX

- Combined pills are very effective. The failure rate when correctly and consistently used is only **0.1%** or 1 per 1000 in the first year of use, but the typical failure rate as commonly used is **1.8%**.
- The failures are mostly due to missed pills, delay in starting the next course, and stoppage of the drug due to side effect or fear complex without taking other contraceptive measures.

NONCONTRACEPTIVE BENEFITS OF OC PILLS

- **Cure of menstrual disorders:** OCs cure dysmenorrhea and ovulation pain. Menorrhagia and metrorrhagia can always be controlled by the use of combined oral contraceptives (COCs). They also make the cycles regular.
- **Protection against cancer:** It has been conclusively proved that OCs directly prevent two common types of genital cancer: Endometrial cancer and ovarian cancer. It also indirectly prevents choriocarcinoma by preventing pregnancy.
  - COCs decrease the ovarian cancer by about 40% and the effect persists for at least 10 years.
  - COCs also lower the risk of endometrial cancer by about 50%; the effect lasts for up to 15 years.
  - They also decrease the risk of colon cancer.
- **Protection against benign tumors and related diseases:**
  - *Benign breast diseases (BBDs):* It is well-documented that BBDs, such as fibrocystic and fibroadenomatosis diseases, are reduced by 50–70% in pill users.
  - *Ovarian functional cysts:* Various studies have shown that low-dose OCs lowers the risk of developing functional ovarian cysts. The risk of follicular cysts goes down by 50% and that of corpus luteum cysts by about 80%.
  - *Fibromyoma of the uterus:* The risk of uterine fibroid is reduced by about 30% in women who have used OCs for 10 years. Low-dose OCs helps reduce fibroids and lessen menstrual flow.
- **Protection against:**
  - *Ectopic pregnancy:* Chance of ectopic pregnancy with its grave consequences is lowered by 50% in low-dose OC users.

- **Pelvic inflammatory diseases:** Several studies have shown that regular pill users are protected from PIDs to the extent of 50%. OCs reduce PIDs by hindering the ascent of STD bacteria (including chlamydia) from the vagina upward by thickening the cervical mucus and lessening uterine motility, as well as by obviating illegal abortions and delivery of unwanted children.
  However, barrier contraceptives protect women better against STDs and HIV/AIDS than OCs do.
- **Anemia and malnutrition:** Pills reduce iron-deficiency anemia by reducing menstrual flow in 60–80% of pill users; they improve nutrition of women by preventing repeated and frequent pregnancies.
- **Endometriosis:** Combined high-dose pills control endometriosis to a good extent when used continuously with increasing doses to produce pseudopregnancy.

❖ **Acne and hirsutism:** OCs are effective in treating acne and hirsutism by increasing sex-hormone-binding globulin and significantly decreasing free testosterone levels. Formulations with desogestrel, drospirenone (DRSP) and cyproterone are especially effective in this respect.
❖ **Premenstrual syndrome:** OCs and pills containing DRSP reduce premenstrual syndrome.
❖ **Polycystic ovarian syndrome (PCOS):** OC pills are highly effective as they regularize the cycles and suppress acne and hirsutism. (OC pills containing cyproterone preferred).

Q. Side effects/risks of OC pills.

INTRODUCTION

As in Previous Answer.

IMPORTANT SIDE EFFECTS/RISKS OF OC PILLS

Breakthrough Bleeding (BTB)

❖ This is slightly more common with the lower dose pills. The women should have two pills a day for 2 or 3 days, which usually controls BTB; if not, EE 0.02 mg may be taken for 7 days along with the pills.
❖ Hypomenorrhea happens sometimes with low-dose pills. The women should be reassured that is not harmful but rather good for health. But if they are not convinced, EE 0.02 mg may be added in the last 7 days for a few cycles.
❖ Amenorrhea is usually temporary and not harmful.
❖ Change to triphasic pills or supplementation with EE for two to three cycles usually cures amenorrhea.

Stroke and Myocardial Infarction

❖ Women who do not smoke, have their blood pressure checked, and do not have hypertension or diabetes are at **no increased risk** of myocardial infarction if they use low-dose COCs, irrespective of their age and duration of OC use.
❖ The risk of hemorrhagic stroke does not increase in women below 35 years of age who do not smoke and are not hypertensive.
❖ Current users of low-dose COCs have a low absolute risk of venous thromboembolic events (VTE) mainly because incidence of VTE is very low in nonpregnant women. Nevertheless,

this risk is three to six times more than nonusers. The absolute risk of VTE attributable to OC use rises with increasing age, recent surgery, and some forms of thrombophilia.
- Progestogens are associated with the increase of low-density lipoprotein cholesterol and a decrease of high-density cholesterol, which increase the risk of atherosclerosis, coronary heart disease and cerebral thrombosis; but estrogens have the opposite effect, and these actions seem relatively balanced in low-dose COCs.

Breast and Cervical Cancer

- There is a small increase in risk of current users of the pill **(relative risk 1.24)**, and the risk reduces gradually over the 10 years after discontinuing use. Breast cancer in current or past OC users is largely localized in the breast—a condition that usually has a better prognosis. The risk of breast cancer is due to the progestogen component of the pills, as the risk is same among users of progestogen-only methods.
- Studies have shown a modest increase in the risk of cervical cancer (1.3–1.8-fold) among women who have used COCs for more than 5 years. However, it is not clear whether the increased risk is due to direct effect of the pill or some characteristics of the pills' users such as age at first intercourse, number of sexual partners, parity, and smoking status.

Liver Tumor

OCs increase the incidence of a rare benign liver tumor, namely, primary hepatocellular adenoma.

Minor Side Effects

Nausea, vomiting may happen initially. Other minor side effects include: Mastalgia, weight gain, and chloasma.

Q. Contraindications for combined OC pills.

INTRODUCTION

As in previous answer.

CONTRAINDICATIONS

Absolute Contraindications

- Active liver disease (hepatitis/tumor)
- Postpartum: Breastfeeding
- Thrombophilia
- Ischemic heart disease
- Complicated migraine
- Pregnancy
- Complicated valvular heart disease
- Breast cancer (current or past history)
- Severe hypertension (systolic >160 or diastolic >100)

- Diabetes mellitus (DM) with vascular complications
- Current history of thromboembolism/stroke/deep vein thrombosis.

Relative Contraindications
- Smoking
- Age more than 35 years
- Mild hypertension
- Uncomplicated DM

Q. Injectable contraceptives.

INTRODUCTION

Progestogen—only injectable contraceptives include:
- Depot medroxyprogesterone acetate (DMPA)
- Norethisterone enanthate (NET EN or Noristerat).

One injection of Depo-Provera remains effective for **3 months**. It is administered in the form of a **150 mg injection** once every 3 months plus or minus 14 days.

One **200 mg NET EN** injection is to be taken **every 2 months**.

Both DMPA and NET EN are highly effective methods of contraception especially in lactating mothers where estrogen is contraindicated.

FAILURE RATE

Pearl Index

Typical failure rate of progestogen—only injectables, as commonly used, is **0.1–0.4%**.

MECHANISM OF ACTION

The injectable contraceptives act by **inhibiting ovulation** in most women. They also work by making **cervical mucus thick** and scanty, thus creating a barrier to sperm penetration, and making the **endometrium less suitable for implantation**.

NONCONTRACEPTIVE BENEFITS

- It cures menstrual troubles like **menorrhagia and dysmenorrhea**
- Medical management of **endometriosis** (pseudopregnancy regimen)
- Prevention and treatment of endometrial hyperplasia
- **DMPA prevents sickling** and the development of abnormal-shaped red blood cells, and lessens episodic bone pain in women suffering from sickle cell diseases; it is thought to be the **best contraceptive for patients of sickle cell anemia**
- DMPA reduces the risk of PID disease and ectopic pregnancy
- DMPA use protects against the risk of endometrial and ovarian cancer
- Injectables are suitable in cases with myoma and endometriosis, as contraception is provided without estrogen effect.

SIDE EFFECTS

- Irregular menstrual bleeding and spotting, as well as temporary amenorrhea, are the most common side effects in DMPA and NET EN users
- **Weight gain:** The average weight gain is 1–3 kg in most cases
- There is a delay of few months in becoming pregnant following discontinuation of the injection
- **Bone density changes:** There is a risk of bone loss among long-term DMPA users leading to osteoporosis; however, this bone loss is reversible on cessation of the contraception.

Combined (estrogen + progesterone) monthly injectable contraceptives (not yet available in India):

- DMPA 25 mg plus estradiol cypionate 5 mg marketed as Cyclofem
- NET EN 50 mg plus estradiol valerate 5 mg marketed as Mesigyna.

Q. Emergency contraception (interceptives).

INTRODUCTION

Agents that do not interfere with fertilization but act on the endometrium to **prevent implantation are called interceptive agents**.

INDICATIONS

- Unplanned, unprotected intercourse
- After rape
- Rupture or tear in the condom at the time of intercourse.

METHODS

Two methods of emergency contraception are available now: (1) Hormonal and (2) Mechanical (IUD).

Hormonal

There are three types of **hormonal** emergency contraception (emergency window: 72 hours):

LNG—Only Pills (Preferred)

- One tablet of 0.75 mg LNG pill should be taken as soon as possible after unprotected intercourse, followed by a same dose taken 12 hours later; both doses must be taken within 72 hours of intercourse.
- Single 1.5 mg dose of LNG (most commonly used) is as effective for emergency contraception as two 0.75 mg doses of LNG taken 12 hours apart.
  Failure rate (pregnancy rate): **0–1%**.

Combined Estrogen and Progestogen Pills (Less Preferred)

- It is also known as the Yuzpe Regimen.
- High-dose pills contain 50 µg of EE and 250 µg LNG (or 500 µg norgestrel).

- Two pills should be taken as soon as possible, but not later than 72 hours of unprotected coitus; this must be followed by two other pills 12 hours later.
- When only low-dose pills containing 30 µg of EE and 150 µg of LNG (300 µg of norgestrel) are available, four pills should be taken as the first dose within 72 hours of unprotected intercourse, followed by four more pills after 12 hours.
- Main side effect is nausea and vomiting. Failure rate: **0–2%**.

Ulipristal Acetate

Ulipristal **(30 mg single dose)** is a selective progesterone receptor modulator (SPRM) recently approved by US Food and Drug Administration (US FDA) for emergency contraception within 120 hours (preferably within 72 hours) after an unprotected intercourse or contraceptive failure.

Mechanical

- IUDs introduced postcoitally can prevent pregnancy very successfully (failure rate = **0.1%**).
- IUDs can be used postcoitally **up to 5 days following sexual exposure**.
- Thus, this method can be used even after 48 hours more delay than the hormonal methods allow.

MECHANISM OF ACTION

They may act through:
- Inhibition or delay of ovulation
- Prevention of implantation in the altered endometrium (interception = main action)
- Prevention of fertilization due to quick transport of sperms or ova
- **They cannot interrupt already established pregnancy (cannot cause an abortion).**

Q. Indications of Medical Termination of Pregnancy (MTP). Add a note on medical method of abortion in first trimester. Complications of surgical evacuation.

INDICATIONS OF MTP

As per India's abortion laws, only qualified doctors under stipulated conditions can perform abortion on a woman in an approved clinic or hospital. The Indian abortion laws fall under the Medical Termination of Pregnancy (MTP) Act, which was enacted by the Indian Parliament in the year 1971. The MTP Act came into effect from April 1, 1972. The MTP Act of India clearly states the conditions under which a pregnancy can be ended or aborted, the persons who are qualified to conduct the abortion:

- Pregnancy would involve serious risk of life or grave injury to physical and/or mental health of the pregnant woman **(therapeutic grounds)**.
  Examples: Certain heart diseases like pulmonary hypertension (Eisenmenger's syndrome), grade 3/4 lesions, malignant hypertension, and psychiatric illness.
- There is a substantial risk of child being born with serious physical and mental abnormalities so as to be handicapped in life **(eugenic grounds)**.

Chapter 9: Contraception

Examples: Chromosomal abnormalities like trisomy 21, 18, 13, etc. congenital anomalies not compatible with life like anencephaly, complex heart diseases, bilateral renal agenesis, etc.
- When pregnancy is caused by rape.
- Pregnancy is caused as result of failure of contraception.
  - Only the consent of the woman is required. The consent of male partner is not needed.
  - MTP in unmarried girls under the age of eighteen requires the consent of a guardian.
  - MTP in lunatics requires the consent of a guardian.
  - Previously, MTP was only till **twenty weeks of gestation,** but after 2021 Amendments, the gestation period upper limit for MTP (with 2 doctors' opinion) has been extended from 20 weeks to **24 weeks in special categories of women (details in the next answer)**

■ METHODS OF FIRST TRIMESTER MTP

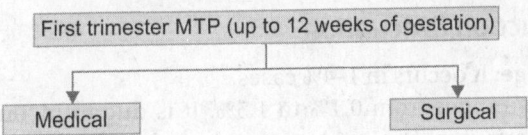

Medical

- It is now officially allowed up to **9 weeks of gestation**
- Drugs used: Mifepristone followed by misoprostol
- Mifepristone (RU486) is a progesterone antagonist
- It acts preferentially on target cells of the endometrium and decidua, counteracting the effect of progesterone, which is essential for establishment and maintenance of pregnancy.
  - It affects the pituitary gonadotropic cells, producing a remarkable decrease of LH secretion, leading to luteolysis
  - It causes softening and ripening of the cervix and produces increased contractibility of the myometrium
  - It causes a marked increase in sensitivity of the uterus to exogenous PGs.

Dose

- Earlier 600 mg orally was used but now recent studies have shown that 200 mg is as effective, so **200 mg is used**. Patient takes this orally on day 1.
- This is followed by **misoprostol tablets (PG E1 analog) 800 µg vaginally or 400 µg orally/sublingual 48 hours later** (day 3). Remaining 400 µg oral/sublingual can be taken after another 12 hours if required
- **Success rate is 96–98%**
- Follow-up visit and USG is required after 14 days to rule out retained products of conception.
- If there are retained products a check curettage is necessary.

Contraindications due to Medical Reasons

- Smoking with age 35 years
- Anemia—hemoglobin <8 g%
- **Suspected/confirmed ectopic pregnancy**/undiagnosed adnexal mass
- **Coagulopathy** or women on anticoagulant therapy

- Chronic **adrenal failure** or current use of systemic corticosteroids
- Uncontrolled hypertension with BP >160/100 mm Hg
- Cardiovascular diseases such as angina, valvular disease, arrhythmia
- **Severe renal, liver, or respiratory diseases**
- Glaucoma
- Uncontrolled seizure disorder
- Allergy or intolerance to mifepristone/misoprostol or other prostaglandins
- **Lack of access to 24-hour emergency services.**

Surgical

- Suction evacuation or manual vacuum aspiration
- Can be done up to 12 weeks of gestation.

Complications of Suction Evacuation

- **Uterine hemorrhage:** It occurs in 1–4% cases.
- **Pelvic infection:** It ranges from 0.1% to 1.5%. It is due to incomplete evacuation and improper aseptic technique. The incidence can be reduced to a great extent by prophylactic use of antibiotic.
- **Cervical injury:** This complication occurs in 0.01–1% cases.
- **Uterine perforation:** This is the most dangerous complication, but fortunately it happens very rarely in 0.1–0.28% cases.
  When perforation occurs or is suspected, the patient should be kept under observation and antibiotic should be started. Usually, she can be discharged in 24-hour time. If there is strong suspicion or actual diagnosis of injury to the intestines or omentum, or if hemorrhage occurs, laparotomy should be performed followed by necessary steps.
- **Retained products:** Incomplete abortion happens in 24% cases
- **Continuation of pregnancy:** In about 1% cases
- **Delayed complications:**
  - Cervical incompetence
  - Uterine synechiae.

Q. 2021 Amendment in MTP Act.

Q. Recent changes in MTP Act.

MTP AMENDMENT ACT, 2021

On 29 January 2020, Government of India first introduced the **MTP Amendment Bill 2020**, which was passed in Lok Sabha on 17 March 2020. A year later, the Bill was placed in Rajya Sabha and was passed on 16 March 2021 as the **MTP Amendment Act, 2021**.

The amendments are as below:
- **Married clause dropped:** The MTP Act earlier permitted termination of the pregnancy by only a married woman in the case of failure of contraceptive method or device. With the amendment, **unmarried women can now seek safe abortion services on grounds of contraceptive failure.**
- **Increase in gestation limit:** Under the MTP Act 1971, the time limit for terminating pregnancy was up to 12 weeks on the advice of one doctor and up to 20 weeks on the

advice of two doctors. Moreover, post 20 weeks terminating pregnancy was not permitted. However, now all women can terminate pregnancy up to 20 weeks on the advice of one doctor and special categories of women (survivors of sexual abuse, minors, victims of rape, incest, disabled women/fetal anomalies) can seek termination **up to 24 weeks.**
- Moreover, women/couples can seek termination of pregnancy, anytime during the gestation period for severe fetal anomalies not compatible with life, as diagnosed by the Medical Boards.
- **Medical Boards:** The amendments mandate constitution of Medical Boards in all the states and union territories for diagnosing substantial fetal anomalies. The Board will decide if a pregnancy may be terminated after 24 weeks and each board will have a gynecologist, radiologist/sonologist, pediatrician and other members notified by the government.
- **Confidentiality:** A registered medical practitioner may only reveal the details of a woman whose pregnancy has been terminated to a person authorized by law. Violation is punishable with imprisonment up to a year, a fine, or both.

MTP Rules, 2021

Following are the revised rules as per the Amendment Act:
- The gestation period upper limit for terminating a pregnancy with **1 doctor's opinion has been extended from 12 weeks to 20 weeks, with the rule being expanded to include unmarried women as well**.
- The gestation period upper limit for termination of pregnancy with **2 doctors' opinion has been extended from 20 weeks to 24 weeks**, for the following special categories:
  - Survivors of sexual assault or rape or incest
  - Minors
  - Change of marital status during the pregnancy (widowhood and divorce)
  - Women with physical disabilities
  - Mentally ill women
  - The fetal anomalies that have substantial risk of being incompatible with life or if the child is born it may suffer from such physical or mental abnormalities to be seriously handicapped
  - Women with pregnancy in humanitarian settings or disaster or emergency
- A state-level Medical Board will determine the request for termination of a pregnancy longer than 24 weeks in the cases of fetal anomalies.

Role of the Medical Board

- To examine the woman and her reports
- To approve or deny the request for termination within 3 days of receiving it
- To ensure that the termination procedure, when advised by the Medical Board, is carried out with all safety precautions along with appropriate counseling within 5 days of the receipt of the request for medical termination of pregnancy.

The Medical Board shall consist of the following:
- A Gynecologist
- A Pediatrician
- A Radiologist or Sonologist
- Other members notified by the State Government or Union Territory.

Q. Long acting reversible contraception (LARC).

DEFINITION

LARC is defined as contraceptive methods that require administration **less than once per cycle or month**.

Included in the category of LARC are:
- Copper intrauterine devices
- Progestogen-only intrauterine systems (LNG IUS/MIRENA)
- Progestogen-only injectable contraceptives
- Progestogen-only subdermal implants

ADVANTAGES

- LARC methods are more cost effective than the combined oral contraceptive pill even at 1 year of use
- IUDs, IUSs and implants are more cost effective than the injectable contraceptives
- There is better patient compliance and increasing the uptake of LARC methods will reduce the numbers of unintended pregnancies.

For, copper intrauterine devices, progestogen-only intrauterine systems [LNG IUS/MIRENA] and progestogen-only injectable contraceptives refer to previous answers (*refer* pages 123–125, 130).

CONTRACEPTIVE IMPLANTS

- The **Norplant system** consists of six silastic capsules each containing 36 mg of LNG.
- These are inserted under the skin in the inside of the upper arm or forearm in most cases, in a fan-shaped manner under local anesthesia.
- It is effective for 5 years.
- **Norplant II or Janelle** has two rods, and remains effective for 5 years.

Norplant prevents pregnancy in three ways:
1. It makes cervical mucus thicker and scantier, preventing sperm penetration
2. LNG suppresses ovulation
3. It depresses the endometrial growth, necessary for implantation of the ovum.

Both Norplant and LNG rod (Norplant II or Jadelle) have a **failure rate of 0.4–0.8%**.

Implanon is a new contraceptive implant.
- It is a single-rod device containing 67 mg of the progestogen 3-ketodesogestrel, also called etonogestrel
- It is effective for 3 years, needs removal after that
- It is placed subcutaneously on the inner side of the upper arm under local anesthesia
- Mechanism of action is similar to Norplant
- NO PREGNANCIES have been reported so far with the use of Implanon.

CHAPTER 10

Miscellaneous

Q. Dermoid cyst.

INTRODUCTION

Dermoid cyst (also called mature cystic teratoma) is the most common benign germ cell tumor of the ovary and also the most common ovarian neoplasm in patients younger than 20 years.

They are commonly composed of multiple cell types derived from one or more of the three germ layers. The word is derived from the Greek teras, meaning monster, which Virchow coined.

However, they may be monodermal and highly specialized.

- It accounts for 10-20% of all ovarian neoplasms. They are bilateral in 15-20% of cases.
- The cyst is moderate in size. The capsule is tense and smooth.
- On cut section there is one area of solid projection called **Rokitansky protuberance**, which is covered with skin with sweat and sebaceous glands. It is here that teeth and bones are found.
- The predominant content of cyst is hair and sebaceous material. There may be clear cerebrospinal fluid (CSF) as well.
- There may be an area of thyroid tissue—struma ovarii, which may be associated with hyperthyroidism.

CLINICAL FEATURES

Symptoms

- Uncomplicated ovarian dermoids tend to be **asymptomatic** and are often discovered incidentally
- They do, however, predispose to **ovarian torsion**, and may then present with acute pelvic pain
- Lump in the lower abdomen
- Dull aching pain/heaviness in lower abdomen
- They are generally moderate in size and not felt per abdomen.

On Pelvic Examination

- The uterus is felt separate from the mass

- A groove is felt between the mass and the uterus
- The lower pole of the cyst is felt through the fornix
- The dermoid cysts because of its fat content may float and may be felt in the anterior fornix (**Krustner's sign**).

INVESTIGATIONS

Radiographic features are described here:

Plain Film X-ray

May show calcific and tooth components with the pelvis.

Pelvic Ultrasound

Ultrasonography (USG) is the preferred modality. Typically an ovarian dermoid is seen as a cystic adnexal mass with some mural components. Most lesions are unilocular.

The spectrum of features includes:
- **Rokitansky nodule**/dermoid plug
- **Tip of the iceberg sign:** echogenic mass with posterior sound attenuation owing to sebaceous material and hair within the cyst cavity (echogenic interface at edge of mass that obscures visualization of deep structures)
- Echogenic shadowing, calcific, or dental components
- Presence of fluid-fluid levels
- **Dot-dash pattern:** Multiple thin, echogenic bands caused by hair in the cyst cavity.

CT Scan

- High sensitivity in the diagnosis of cystic teratomas though is not routinely recommended for this purpose.
- Typically computed tomography (CT) images demonstrate fat (areas with very low Hounsfield values), fat fluid level, calcification (sometimes tooth), Rokitansky protuberance and tufts of hair. The presence of most of the above is diagnostic of ovarian cystic teratomas in 98% of cases. Whenever the size exceeds 10 cm or soft tissue plugs and cauliflower-appearance with irregular borders is seen, malignant transformation should be suspected.

Pelvic MRI

Magnetic resonance imaging (MRI) evaluation usually tends to be reserved for difficult cases, but is exquisitely sensitive to fat components. Enhancement is also able to identify solid invasive components.

COMPLICATIONS

- Torsion is the most common (15–20%) cases
- Rupture is rare (1%)
- Rarely, within some mature teratomas certain elements (most commonly squamous components) undergo malignant transformation (1–2%).

Chapter 10: Miscellaneous

■ TREATMENT AND PROGNOSIS

- They are slow growing (1–2 mm a year) and therefore some advocate nonsurgical management. Larger lesions are often surgically removed. Many recommend initial serial follow-up for lesions under 7 cm to monitor growth, beyond which a resection is advised.
- **Ovarian cystectomy leaving behind the healthy ovarian tissue is the operation of choice.** If the tumor is very big then oophorectomy may be required.
- Laparotomy or laparoscopy can be done. Laparoscopy is preferred nowadays.

Q. Mention complications of benign ovarian cysts and clinical features and management of torsion of ovarian tumor.

Q. Differential diagnosis and management of ovarian torsion.

■ COMPLICATIONS OF BENIGN OVARIAN CYSTS

- Torsion
- Infection
- Rupture
- Intracystic hemorrhage
- Pseudomyxoma peritonei
- Malignancy.

The torsion is more common in tumors with:
- Moderate size (too big and too small tumors will not undergo torsion)
- Moderate weight
- Free mobility
- Long pedicle.

Dermoid cyst has the maximum risk of torsion among all ovarian tumors.

Predisposing Factors for Torsion

- Trauma
- Coitus
- Heavy physical exercises

Two groups of women show a particular tendency to be affected by ovarian torsion:
1. Women in their mid 20s and
2. Women who are postmenopausal.

Approximately 20% of cases of torsion occur during pregnancy.

■ CLINICAL FEATURES

Symptoms

- Classically, the patient presents with the **sudden onset** (commonly during exercise or other agitating movement) of **severe, unilateral lower abdominal pain** that worsens intermittently over many hours.
- A minority of them, however, complain of mild pain that follows a more prolonged time course

- The pain usually is localized over the involved side, often radiating to the back, pelvis, or thigh. Approximately 25% of patients experience bilateral lower quadrant pain. The pain is described as sharp and stabbing or less frequently, crampy
- The patient may also complain of lump in the abdomen
- The lump may also be present before the pain
- Nausea and vomiting occur in approximately 70% of patients
- A history of previous episodes may be elicited, possibly attributable to partial, spontaneously resolving torsion. Fever may occur as a late finding as the ovary becomes necrotic.

Physical Examination

- General condition usually remains unaffected except the patient is in agony and pain
- The physical examination, like the history, is typically nonspecific and is highly variable
- A unilateral, tender, tense cystic mass with restricted mobility, in the hypogastrium, and arising from pelvis
- However, the absence of such a finding does not exclude the diagnosis and the absence of tenderness cannot be used to rule out torsion
- Pelvic examination reveals the mass felt separate from the uterus
- Peritoneal findings are infrequent and indicate advanced disease if present.

DIFFERENTIAL DIAGNOSIS

- Appendicitis
- Diverticulitis
- Ruptured ectopic pregnancy
- Endometriosis
- Torsion of subserous pedunculated fibroid
- Bowel obstruction
- Mesenteric ischemia
- Nephrolithiasis
- Pelvic inflammatory disease
- Urinary tract infection.

FATE

- A partial torsion may untwist spontaneously
- In complete torsion, there is obstruction of both venous and arterial system leading to venous congestion and extravasation of blood inside the cyst
- The cyst may rupture or become gangrenous and the omentum or intestine may get adhered to it.

INVESTIGATIONS

Ultrasonography and color Doppler are the investigation of choice and should be the first examination performed.
- Typically, the affected ovary is enlarged.
- It can show morphologic changes in the ovary and can help in determining whether blood flow is impaired.

Chapter 10: Miscellaneous

- Normal Doppler imaging must not, however, be used as a basis for excluding the diagnosis.
- Color Doppler sonography may be helpful in predicting viability of adnexal structures by depicting blood flow within the twisted vascular pedicle and presence of central venous flow.

Rarely, computed tomography (CT) or MRI is needed to make a definitive diagnosis.

The CT or MRI can serve as a secondary modality when ultrasonographic findings are nondiagnostic.

TREATMENT

- Outpatient care has no role. Patient should be admitted
- Pain medication may be given to a patient who presents with abdominal pain
- The use of nonsteroidal anti-inflammatory drugs and opioids is acceptable
- Surgery: Laparotomy or laparoscopy. Laparoscopy is preferred
- Patients with either a suspected or confirmed diagnosis of ovarian torsion should be admitted. Laparoscopy can be used for both confirmation of the diagnosis and treatment
- The exact surgery depends on the viability of the tissue
- **Detorsion to be tried first.** If the ovaries and tubes look healthy then the cystectomy can be performed
- If there is necrosis then oophorectomy or salpingo-oophorectomy must be done.

Q. Cervical erosion (ectopy).

DEFINITION

Normally, the endocervical canal is lined with columnar epithelium and the ectocervix with squamous epithelium. These connect at the squamocolumnar junction (SCJ). **In cervical erosion, the columnar epithelium may extend further down and protrude on the ectocervix.** It may also undergo squamous metaplasia and transform to stratified squamous epithelium.

CAUSES OF CERVICAL EROSION

Excess Estrogen Level

Cervical erosion is believed to be a response to high levels of circulating estrogen in the body.

- *In pregnancy:* Cervical erosion is a very common finding during pregnancy
  - It can cause mild bleeding during pregnancy, usually during sexual intercourse when the penis touches the cervix. The erosion disappears spontaneously 3–6 months after childbirth
- *In women on birth control pills*
- *At birth and puberty:* Cervical erosion is found in at least one-third of all female babies. It is a response to the maternal estrogen that the babies are subjected to while still in the uterus. The erosion disappears as the influence decreases in few days but can reappear at puberty
- *In women on hormone replacement therapy (HRT):* HRT in menopause mainly consists of replacement of estrogen in the body through pills, patches, creams, etc. This estrogen can cause cervical erosion.

Infections

The theory that infection is the cause of cervical erosion is discarded. Infection does not cause cervical erosion but it is rather the other way around—the changed cells of cervical erosion are more susceptible to various bacteria and fungi and tend to get infected very easily.

Miscellaneous Causes

It is believed by many that chronic infection of the vagina, vaginal douching, and chemical contraceptions like antisperm gels can change the normal level of acidity of the vagina and cause cervical erosion. But these theories are yet to be proved.

■ PATHOGENESIS

- ❖ The columnar epithelium of endocervix replaces the squamous epithelium
- ❖ Usually single layer (flat type)
- ❖ Hyperplastic and folds inwards → follicular erosion
- ❖ Folds inwards and outwards → papillary erosion
- ❖ During healing the SCJ moves toward the external os:
  - ▹ The squamous epithelium grows beneath the columnar epithelium which gradually disintegrates
  - ▹ Squamous metaplasia of columnar cells.

■ CLINICAL FEATURES

Symptoms

- ❖ Asymptomatic.
- ❖ *Increased vaginal discharge:* Usually copious, clear or cloudy and slippery to the touch. If infections occur, there may be pus cells making the discharge mucopurulent. Infections can also cause the vaginal discharge to have a foul smell.
- ❖ *Bleeding:* Contact with the columnar cells of cervical erosion can cause the fragile tissue to break causing bleeding. This is usually seen after sexual intercourse or even after passing hard stool.
- ❖ *Other symptoms of cervical erosion:* Many symptoms like backache, chronic ill health, and even infertility have been said to be due to cervical erosion. But it is more likely that these are the symptoms of chronic pelvic infection which may be the result or cause of cervical erosion.

Signs

On examination:
- ❖ The area of cervical erosion is seen as a **bright, red surface** surrounding and beyond the external os. It extends inside the cervix
- ❖ The margin is well defined and the whole area may be smeared with cervical discharge
- ❖ It feels soft but a little granular to the touch of the examining finger
- ❖ It can bleed a little during examination. It can look like and be mistaken for cervical cancer.

Chapter 10: Miscellaneous

DIFFERENTIAL DIAGNOSIS
- Ectopion
- Early cancer
- Primary sore of syphilis
- Tubercular ulcer.

INVESTIGATIONS
- PAP smear (cytology) to exclude dysplasia and malignancy
- In doubtful cases, a cervical biopsy should be done.

TREATMENT
During pregnancy, the treatment should be withheld till 12 weeks postpartum.
- If the cervical erosion has no symptoms and is discovered on routine examination, treatment is not required
- If symptoms are present, however, active treatment becomes necessary. The aim of the treatment is to destroy the columnar cells so that normal squamous cells can grow in their place:
  - *Electrocautery*: The cells are burned off by using heat generated by electric current
  - *Diathermy*: High temperatures are applied to the area of cervical erosion so the cells are damaged
  - *Cryocautery*: Extreme cold generated by the application of nitrous oxide gas
  - Laser vaporization.
- **Infections:** These should also be controlled by antibiotics
- **Postoperative advice:** The area of cervical erosion takes 6–8 weeks to heal. So the patient is asked to avoid sex or use tampons during this period to avoid any injury.

Q. Define menopause. What are the various symptoms? Add a note on HRT.

DEFINITION
Menopause is defined as the permanent cessation of menses and is physiologically correlated with the decline in estrogen secretion resulting from the permanent loss of follicular/ovarian function.

The clinical diagnosis is confirmed following **stoppage of menses for 1 year** without any other pathology. So the woman is declared to have attained menopause only retrospectively.
- The time of menopause is determined genetically and occurs at the median age of 51 years in West and 47 years in India, range being 45–55 years.
- **Premature ovarian failure is defined as menopause occurring spontaneously before 40 years of age.**
- **Delayed menopause is when the menopause occurs after the age of 55 years.**

MENOPAUSAL SYMPTOMS
- Hot flushes/vasomotor symptoms
  - The classic symptom associated with *estrogen deficiency is the hot flash, also known as hot flush*

- This symptom is described as "recurrent, transient periods of flushing, sweating and a sensation of heat, often accompanied by palpitation, feeling of anxiety, and sometimes followed by chills"
- The entire episode usually lasts 1–3 minutes and may recur as many as 30 times per day, although 5–10 times per day is probably more common
- Hot flashes are experienced by at least half of all women during natural menopause and even more women after surgical menopause
- In severe cases, hot flashes may be accompanied by fatigue, anxiety, irritability, depression, and memory loss. These sensations, if occurring at night, are called as "night sweats" and can lead to interruption of sleep patterns
- Physiologically, *hot flashes correspond to marked, episodic increase in the frequency, and intensity of gonadotropin-releasing hormone (GnRH) pulses* from the hypothalamus and not due to increased GnRH secretion

❖ *Urogenital atrophy:* Vaginal dryness, dyspareunia, recurrent vulvovaginal infections, and urinary tract infections and stress urinary incontinence (SUI)
❖ Mood swings, irritability, depression, and insomnia
❖ Decreased libido
❖ Memory loss/cognitive decline
❖ *Osteoporosis:* Defined as the reduction in the quantity of bone, leading to enhanced susceptibility to fractures. Bones associated with postmenopausal fractures:
  - Spinal vertebra
  - Radius
  - Neck of femur.

HORMONE REPLACEMENT THERAPY

Based on the results of **Women's Health Initiative (WHI) trial**, the following are now the accepted indications for HRT:
❖ Menopausal symptoms such as hot flushes, vaginal dryness, mood swings, irritability, etc.
❖ Prevention and treatment of osteoporosis
❖ Decreased libido.

The HRT is not given for primary prevention of heart disease.

The current recommendation is to use HRT at the **lowest effective dose for a short period of time.**

The different hormones used are:
❖ **Estrogen (E) and progesterone (P) combination:**
  - The principle hormone used/needed is estrogen
  - As unopposed estrogen is a risk factor for endometrial hyperplasia and cancer; in women with *intact uterus both E + P should be given.*
  - In hysterectomized women, only E can be given.
  - The most commonly prescribed oral estrogen is conjugated equine estrogen (CEE). The dose used generally 0.625–1.25 mg/day. Low dose 0.3 mg can also be used.
  - The most common progestin is medroxyprogesterone acetate (MPA) 2.5–5 mg/day. Micronized progesterone 100–200 mg/day or dydrogesterone 5–10 mg/day can also be used.
  - Levonorgestrel-releasing intrauterine system (LNGIUS) (MIRENA) can also be inserted. It has no systemic side effects of progesterone.

- ❖ **Testosterone:**
  - ▷ The most common indication for androgens is loss of libido.
  - ▷ Testosterone by peripheral conversion to estrogen will also relieve the hot flushes.
- ❖ **Tibolone (1.25–2.5 mg/day):**
  - ▷ It is considered as designer HRT. It is a selective tissue estrogen activity regulator (**STEAR**)
  - ▷ It has estrogenic, progestogenic, and androgenic properties.
- ❖ **Selective estrogen receptor modulators (SERMs):**
  - ▷ Raloxifene is a SERM, which binds with higher affinity to estrogen alpha-receptor than the beta-receptors
  - ▷ Clinically, raloxifene produces an effect similar to estrogen on skeletal and cardiovascular system, while behaving as an estrogen antagonist in the uterus and breast
  - ▷ Raloxifene maintains a favorable lipid profile and does not exert a proliferative effect on the endometrium
  - ▷ Effects on bone remodeling are similar to those of estrogen; there is a decrease in the incidence of fractures. Raloxifene is useful in decreasing the risk of osteoporosis
  - ▷ Unfortunately, raloxifene does not relieve hot flushes and can even worsen them
  - ▷ There is increased incidence of venous thromboembolism (VTE).

Types of HRT

- ❖ **Estrogen-only HRT** usually recommended ONLY for women who have undergone hysterectomy. There is no need to take progestogen because there is no risk of endometrial cancer.
- ❖ **E+P: Cyclical HRT** is known as sequential HRT, is often recommended for women who have menopausal symptoms but still have their periods.
  There are two types of cyclical HRT:
  1. Monthly HRT—estrogen every day and progestogen for the last 12–14 days
  2. Three monthly HRT—estrogen every day and progestogen for 12–14 days, every 13 weeks.
- ❖ **Continuous combined HRT:** It is usually recommended for women who are postmenopausal. It involves taking estrogen and progestogen every day without a break.

Various ways in which HRT can be taken:
- ❖ **Tablets**
- ❖ **Transdermal patch:** Patches are available containing 17 beta-estradiol which release 40–80 µg of estrogen/day. The patch to be applied below the waistline and to be changed twice a week
- ❖ **Subdermal implants:** Under local anesthetic, small pellets of estrogen are inserted subcutaneously over the anterior abdominal wall or buttock or thigh. Can be kept for 6 months
- ❖ **Percutaneous estrogen gel:** Delivers **1 mg of estradiol/day when applied to the skin**
- ❖ **Local estrogen vaginal cream** (for urogenital atrophy): For vaginal dryness, atrophic vaginitis. It also reduces frequency, urgency, and recurrent infections. Conjugated equine vaginal estrogen cream 1.25 mg daily is very effective.

■ CONTRAINDICATIONS OF HRT

- ❖ Active liver disease (hepatitis/tumor)
- ❖ Undiagnosed vaginal bleeding

- Thrombophilias
- Ischemic heart disease (IHD)/coronary artery disease (CAD)
- Complicated migraine
- Complicated valvular heart disease
- Breast and ovarian cancer (current or past history)
- Severe hypertension (systolic >160 or diastolic >100)
- Diabetes mellitus (DM) with vascular complications
- History of thromboembolism/stroke/deep vein thrombosis (DVT).

SIDE EFFECTS

- Fluid retention and bloating
- Breast tenderness
- Nausea
- Leg cramps
- Headaches
- Acne.

RISKS OF HRT

- Breast cancer (marginal increase in risk of breast cancer):
  - Using HRT for 5 years would only increase the average risk from 1% to 1.6%
  - Risk appears to return to normal within 5 years of stopping taking HRT.
- Ovarian cancer:
  - The HRT slightly increases the risk of developing ovarian cancer
  - When HRT is stopped, risk returns to normal over the course of a few years.
- Increased risk of coronary heart disease [relative risk (RR) 1.29] and VTE.
- The risk of stroke is increased in women who smoke and are overweight. Women starting HRT and aged below 60 are not at an increased risk of stroke. Combined HRT **does not** increase the risk of endometrial cancer.

Q. Features of Turner's syndrome.

INTRODUCTION

Turner's syndrome occurs in about 1 in 2,500 newborn girls worldwide.

FEATURES OF TURNER SYNDROME (45 XO)

- Short stature
- Broad chest, widely spaced nipples (shield chest)
- Congenital lymphedema
- Cubitus valgus
- Webbed posterior neck
- High arched palate
- Ovarian dysgenesis and infertility (90%)
- Aortic coarctation or bicuspid aortic valves

- Normal intelligence
- Hypoplastic uterus (due to lack of estrogen).

INVESTIGATIONS

- Sex chromatin study negative
- Karyotype is 45 XO
- Sr E2 is very low
- Very high follicle-stimulating hormone (FSH) and luteinizing hormone (LH).

TREATMENT

The primary treatments include hormone therapies:
- **Growth hormone:** It is recommended for most girls with Turner syndrome. The goal is to increase height as much as possible
- Growth hormone treatment is usually given several times a week as injections of somatropin
- **Estrogen therapy:** Most girls with Turner syndrome need to start estrogen and related hormone therapy in order to begin puberty and achieve adult sexual development
- Estrogen replacement therapy usually continues throughout life, until a woman reaches the average age of menopause. Cyclical estrogen and progesterone therapy can also lead to regular menstruation in these patients.

Pregnancy and fertility treatment:
- Some women with Turner syndrome can become pregnant with IVF and donor oocyte.
- This requires a specially designed hormone therapy to prepare the uterus for pregnancy.

Q. PCPNDT Act.

INTRODUCTION

Pre-Conception and Pre-Natal Diagnostic Techniques (PCPNDT) Act, 1994 is an Act of the Parliament of India enacted to stop female feticides and stop the declining sex ratio in India. The act has banned prenatal sex determination.

Sex selection is any act of identifying the sex of the fetus and elimination of the fetus if it is of the unwanted (female) sex.

OBJECTIVE

The main purpose of the Act is to ban the use of sex selection techniques after conception and prevent the misuse of prenatal diagnostic technique for sex selective abortions.

SALIENT FEATURES

Offences under this Act include conducting or helping in the conduct of prenatal diagnostic technique in the unregistered units, sex selection on a man or woman, conducting PND test for any purpose other than the one mentioned in the act, sale, distribution, supply, renting, etc., of any ultrasound machine or any other equipment capable of detecting sex of the fetus.

MAIN PROVISIONS

- The Act provides for the prohibition of sex selection, before, or after conception.
- It regulates the use of prenatal diagnostic techniques, like ultrasound and amniocentesis by allowing them their use only to detect: *genetic/chromosomal abnormalities, metabolic disorders, certain congenital malformations, hemoglobinopathies and sex-linked disorders.*
- No laboratory or clinic will conduct any test including USG for the purpose of determining the sex of the fetus.
- No person, including the one who is conducting the procedure as per the law, will communicate the sex of the fetus to the pregnant woman or her relatives by words, signs, or any other method.
- Any person who puts an advertisement for prenatal and preconception sex determination facilities in the form of a notice, circular, label, wrapper or any document, or advertises in electronic or print form or engages in any visible representation made by means of hoarding, wall painting, signal, light, sound, smoke, or gas, can be imprisoned for up to 3 years and fined ₹10,000.
- The Act mandates compulsory registration of all diagnostic laboratories, all genetic counseling centers, genetic laboratories, genetic clinics, and ultrasound clinics.

AMENDMENT IN 2003

Pre-Natal Diagnostic Techniques (Regulation and Prevention of Misuse) Act, 1994 (PNDT), was amended in 2003 to the Pre-Conception and Pre-Natal Diagnostic Techniques (Prohibition of Sex Selection) Act, PCPNDT Act to improve the regulation of the technology used in sex selection.

Implications of the amendment are:
- Amendment of the Act mainly covered bringing the technique of preconception sex selection within the ambit of the Act
- Bringing ultrasound within its ambit
- Provision for more stringent punishments
- Empowering appropriate authorities with the power of civil court for search, seizure, and sealing the machines and equipment of the violators
- Regulating the sale of the ultrasound machines only to registered bodies.

SECTION 2

Obstetrics

Section Outline

11. Placental Functions and Physiological Changes
12. Antenatal Care and Tests for Fetal Well-being
13. Labor
14. Malpresentations and Malposition
15. Abortions/Miscarriages
16. Ectopic Pregnancy
17. Preeclampsia/Eclampsia
18. Antepartum Hemorrhage and Postpartum Hemorrhage
19. Medical and Surgical Disorders
20. Preterm, Intrauterine Growth Restriction and Postdatism
21. Puerperal Sepsis
22. Obstructed Labor and Rupture Uterus
23. Vesicular Mole and Liquor Disorders
24. Twins
25. Induction of Labor and Operative Delivery
26. Previous Lower Segment Cesarean Section/Vaginal Birth After Cesarean
27. Miscellaneous

CHAPTER 11

Placental Functions and Physiological Changes

Q. Functions of placenta.

PLACENTAL FUNCTIONS

1. Transfer of nutrients from the mother to the fetus by the following mechanisms:
   - Simple diffusion
   - Facilitated diffusion
   - Active transport
   - Endocytosis
   - Exocytosis
   - Leakage.

   This is responsible for the following functions:
   - **Respiratory function:** By intake of oxygen and output of carbon dioxide by simple diffusion across the fetal membrane. The O_2 supply to the fetus is at the rate of 5 mL/kg/min and this is achieved with **cord blood flow of 165–330 mL/min**.
   - **Excretory function:** By simple diffusion of waste products (e.g., urea, uric acid, creatinine) from fetal to maternal circulation.
   - **Nutritive function:**
     - **Glucose: Facilitated diffusion with help of GLUT 1**.
     - **Lipids:** Direct transfer.
     - **Amino acids: Active transport (ATPase)**.
     - **Water and electrolytes:** Na, K, Cl by simple diffusion; Ca, Fe, phosphorus by active transport. Water soluble vitamins are actively transferred while fat soluble vitamins are slowly transferred.
     - **Hormones:** Insulin, steroids from the adrenals, thyroid, chorionic gonadotropin or placental lactogen cross the placenta at a very slow rate. Parathormone and calcitonin do not cross the placenta.

2. **Endocrine function:** Placenta produces **protein hormones** [human chorionic gonadotropin (hCG), human placental lactogen (hPL), pregnancy-specific beta 1-glycoprotein (PS beta 1G), pregnancy-associated plasma protein-A (PAPP-A)] and **steroidal hormones** (estrogen and progesterone).

3. **Enzymatic function:** Placenta secretes many enzymes such as diamine oxidase, oxytocinase, phospholipase A2.

4. **Barrier function:** To protect the fetus from toxic effects of substances in the maternal blood. Most substances with high molecular weights (>500 Dalton) are held up. Antibodies and antigens cross the placenta in both directions. Maternal infections such as viral (rubella, chickenpox, measles, mumps, poliomyelitis), bacteria (tubercle bacillus, *Treponema pallidum*), protozoa (*Toxoplasma gondii*, malarial parasites) can cross the placental barrier and affect the fetus. Most drugs can cross the placenta and affect the fetus.
5. **Immunological function:** The fetus and the placenta contain paternally determined antigens which can lead to immunological rejection. The placenta has some role in preventing such a rejection. Placental hormones have got some immunosuppressive effect. There is production of **blocking antibodies** by mother in response to **TLX (trophoblast lymphocyte cross-reactive)** antigen which protect the fetus from rejection.

Q. Amniotic fluid.

INTRODUCTION

Amniotic fluid surrounds the fetus everywhere except at its attachment with the body stalk. The fluid is completely replaced in **every 3 hours**.

SOURCE

- Transudation of maternal serum across placenta.
- Transudation of fetal circulation across the umbilical cord or placental membranes.
- Secretion from amniotic epithelium.
- Transudation of fetal plasma through nonkeratinized fetal skin before 20 weeks.
- Fetal urine: **400–1200 mL/day** at term.
- Fetal lung fluid.

REMOVAL

- Fetus swallows 400–700 mL of fluid per day.
- Intramembranous absorption of water and solutes (200–500 mL/day) from the amniotic compartment to fetal circulation through the fetal surface of the placenta.

VOLUME

This is related to gestational age.

Gestational age (weeks)	Volume (mL)
12	50
20	400
36–38	1000
40	800
43	200

PHYSICAL FEATURES

- Faintly alkaline

- Low specific gravity 1.010
- An osmolarity of 250 mOsmol/L is suggestive of fetal maturity
- **Pale straw color** due to exfoliated lanugo and epidermal cells from the fetal skin.

Color of amniotic fluid	Clinical importance
Colorless	Preterm
Straw colored	Term
Meconium stained	Fetal distress
Golden	Rh incompatibility
Amber/saffron	Postdatism
Blood stained	Abruptio placentae
Tobacco juice	Intrauterine fetal death (IUFD)
Purulent	Chorioamnionitis

■ COMPOSITION

- **98–99% water**
- 1–2% solids (proteins, glucose, lipids, NPN, urea, uric acid, Na, K, Cl).

■ FUNCTIONS

Main function = **protect the fetus**
- Shock absorber
- Maintains even temperature
- Allows free movements of fetus and prevents adhesions
- During labor, bag of water helps in cervical dilatation
- Flushes the birth canal and by its bactericidal action protects fetus and prevents ascending infection to the uterus.

■ CLINICAL IMPORTANCE

- Study of amniotic fluid provides useful information about fetal well-being and maturity
- Amniotic fluid index (AFI) is used for fetal well-being and to diagnose poly and oligohydramnios
- ARM and drainage of liquor is a method for induction of labor.

Q. Tabulate the important physiological changes during pregnancy.

Q. Cardiovascular changes during pregnancy.

■ INTRODUCTION

During pregnancy there are progressive anatomical, physiological, and biochemical changes in all systems of the body. It is a phenomenon of **maternal adaptation** to increasing demands of growing fetus.

PHYSIOLOGICAL CHANGES IN PREGNANCY

1. Hematological Changes

Blood volume (mL)	Increased	+30–40%
Plasma volume (mL)	Increased	+40–50%
RBC volume (mL)	Increased	+20–30%
Total Hb (g)	Increased	+20%
Hb (g%) PCV (%)	Decreased	–20%

(PCV: packed cell volume)

2. Plasma Protein Changes in Pregnancy

Total protein (g)	Increased	+20–30%
Plasma protein concentration (g%)	Decreased	–10%
Albumin (g%)	Decreased	–30%
Globulin (g%)	Slight increase	+5%
Albumin/globulin ratio	Decreased	–

3. Blood Coagulation Factors

Increased	Decreased	Unaffected
Fibrinogen (+50%)	Factor XI	Clotting time
ESR (4 times)	Factor XIII	Bleeding time
Factor IX	Platelet count	
X		
VIII		
VII		
II		

(ESR: erythrocyte sedimentation rate)

Platelet count slightly decreases during pregnancy; however, there is no decline in platelet function.

4. Respiratory System Changes in Pregnancy

Increased	Decreased	Unaffected
Tidal volume	Functional residual capacity	Respiratory rate
Minute ventilation	Expiratory reserve volume	Vital capacity
Minute O_2 uptake Inspiratory capacity	Residual volume Total lung capacity	Inspiratory reserve volume

5. Renal Changes in Pregnancy

Increased	Decreased
• Renal blood flow (+50%) • GFR (+50%) • Creatinine clearance • Glucosuria • Aminoaciduria	• S creatinine • S BUN • S uric acid plasma osmolality • S $Na^+/K^+/Cl^-$

(S: serum; BUN: blood urea nitrogen; GFR: glomerular filtration rate)

- ❖ S aldosterone increases in pregnancy.
- ❖ S ADH (antidiuretic hormone) remains unchanged in pregnancy.

6. Cardiovascular Changes

Anatomical Changes

- ❖ Due to elevation of diaphragm because of gravid uterus, the heart is pushed upwards and outwards with slight rotation to the left
- ❖ The apex beat is shifted to the 4th intercostal space about 2.5 cm outside the midclavicular line
- ❖ Systolic murmur can be heard in pulmonary or apical area
- ❖ **Mammary murmur:** Continuous hissing murmur in tricuspid area in left 2nd and 3rd intercostal space (due to increase in blood flow through internal mammary vessels)
- ❖ S3 and rarely S4 may be auscultated
- ❖ *2D echo:* Increase in left ventricular end diastolic diameter. Increase in left and right atrial diameters
- ❖ *ECG:* Left axis deviation.

Cardiac Output (CO)

- ❖ **Cardiac output increases by 40% during pregnancy**
- ❖ The cardiac output begins to rise from 5th week of gestation and reaches its peak at **30–32 weeks** and then remains static till term.
- ❖ So the maximum risk of a heart disease patient to have cardiac failure **during pregnancy** is at **32 weeks**.
- ❖ CO increases by 50% during each uterine contraction in labor and there is **80% increase in CO immediately postpartum** (as the uterus contracts, blood from uterus is pushed back into the maternal system, also known as **autotransfusion**).
- ❖ Therefore, the risk of cardiac failure is maximum in the immediate postpartum period (followed by intrapartum). *To avoid this, diuretics should be given after placental delivery to heart disease patients.*
- ❖ CO returns to prelabor value by one hour following delivery and to prepregnant levels by another **4-week time**.

Hemodynamic Changes during Pregnancy

Parameter	Nonpregnant	Pregnancy near term	Change
Cardiac output (L/min)	4.5	6.26	+40%

Contd...

Contd...

Parameter	Nonpregnant	Pregnancy near term	Change
Stroke volume (mL)	65	75	+27%
Heart rate (per minute)	70	85	+17%
Blood pressure	Unaffected or midpregnancy drop of diastolic pressure by 5–10 mm Hg		
Venous pressure	10 cm (femoral)	20–25 cm water	+100%
Colloid oncotic pressure (mm Hg)	20	18	–14%
Systemic vascular resistance (SVR)			–21%
Pulmonary vascular resistance (PVR)			–34%

Blood Pressure

- Systemic vascular resistance (SVR) decreases by 21% due to smooth muscle relaxing effect of:
  - Progesterone
  - Nitric oxide (NO)
  - Prostaglandins (PG)
  - Atrial natriuretic peptide (ANP)
- BP (CO × SVR) is decreased
- There is decrease in diastolic BP and mean arterial pressure (MAP) by 5–10 mm Hg.

Venous Pressure

- Antecubital venous pressure remains unaffected
- Femoral venous pressure (normal = 8–10 cm of water) is markedly raised (pressure of gravid uterus on common iliac veins) to about 25 cm of water during pregnancy in lying down position and to about 80–100 cm water in standing position.

Central Hemodynamics

No significant change in central venous pressure (CVP), mean arterial pressure (MAP), and pulmonary capillary wedge pressure (PCWP).

Regional Distribution

- In nonpregnant state uterine blood flow is about 50 mL/min.
- Uteroplacental blood flow increases progressively during pregnancy, ranging from approximately 700–900 mL/min near term.

The increase is due to vasodilatation effect of:
- Progesterone
- NO
- PG
- ANP
- Pulmonary blood flow (normal = 6000 mL/min) is increased by 2500 mL/min
- Renal blood flow (normal = 800 mL/min) increases by 400 mL/min.

CHAPTER 12

Antenatal Care and Tests for Fetal Well-being

Q. Biophysical profile (BPP).

■ INTRODUCTION

The biophysical profile score is a method used to assess the well-being of a fetus at increased risk for death or damage in utero.
- Evaluates the fetus for the presence of five parameters using ultrasound and an electronic fetal heart rate (FHR) monitor.
- A score of 2 points is given for each parameter that meets criteria.
- **Nonstress test (NST) is performed.**
- The ultrasonography (USG; to evaluate 4 parameters) is continued until all criteria are met or 30 minutes have elapsed.
- The points are then added for a maximum score of 10 (see next page).
- **It is a highly reliable test for fetal well-being. The BPP has a false-negative mortality rate (number of fetal deaths that occur within 1 week of a normal test result) of only 0.6–0.77 deaths per 1000 tests.**

■ INDICATIONS

- Nonreactive NST
- **High-risk pregnancy** [preeclampsia, intrauterine growth restriction (IUGR), postdatism, diabetes, etc.].

Components and their Scores for the Biophysical Profile (Manning's Score)

Component	Score 2	Score 0
Nonstress test (NST)	≥2 accelerations of ≥15 beats/min for ≥15 seconds in 20–40 minutes, i.e., reactive NST	0 or 1 acceleration in 20–40 minutes
Fetal breathing	≥1 episode of rhythmic breathing lasting >30 seconds within 30 minutes	<30 seconds of breathing in 30 minutes
Fetal movement	≥3 discrete body or limb movements within 30 minutes	<3 discrete movements

Contd...

Contd...

Component	Score 2	Score 0
Fetal tone	≥1 episode of extension of a fetal extremity with return to flexion or opening or closing of hand within 30 minutes	No movements or no extension/flexion
Amniotic fluid volume	Single vertical pocket >2 cm	Largest single vertical pocket ≤2 cm

Modified BPP = NST and amniotic fluid index (AFI)

Biophysical Profile Score, Interpretation and Pregnancy Management

Biophysical profile score	Interpretation	Recommended management
10	Normal, nonasphyxiated	No fetal indication for intervention; repeat test weekly except in diabetic patient and post-term pregnancy (twice weekly)
8, Normal fluid	Normal, nonasphyxiated fetus	No fetal indication for intervention; repeat testing per protocol
8, Oligohydramnios	Chronic fetal asphyxia suspected	Deliver if ≥37 weeks, otherwise repeat testing
6	Possible fetal asphyxia	• If amniotic fluid volume abnormal, deliver • If normal fluid at >36 weeks with favorable cervix, deliver • If repeat test ≤6, deliver • If repeat test >6, observe and repeat per protocol
4	Probable fetal asphyxia	Repeat testing same day; if biophysical profile score ≤6, deliver
0–2	Almost certain fetal asphyxia	Deliver

Q. What are the various tests for fetal well-being/fetal surveillance? Add a note on NST/cardiotocography.

Methods for Assessment of Fetal Well-being

Antepartum	Intrapartum	Postpartum
• Nonstress test (NST) • Biophysical profile (BPP) • AFI • Vibroacoustic stimulation test (VAST) • Contraction stress test/oxytocin challenge test (CST/OCT) • Fetal kick count • Color Doppler USG	• CTG (cardiotocography) • Fetal heart rate (Doppler) • Fetal scalp electrode monitoring • Fetal pulse oximetry • Fetal scalp pH monitoring	• Apgar score • Umbilical cord pH

■ NONSTRESS TEST (NST)

Introduction

NST is a test for fetal well-being done in the antenatal period. The patient is **not in labor,** so there are **no contractions** and hence the name, nonstress test (as labor and contractions are considered as a stress for the fetus).

In NST, a continuous electronic monitoring of FHR is done along with fetal movements. With **fetal movements there should be acceleration in FHR,** which if present, indicates a healthy fetus. The accelerations in FHR with movements are **reflex mediated.**

Important Indications

High-risk pregnancies like:
- Diabetes
- Preeclampsia
- IUGR
- Decreased fetal movements
- Postdatism.

Testing should be started **after 30 weeks of gestation**. Reactive NST is valid **for 7 days** and hence frequency of testing should be weekly except in cases of **postdatism and maternal diabetes where a biweekly test is recommended**.

Interpretation

- **Bradycardia:** The baseline FHR <110 beats/min.
- **Tachycardia:** The baseline FHR >160 beats/min.

Beat-to-Beat Variability

- Normal beat-to-beat variability should be **6–25 beats/min**.
- Diminished beat-to-beat variability can be an ominous sign and may indicate a seriously compromised fetus.
- Loss of beat-to-beat variability along with deceleration is associated with fetal academia.

Reactive (Reassuring) NST (Fig. 12.1)

Two or more accelerations of ≥15 beats/min above the baseline, lasting for ≥15 seconds are present in 20–40 minutes observation period.

Nonreactive (Nonreassuring) NST

Presence of less than two FHR accelerations within a 20–40 minute testing period.

The false-positive rate (healthy fetus but nonreactive NST) **of nST is 50%** whereas the **false-negative rate** (number of fetal deaths that occur within 1 week of a normal test result) is **1.4–1.8 per 1000 tests.**

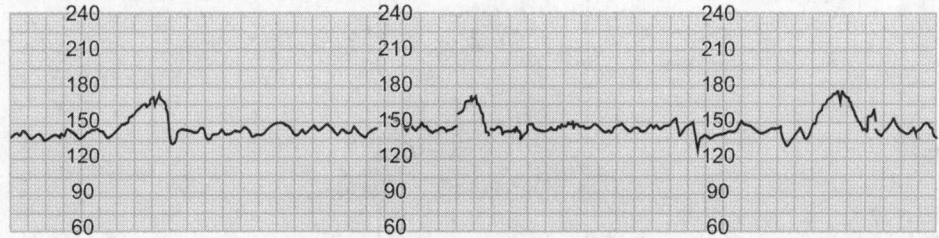

Fig. 12.1: Reactive nonstress test (NST).

CARDIOTOCOGRAPHY (CTG)

Introduction

The difference between NST and cardiotocography (CTG) is that in NST there are no contractions whereas **CTG is done during labor so the fetal heartbeat (cardio) and the uterine contractions (-toco-) both are recorded. So CTG is an intrapartum fetal monitoring test**.

Interpretation

The interpretations are same as NST. There are three types of decelerations:
1. Early decelerations are due to **head compression** (stimulation of vagus nerve).
2. Late decelerations are due to **uteroplacental insufficiency (fetal distress/hypoxia)**.
3. Variable decelerations are due to **cord compression** (oligohydramnios in labor).

Features of Early Fetal Heart Rate Deceleration

Characteristics include gradual decrease in the heart rate with both onset and recovery coincident with the onset and recovery of the contraction **(Fig. 12.2)**.

Features of Late Fetal Heart Rate Deceleration

Characteristics include gradual decrease in the heart rate with the nadir and recovery occurring after the end of the contraction. The nadir of the deceleration occurs 30 seconds or more after the onset of the deceleration **(Fig. 12.3)**.

Features of Variable Fetal Heart Rate Deceleration

Characteristics include abrupt decrease in the heart rate with onset commonly varying with successive contractions. The decelerations measure ≥15 beats/min for 15 seconds or longer with an onset to nadir phase of less than 30 seconds. Total duration is less than 2 minutes **(Fig. 12.4)**.

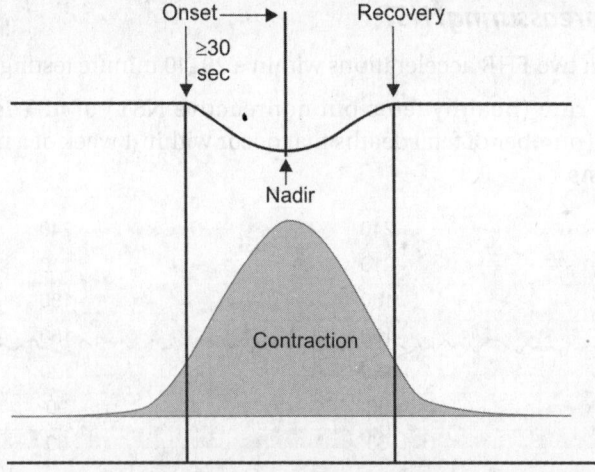

Fig. 12.2: Early deceleration.

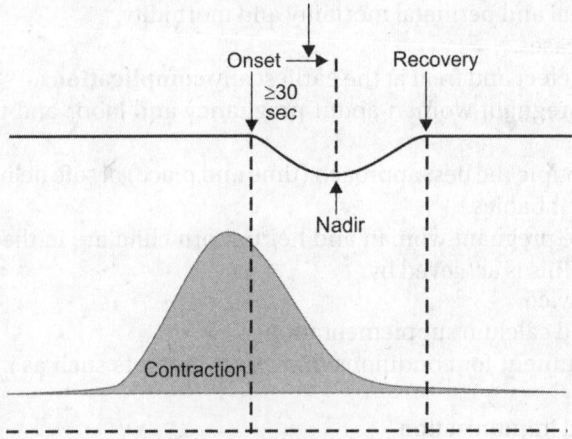

Fig. 12.3: Late deceleration.

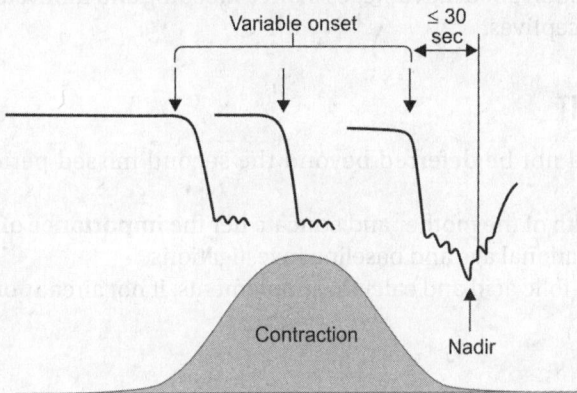

Fig. 12.4: Variable deceleration.

Q. Components of antenatal care.

Q. Define antenatal care, components at first visit and schedule for subsequent visit in ideal set-up for uncomplicated pregnancy.

■ DEFINITION

Antenatal care (ANC) is the **systematic supervision** (care, examination and advice) of the woman during pregnancy.
ANC comprises of:
❖ Careful **history taking and examination**
❖ **Advice** to pregnant women.

■ AIMS AND OBJECTIVES

1. *The primary aim of ANC is* to promote and protect the health of women and the unborn fetus during pregnancy so as to achieve at the end, **a normal pregnancy and healthy mother and a healthy baby**.

2. To reduce maternal and perinatal mortality and morbidity.
3. Screen high-risk cases.
4. To prevent or to detect and treat at the earliest any **complications**.
5. To **educate** the pregnant women about pregnancy and labor and the complications of pregnancies.
6. To discuss with couple the best approach (time and place) of safe delivery and the best way of bringing up their babies.
7. To ensure that the pregnant woman and her unborn child are in the best possible health prior to delivery. This is achieved by:
    - Nutritional advice
    - Iron, folate and calcium supplementation
    - Providing treatment for conditions that affect mothers such as malaria, tuberculosis, HIV, etc.
    - Tetanus toxoid immunization
    - Providing voluntary HIV testing and counseling.
8. Providing information about advantages of breastfeeding and motivate for family planning and use of contraceptives.

AT THE FIRST VISIT

The first visit should not be deferred beyond the second missed period, ideally must be earlier.
- To assess the health of the mother and educate her the **importance of regular follow-up**
- To assess the gestational age and baseline investigations
- To start with iron, folic acid and calcium supplements, if not already on it.

History Taking

Ask about:
- Full name
- Husband's name
- Age (extremes of age is obstetric risk factor)
- Address
- Age of marriage
- Gravida and parity
- Religion
- Occupation of the patient and the husband (gives idea about her **physical activity, stress, occupational hazard** and socioeconomic condition. To anticipate complications of **anemia, prematurity, IUGR, etc., associated with low social status**)
- *Period of gestation:* Ask about the first day of the last **normal** menstrual period (LNMP) and assign the expected date of delivery (EDD) and also inquire about the past menstrual cycle
- *Habits:* Smoking/chewing tobacco, alcohol, etc. and other addictions
- *Complaints:* Bleeding or spotting since becoming aware of being pregnant, pain in abdomen, nausea, vomiting, sleep, appetite, bowel habit, etc.
- *History of present pregnancy:* Trimester wise complaints or complications noted. Medications, supplements, immunization, number of previous antenatal visits (booking status) noted

- *Obstetric history:* To know about any **antenatal, intrapartum and postpartum complications** of previous pregnancies:
  - Number and type of previous pregnancies (miscarriage, ectopic pregnancy, preterm/post-term delivery)
  - Previous deliveries and any complication or procedure related to the previous deliveries (cesarean section and its indication, forceps or vacuum extraction, manual removal of the placenta)
  - Date (month, year) and outcome of each event (live birth, still birth, abortion, ectopic, twins, hydatidiform mole, child with any abnormality, neonatal and infant death)
  - Birth weight if known and sex of children
  - Special maternal complications, events and interventions (e.g., blood transfusion) in previous pregnancies

Past Medical and Surgical History

Ask about history of specific diseases and conditions, including: Tuberculosis, cardiovascular diseases, hypertension, chronic renal disease, epilepsy, diabetes mellitus, reproductive tract infections/sexually transmitted infections (RTIs/STIs)/HIV-AIDS, malaria, hepatitis and other liver diseases, any allergies, other chronic diseases, surgeries, blood transfusion, current use of medicines.

Family History

Family history of tuberculosis, hypertension, diabetes mellitus and any hereditary disease to be enquired.

Physical Examination

Perform routine physical examination and particularly pay attention to the following:
- *Build*: Average/thin/obese
- *Nutrition*: Good/average/poor
- Height and weight (kilograms) for setting a baseline for further monitoring of appropriate weight gain
- Pallor/signs of anemia (pale complexion, fingernails, conjunctiva, oral mucosa, tip of tongue and shortness of breath)
- Glossitis, stomatitis, icterus
- *Neck*: Lymph nodes, neck veins, thyroid enlargement
- *Edema feet*: Examine both legs, medial malleolus and lower 1/3rd of tibia
- Pulse and blood pressure for detecting hypertension
- Chest and heart auscultation for detecting underlying cardiovascular and respiratory diseases
- Obstetric examination
  - Inspection
  - Symphysis-fundal height
  - Palpation: Various grips to determine lie and growth
  - Auscultation of fetal heart structures (FHS) from 20 weeks onward
- Breast exam for inverted nipple, which can impact breastfeeding
- External genitalia for vaginal discharge
- Pap smear maybe taken.

INVESTIGATIONS

Perform the following tests:
- *Routine urine analysis:* Protein, sugar, pus cells
- *Blood:* Blood group typing (ABO and Rh), hemoglobin, venereal disease research laboratory (VDRL), blood sugars, thyroid-stimulating hormone (TSH) and HIV (after consent and counseling) and hepatitis B surface antigen (HBsAg)
- Pap smear is routinely done at many clinics.

Special Investigations

- **Dual marker test at 11–13 weeks or triple or quadruple marker test at 16–18 weeks** as a screening tests for trisomy
- **Hb electrophoresis:** to detect thalassemia
- USG:
  - USG in first trimester helps to detect:
    - Viable intrauterine pregnancy
    - Rule out ectopic pregnancy
    - Accurate dating
    - Number of fetuses
    - Any uterine and adnexal pathology
  - **Nuchal translucency (NT) scan at 11–13 weeks of gestation. NT >3 mm is a marker for Down's syndrome and requires further investigations.**
  - Anomaly/malformation scan at 18–20 weeks of gestation.

Repetition of Investigations

- Hemoglobin should be repeated at 28 weeks and 36 weeks.
- Blood sugars fasting and postprandial at 26–28 weeks. **DIPSI test is preferred for GDM screening between 24–28 weeks**.
- Urine checked for sugars and proteins at every antenatal visit.

SUPPLEMENTS

- Folic acid 400 mcg is recommended (ideally to be started one month before conception) throughout the pregnancy, especially in first trimester to prevent neural tube defect (NTD) and later megaloblastic anemia
- *Iron:* There is an increase in iron requirement during pregnancy which cannot be met with dietary supplementation. Hence all pregnant mothers need iron therapy starting from 12–16 weeks onward. One tablet containing 60 mg elemental iron to be taken every day, if hemoglobin is above 10 g%. The dose is increased to 2–3 tablets in cases of anemia
- *Multivitamins:* Vitamin B complex, D supplementation should also ideally be recommended
- *Calcium:* As calcium requirement is doubled in pregnancy, patient should be advised to take at least one tablet of 500 mg calcium.

Chapter 12: Antenatal Care and Tests for Fetal Well-being

■ IMMUNIZATION

Tetanus: Immunization protects both mother and neonate. In unprotected women 0.5 mL tetanus toxoid (TT) is given IM at 4–6 weeks interval for two such, the first dose between 16 and 24 weeks. If immunized in the past, a booster dose of 0.5 mL IM is given in last trimester.

Recent Advances

Td (tetanus & diphtheria) vaccine is preferred over TT.

CDC recommends that women should get **Tdap vaccine** (tetanus, diphtheria and pertussis) during the early part of the **3rd trimester** of every pregnancy. By doing so, she helps protect her baby from whooping cough in the first few months of life.

It is also advisable to give **influenza** (H1N1/swine flu) vaccination.

■ DIETARY ADVICE

Increase in calorie requirement is about **300 kcal** over nonpregnant state during second half of pregnancy. There is also an increase in requirement of protein, iron and calcium. The patient is to be advised to eat balanced healthy diet. Women with normal BMI should eat to maintain the scheduled weight gain of 11–12 kg in pregnancy.

■ IMPORTANT INSTRUCTIONS

Patient is to be motivated and persuaded to attend antenatal checkup on schedule date of visit. To report early and immediately in cases of:
- Pain in abdomen
- Bleeding per vagina, even if slight
- Gush of watery fluid per vaginam [suggestive of premature rupture of membranes (PROM)]
- Decrease or absent fetal movements
- Untoward symptoms such as intense headache, epigastric pain, vomiting and scanty urination.

■ FREQUENCY OF VISITS

Generally, checkup is done at interval of:
- 4 weeks up to 28 weeks, then
- 2 weekly up to 36 weeks and then
- Weekly till delivery.

In developing countries, **WHO had initially recommended at least four visits**:
- Second trimester 16–18 weeks
- 24–28 weeks
- 32 weeks
- 36 weeks.

RECENT ADVANCES

2016 WHO ANC Model

WHO now recommends 8 ANC contacts (visits)

2016 WHO ANC model
First trimester • Contact 1: up to 12 weeks **Second trimester** • Contact 2: 20 weeks • Contact 3: 26 weeks **Third trimester** • Contact 4: 30 weeks • Contact 5: 34 weeks • Contact 6: 36 weeks • Contact 7: 38 weeks • Contact 8: 40 weeks

CHAPTER 13

Labor

Q. What are the stages of labor? Differences between true and false labor.

■ DEFINITION
Series of events that take place in genital organs in an effort to expel the viable products of conception out of womb through vagina into outer world is called as labor.

■ STAGES OF LABOR
Labor has four stages:

First Stage of Labor
- Begins with **regular uterine contractions and ends with complete cervical dilatation at 10 cm**
- Traditionally, divided into a **latent phase** (till cervix is 3–4 cm dilated) and an **active phase** (4–10 cm)
- **As per WHO 2020 Labor Care Guide, active phase is cervical dilatation of 5 cm or more**
- The latent phase begins with mild, irregular uterine contractions that soften and shorten the cervix
- Contractions become progressively more rhythmic and stronger
- The active phase usually begins at about 4 cm of cervical dilation and is characterized by rapid cervical dilation and descent of the presenting fetal part
- Its average duration is 12 hours in primigravida and 6 hours in multiparous woman.

Second Stage of Labor
- Begins with complete cervical dilatation and ends with the **delivery of the fetus**
- In nulliparous women, the second stage should be considered prolonged if it exceeds 3 hours if regional anesthesia is administered or 2 hours in the absence of regional anesthesia
- In multiparous women, the second stage should be considered prolonged if it exceeds 2 hours with regional anesthesia or 1 hour without it.

Third Stage of Labor

❖ The period between the delivery of the fetus and the **delivery of the placenta** and fetal membranes.
❖ Delivery of the placenta often takes less than 10 minutes, but the third stage may last as long as 30 minutes.
❖ The duration is reduced to 5 minutes with active management of third stage of labor (AMTSL).

Fourth Stage of Labor

At least 1 hour observation after the expulsion of placenta and membranes. General condition of the mother and behavior of uterus are carefully to be monitored.

Differences between True and False Labor

True labor	False labor
Contractions occur at regular intervals	Contractions occur at irregular intervals
Intervals gradually shorten	Intervals remain long
Intensity gradually increases	Intensity remains unchanged
Discomfort is in the back and abdomen	Discomfort is chiefly in the lower abdomen
Progressive effacement and dilatation of cervix	**Cervix does not dilate**
Discomfort is not stopped by sedation	Discomfort usually is relieved by sedation
Associated with show and formation of bag of forewaters	Not associated
Associated with descent of the presenting part	No descent

Q. Partogram/partograph.

DEFINITION

Partogram is a composite graphical record of key data (maternal and fetal) during labor entered against time on a single sheet of paper.

It provides an accurate record of the progress of labor and any delay or deviation from normal may be detected quickly and treated accordingly. It was first devised by **Freidman in 1954**.

COMPONENTS

❖ **Patient identification:** Name, gravida, and parity
❖ **Time:** It is recorded at an interval of one hour. Zero time for spontaneous labor is time of admission in the labor ward and for induced labor is time of induction
❖ **Fetal heart rate:** It is recorded at an interval of **thirty minutes**
❖ State of membranes and color of liquor: "I" designates intact membranes, "C" designates clear, and "M" designates meconium stained liquor
❖ **Cervical dilatation** and descent of head
❖ *Uterine contractions:* Squares in vertical columns are shaded according to duration and intensity
❖ Drugs and fluids given to patient during labor
❖ *Blood pressure:* It is recorded in vertical lines at an interval of 4 hours

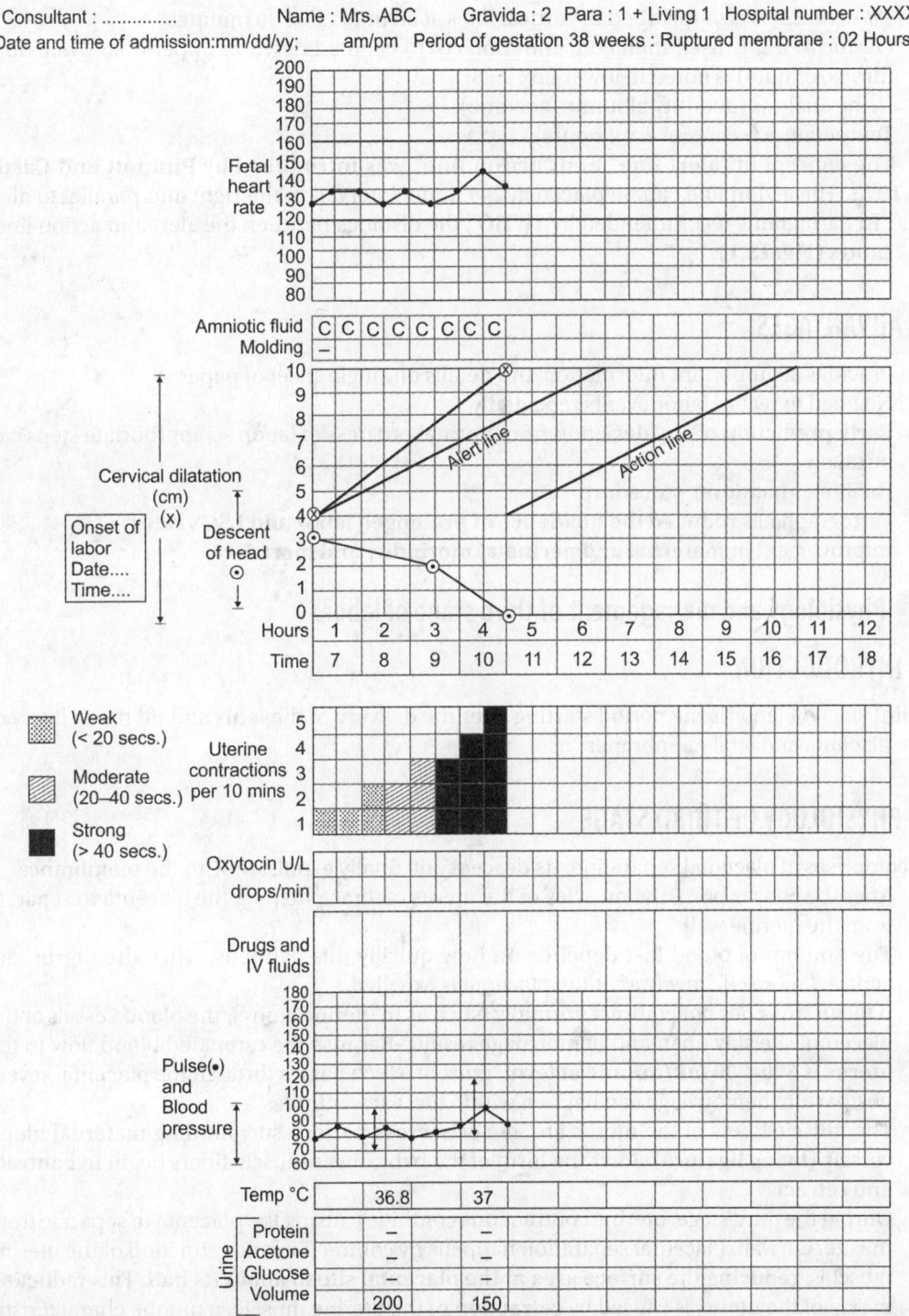

Fig. 13.1: Partograph (modified WHO) representing graphically the important observations in labor. The cervical dilatation and descent of head are shown in relation to alert and action lines. Intensity and duration of uterine contraction are shown with shades.

- *Pulse rate:* It is also recorded in vertical lines at an interval of 30 minutes
- *Oxytocin:* If it is used then concentration (U/L) is noted down in upper box; while dose (drops/minute) is noted in lower box
- Urine analysis (quantity albumin, acetone)
- Temperature record (every 2 hours).

The concept of **"alert line" and "action line" was introduced by Philpott and Castle in 1972**. The action line can be placed at 2–4 hours interval, to the right and parallel to alert line. In partograms recommended by **"WHO"**, the distance between the alert and action lines is **4 hours (Fig. 13.1)**.

ADVANTAGES

- Provides all important information and details on single sheet of paper
- No need to record labor events repeatedly
- **Early prediction** of any deviation from normal progress of labor, so appropriate steps can be taken
- Facilitates handover procedure
- Partograph has **reduced the incidence of prolonged labor and LSCS rates**
- Improvement in **maternal and perinatal morbidity and mortality**.

Q. Physiology and management of third stage of labor.

INTRODUCTION

Third stage of labor is the period starting after the delivery of the fetus and till the delivery of the placenta and fetal membranes.

PHYSIOLOGY OF THIRD STAGE

It comprises of placental separation, its descent and finally expulsion with the membranes.

- After the baby is born, the muscles of the uterus contract, helping the placenta to separate from the uterine wall
- The amount of blood lost depends on how quickly this happens, since the uterus can contract more effectively after the placenta is expelled
- If the uterus does not contract normally (such as in uterine atony), the blood vessels at the placental site stay open and hemorrhage results. Because the estimated blood flow to the **uterus is 500–800 mL/minute at term**, most of which passes through the placenta, severe postpartum hemorrhage can happen within just a few minutes
- The muscle fibers of the uterus are in a **crisscross pattern** surrounding maternal blood vessels **(living ligature)**. After the birth of the baby, these muscle fibers begin to **contract and retract**
- During the third stage, uterine contractions continue causing the placenta to separate from the uterine wall. Placental separation happens by contraction and retraction of the uterine muscles, **reducing the surface area at the placental site to about its half**. This reduction in size of the uterus is caused by **retraction** of the uterine muscle, a unique characteristic that helps maintain its shortened length after each contraction. As the placental area becomes smaller, the placenta begins to separate from the uterine wall because, unlike the uterus, it is not elastic and cannot contract and retract

- A shearing force is instituted between the placenta and the placental site which brings about the separation
- The plane of separation runs through **deep spongy layer of decidua basalis**
- At the area where the placenta separates from the uterus, a clot forms. This clot—known as a retroplacental clot—collects between the uterine wall and the placenta, and it further promotes separation.

Methods of Placental Separation

There are two ways of placental separation **(Figs. 13.2A and B)**:
1. **Schultze (more common)**
2. **Matthews Duncan.**

Schultze Mechanism

By far the most common mechanism of placental expulsion.
- Delivery of the placenta with the fetal side presenting. Results when separation begins **centrally** with corresponding formation of a central retroplacental clot, which weights the placenta so the central portion descends first.
- This then inverts the placenta and amniotic sac and causes the membranes to peel off the remainder of the decidua and trail behind the placenta. Bleeding associated with Schultze mechanism is not visible until the placenta and membranes are delivered, since the inverted membranes hold and catch the blood.

Duncan Mechanism

Delivery of the placenta with the maternal side presenting. Results when separation first takes place at the **margin or periphery of the placenta**. The placenta descends sideways and the amniotic sac, therefore, is not inverted but trails behind the placenta for delivery. Blood escapes between the membranes and uterine wall and is visible externally.

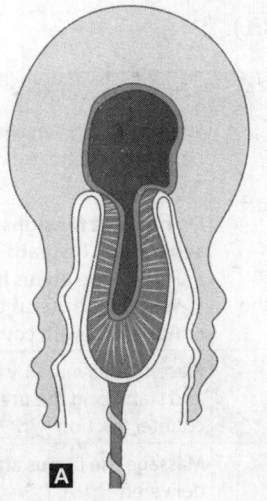
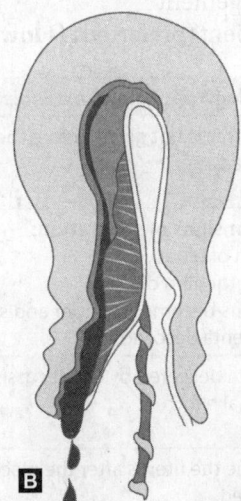

Figs. 13.2A and B: Types of separation of the placenta: (A) Schultze method; (B) Matthews Duncan method.

Memory aid for remembering Schultze vs Duncan: It is based on the appearance of the two different sides of the placenta. Fetal side is shiny and glistening because it is covered by membranes, therefore **"shiny Schultze"**. Maternal side is rough and red-looking, thus **"dirty Duncan"**. Remember: **SSC = Shiny Schultze Central**.

Expulsion and Control of Bleeding

- After complete separation, the placenta is pushed into the flabby lower segment or upper vagina by effective contraction and retraction of uterus
- Thereafter, it is expelled out either by voluntary contraction of abdominal muscles or by manual procedure
- The placental site is rapidly covered by a fibrin net and clots form
- The muscle fibers of the uterus (interlacing intermediate layer of myometrium) compress the blood vessels where the placenta was attached, helping to control bleeding at the placental site **(living ligature principal of hemostasis)**
- Also, thrombosis occurs to occlude the torn sinuses
- **Apposition of walls of uterus (myotamponade)** also contribute.

■ LENGTH OF THIRD STAGE

- Fifty percent of placental deliveries occur within 5 minutes, and 90% are delivered within 15 minutes
- When the third stage of labor lasts longer than 30 minutes, PPH occurs six times more often than it does among women whose third stage lasted less than 30 minutes.

■ MANAGEMENT OF THIRD STAGE

Third stage is the most crucial stage of labor. Its most important and most dangerous complication is PPH.

Two methods of management are:
1. Expectant management
2. Active management (preferred) **(Flowchart 13.1)**.

	Physiologic (expectant) management	*Active management*
Uterotonic	Uterotonic is not given before the placenta delivered	Uterotonic is given within one minute of the baby's birth (after ruling out the presence of a second baby)
Signs of placental separation	Wait for signs of separation: • Gush of blood • Lengthening of cord • Uterus becomes rounder and smaller as the placenta descends	Do not wait for signs of placental separation. Instead: • Palpate the uterus for a contraction • Wait for the uterus to contract • Apply CCT with counter traction
Delivery of the placenta	Placenta delivered by gravity assisted by maternal effort	Placenta delivered by CCT while supporting and stabilizing the uterus by applying counter traction
Uterine massage	Massage the uterus after the placenta is delivered	Massage the uterus after the placenta is delivered

Contd...

Contd...

	Physiologic (expectant) management	Active management
Advantages	• Does not interfere with normal labor process • Does not require special drugs/supplies • May be appropriate when immediate care is needed for the baby (such as resuscitation) and no trained assistant is available • May not require a birth attendant with injection skills	• Decreases length of third stage • Decrease likelihood of prolonged third stage • Decreases average blood loss • Decreases the number of PPH cases • Decreases need for blood transfusion
Disadvantages	• Length of third stage is longer compared to AMTSL • Blood loss is greater compared to AMTSL • Increased risks of PPH	• Requires uterotonic and items needed for injection/injection safety • Requires a birth attendant with experience and skills giving injections and using CCT

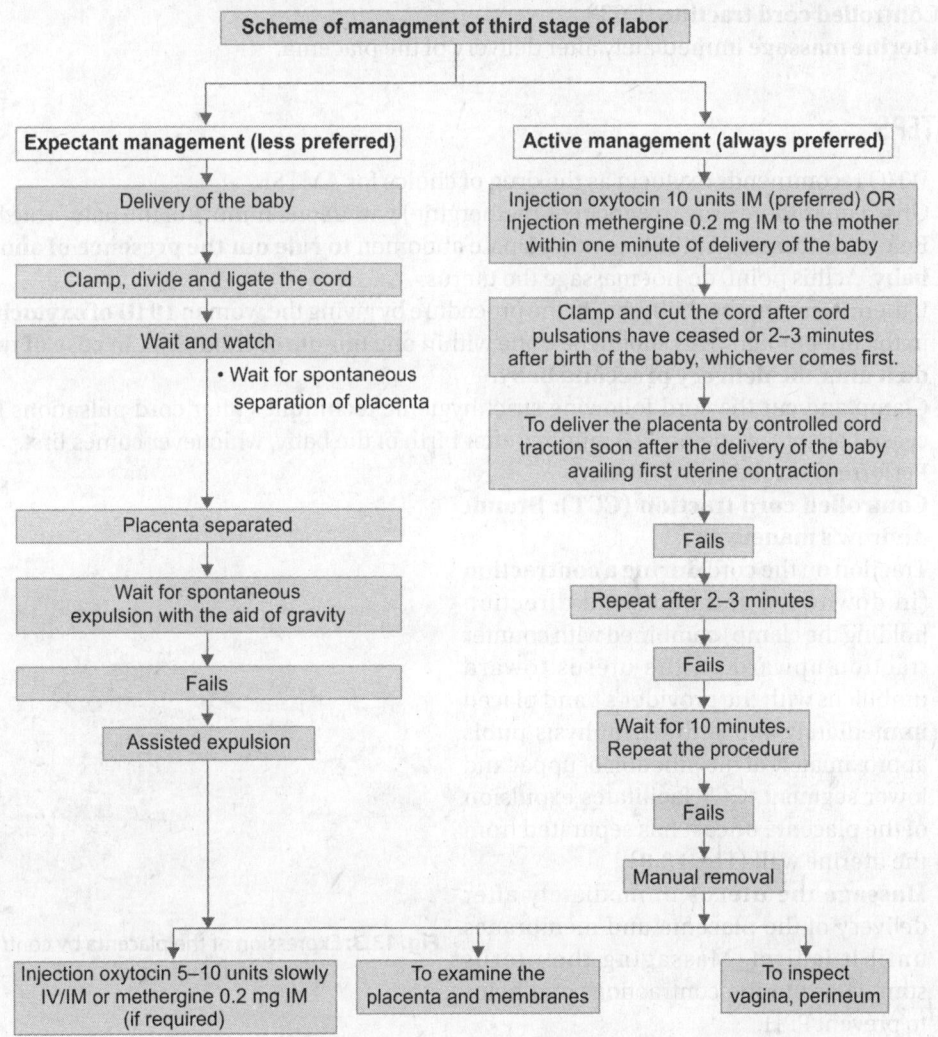

Flowchart 13.1: Scheme of management of third stage of labor.

Q. Active management of the third stage of labor (AMTSL).

INTRODUCTION

Third stage of labor is the period starting after the delivery of the fetus and till the delivery of the placenta and fetal membranes.

DEFINITION

Active management of the third stage of labor (AMTSL): A combination of actions performed during the third stage of labor to **prevent PPH**. AMTSL speeds delivery of the placenta by increasing uterine contractions and prevents PPH by minimizing uterine atony.

The components of AMTSL are:
- Administration of a **uterotonic drug** at the time of delivery of the **anterior shoulder or afterward within one minute after the baby is born (oxytocin is the uterotonic of choice)**
- **Controlled cord traction** (CCT)
- **Uterine massage** immediately after delivery of the placenta.

STEPS

1. WHO recommends oxytocin as the drug of choice for AMTSL.
2. Give a uterotonic drug (oxytocin or methergine) within one minute of the baby's birth.
3. Before performing AMTSL, gently palpate abdomen **to rule out the presence of another baby**. At this point, do not massage the uterus.
4. If there is not another baby, begin the procedure by giving the woman **10 IU of oxytocin IM** in the upper thigh. This should be done within one minute of childbirth. **In case of twins, do it after the delivery of second baby.**
5. Clamp and cut the cord following strict hygienic techniques after cord pulsations have ceased or approximately 2–3 minutes after birth of the baby, whichever comes first.
6. Perform controlled cord traction.
   Controlled cord traction (CCT): Brandt Andrew's maneuver
   Traction on the cord **during a contraction** (in downward and backward direction holding the clamp) combined with counter traction upward on the uterus toward umbilicus with the provider's hand placed immediately above the symphysis pubis approximately at the junction of upper and lower segment. CCT facilitates expulsion of the placenta once it has separated from the uterine wall **(Fig. 13.3)**.
7. **Massage the uterus** immediately after delivery of the placenta and membranes until it is firm. Massaging the uterus stimulates uterine contractions and helps to prevent PPH.

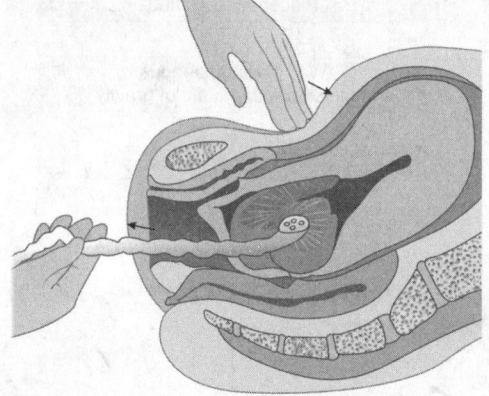

Fig. 13.3: Expression of the placenta by controlled cord traction.

8. Examine the placenta and membranes to ensure they are complete. A small amount of placental tissue or membranes remaining in the woman can prevent uterine contractions and cause PPH.
9. Gently separate the labia and inspect the lower vagina and perineum for lacerations that may need to be repaired to prevent further blood loss. Suture the episiotomy.
10. Perform a comprehensive examination of the woman and newborn one and six hours after childbirth. During the first two hours after the delivery of the placenta, monitor the woman at least every 15 minutes (more often if needed) to:
    - Palpate the uterus to check for firmness
    - Massage the uterus until firm (ask the woman to call for help if bleeding increases or her uterus gets soft)
    - Check for excessive vaginal bleeding.

ADVANTAGES

AMTSL decreases:
- **Incidence of PPH by up to 60%**
- Duration of third stage of labor
- Percentage of third stages of labor lasting longer than 30 minutes
- Need for blood transfusion
- Need for uterotonic drugs to manage PPH.

DISADVANTAGE

The only disadvantage is **slightly increased incidence (1-2%) of retained placenta** and consequent manual removal of placenta. This is more likely to happen when methergine is used for AMTSL.

Q. Management of first stage of normal labor.

INTRODUCTION

First stage of labor starts from onset of true labor pains (regular uterine contractions) and ends with complete cervical dilatation at 10 cm.

GENERAL CONSIDERATIONS

- Labor events have got great psychological, emotional, and social impact to the woman
- Throughout labor, the patient is given **encouragement and emotional support**
- **Privacy** must be maintained
- She is explained about the events from time to time
- Comfortable environment, skill and confidence of the caregiver and the emotional support are all essential.

Management of normal labor aims at *maximal observation with minimal active intervention.* The idea is to maintain the normalcy and to detect any deviation from the normal at the earliest possible moment.

ANTISEPTICS AND ASEPSIS

Strict asepsis has to be maintained. Antiseptic and aseptic precautions are to be taken during vaginal examination and during conduction of delivery.

PATIENT CARE

Shaving or hair clipping of the vulva is done.

The vulva and the perineum are washed liberally with soap and water and then with 10% Dettol solution or Hibitane (chlorhexidine) 1 in 2000.

VAGINAL EXAMINATION IN LABOR

First vaginal examination should be done by a **senior doctor** to be more reliable and informative and it is to be done taking all aseptic precautions.

Complete examination should be done before fingers are withdrawn. The following information is to be noted and recorded carefully:
- Cervical **dilatation** in centimeters
- Degree of **effacement** of cervix
- Status of **membranes** and if ruptured—color of the liquor: clear/meconium stained/blood stained
- Presenting part and its position
- Caput or molding of the head
- **Station** of the head in relation to ischial spines
- Assessment of the **pelvis** especially in primigravida is to be done and presence of vulval varicosity, if any, is to be noted.

Indications of Vaginal Examinations

Vaginal examinations should be restricted to a minimum.
- *At the onset of labor*: To confirm the onset of labor
- *The progress of labor* can be judged on periodic examinations at an interval of 3–4 hours
- *Following rupture of the membrane* to exclude cord prolapse especially where the head is not yet engaged
- *Whenever any interference is contemplated*
- To confirm the actual coincidence of bearing down efforts with complete dilatation of the cervix and to *diagnose precisely the beginning of second stage*.

FIRST STAGE MANAGEMENT

Principles

- Noninterference with watchful expectancy so as to prepare the patient for natural birth
- To monitor carefully the progress of labor, maternal conditions, and fetal well-being so as to detect any intrapartum complication early.

Preliminaries

- Enquiry is to be made about the onset of labor pains or leakage of liquor

- ❖ Thorough general and obstetrical examinations including vaginal examinations are to be carried out and recorded
- ❖ Records of antenatal visits, investigation reports, and any specific treatment given are to be reviewed.

Actual Management

- ❖ **General:** Encouragement, emotional support, and assurance are given. *Constant supervision* is ensured.
- ❖ **Bowel:** An enema with soap and water or glycerin suppository is traditionally given in early stage.
- ❖ **Rest and ambulation:** If the membrane is intact, the patient is allowed to walk about. This attitude prevents vena cava compression and encourages descent of the head. Ambulation can reduce the duration of labor, need of analgesia.
  If, however, labor is monitored electronically or analgesic drug (epidural analgesia) is given, she should be in bed.
- ❖ **Diet:** There is delayed emptying of the stomach and low pH of the gastric contents in labor.
  So food is withheld during active labor **(to prevent Mendelson's syndrome)**. Fluids in the form of plain water or fruit juice may be given in early labor.
  Intravenous fluid with ringer solution is started where any intervention is anticipated or the patient is under regional anesthesia.
- ❖ **Bladder care:** Patient is encouraged to pass urine by herself (bed pan can be given) as full bladder often inhibits uterine contraction and may lead to infection.
  If the patient fails to pass urine especially in late first stage, catheterization is to be done with strict aseptic precautions.
- ❖ **Relief of pain:** Different options include—pethidine injections IM, Entonox inhalation (a mix of nitrous oxide 50% and oxygen 50%) and **epidural analgesia (considered the best and safe and should be offered if facilities are available)**.
- ❖ Assessment of progress of labor and **partograph** recording:
  - ▷ **Pulse** is recorded every 30 minutes.
  - ▷ **Blood pressure** is recorded at every four hours.
  - ▷ **Temperature** is recorded every two hours.
  - ▷ **Urine output** is recorded for volume, protein or acetone. Any drug (oxytocin or other) when given is recorded in the partograph.
  - ▷ **Abdominal palpation:**
    - ♦ *Uterine contractions:* As regard the frequency, intensity, and duration are assessed. *The number of contractions in 10 minutes and duration of each contraction in seconds are recorded in the partograph.* Partograph is charted every half an hour.
    - ♦ *Pelvic grip:* Gradual disappearance of poles of the head which were felt previously, usually occurs in labor. Abdominal palpation for descent of the fetal head in terms of fifths felt above the brim is to be used.
    - ♦ Shifting of the maximal intensity of the fetal heart beat downward and medially.
  - ▷ **To note the fetal well-being:**
    - ♦ Fetal heart rate (FHR) noted every half an hour in the first stage and every 15 minutes in second stage or following rupture of the membranes. *To be of value, the observation should be made immediately following uterine contraction. The count should be made for 60 seconds.*

- Ordinary stethoscope is quite suitable. Doppler, however, is helpful in the case of obesity and polyhydramnios.
- Normal fetal heart rate ranges from 110–160 per minute.

❖ **Continuous electronic fetal monitoring/CTG:** Recording of fetal heart rate and uterine contraction. It is commonly used for high-risk pregnancies.
❖ **Vaginal examination:** (To get information as mentioned above).

To Watch for Maternal and Fetal Distress

Evidence of Fetal Distress

❖ **Loss of beat-to-beat variability**
❖ **Decelerations**
❖ **Tachycardia**
❖ **Bradycardia.**

Evidence of Maternal Distress

❖ Tachycardia (>100 beats/minute)
❖ Anxious look with sunken eyes
❖ Dehydration, dry tongue, acetone smell in breath
❖ Hot, dry vagina often with offensive discharge
❖ Scanty high colored urine with presence of acetone.

Q. Types of Pelves.

Q. Caldwell-Moloy Classification.

CALDWELL-MOLOY CLASSIFICATION OF PELVIC TYPES (1933)

Four types of female pelves were described. Actually, the majority of pelves are of mixed types:
1. **Gynecoid pelvis (50%):**
   - It is the normal female type
   - Shape: Round. Inlet is slightly transverse oval
   - Sacrum is wide with average concavity and inclination
   - Side walls are straight or slightly divergent, with blunt ischial spines
   - Sacro-sciatic notch is wide
   - Bituberous diameter: Normal
   - Subpubic angle is 85–100 degrees
   - No difficulty in vaginal delivery.
2. **Anthropoid pelvis (25%):**
   - It is ape-like type.
   - Shape: Anteroposteriorly oval. All anteroposterior diameters are long
   - Side walls: Straight or divergent, with blunt (non prominent) ischial spines
   - All transverse diameters are short
   - Sacrum is long and narrow
   - Sacrosciatic notch is wide

- Bituberous diameter: Normal or short
- Subpubic angle is narrow
- More incidence of face to pubis delivery (vertex-occipito-posterior).
3. **Android pelvis (20%):**
   - It is a male type
   - Inlet is triangular or heart-shaped with anterior narrow apex
   - Side walls are converging (funnel pelvis) with projecting ischial spines
   - Sacro-sciatic notch is narrow and deep
   - Bituberous diameter: Short
   - Subpubic angle is narrow <90°
   - More chances of DTA, difficult delivery, perineal injuries.
4. **Platypelloid pelvis (5%):**
   - It is a flat female type
   - Shape: Transversely oval
   - All anteroposterior diameters are short
   - All transverse diameters are long
   - Side walls: Divergent, with blunt (non-prominent) ischial spines
   - Sacro-sciatic notch is narrow and small
   - Bituberous diameter: wide
   - Subpubic angle is very wide.

CHAPTER 14

Malpresentations and Malposition

Q. Etiology of breech and types of breech.

■ INTRODUCTION

Breech is the **most common malpresentation.** The lie is longitudinal and the podalic pole presents at the pelvic brim.

■ ETIOLOGY

Fetal

- **Prematurity (most common cause)**
- Multiple pregnancy
- Hydrocephalus (big head can fit well in the fundus)
- Polyhydramnios/oligohydramnios
- Trisomies, anencephaly and myotonic dystrophy.

Maternal

- Congenital malformation of the uterus
- Multiparity
- Chronic pelvic disease (CPD)
- Uterine fibroid/pelvic tumors
- Past history.

Placental

- Placenta previa
- Cornu-fundal attachment of placenta
- Short cord.

Prevalence of Breech Presentation by Gestational Age

Gestational age (weeks)	Breech (%)
28	24
30	17
32	11
34	6
36	5
37–40	4

■ TYPES OF BREECH

Complete

Thighs are flexed at the hips and legs are flexed at the knees (full-flexed attitude). So the presenting part comprises the buttocks, external genitalia and two feet. It is usually or more commonly seen in multipara.

Incomplete

- **Frank breech:** Thighs are flexed at the hips and legs are extended at the knees. The presenting part consists of external genitalia and buttocks. It is **commonly seen in primigravidas** (70%) due to tight abdominal wall, good uterine tone and early engagement.
- **Footling presentation:** Both the thighs and the legs are partially extended bringing the legs at the pelvic brim.
- **Knee presentation:** Thighs are extended but the knees are flexed, bringing the knees to the pelvic brim.

Q. Complications in breech presentation.

■ INTRODUCTION

Breech is the most common malpresentation. The lie is longitudinal and the podalic pole presents at the pelvic brim.

■ COMPLICATIONS

Maternal

- Increased frequency of LSCS and operative vaginal delivery.
- Genital tract trauma.
- Anesthesia complications.

Fetal

The corrected **perinatal mortality** (excluding congenital abnormalities) is **5–35/1000 births**. The fetal mortality is **least in frank breech and maximum in footling presentation** due to higher occurrence of cord prolapse.

- ❖ Intrapartum fetal death
- ❖ **Intracranial hemorrhage:** Compression followed by decompression of unmolded head leads to tear of tentorium cerebelli. This is more in preterm babies.
- ❖ **Birth asphyxia is** due to:
  - ▷ Cord compression after buttocks is delivered and when the head enters the pelvis.
  - ▷ Retraction of the placental site
  - ▷ Premature attempt at respiration when the head is still inside
  - ▷ Delayed delivery of the head
  - ▷ **Cord prolapse**.
- ❖ **Birth injuries are** usually inflicted during manipulative deliveries:
  - ▷ Hematoma: Sternomastoid/thighs
  - ▷ **Fractures:** Femur/humerus/clavicle/odontoid process. There may be dislocation of the hip joint, mandible, C5 and C6 vertebrae.
  - ▷ **Visceral injuries:** Rupture of liver, kidneys, adrenals, lungs and testicular hemorrhage.
  - ▷ Nerve: Medullary coning, spinal cord injury, **brachial plexus** stretching leading to Erb's/Klumpkes paralysis
  - ▷ Long term neurological damage.

Q. External cephalic version (ECV).

Q. Mention complications of ECV and what are the indications of LSCS for breech presentation?

INTRODUCTION

External cephalic version (ECV) is a procedure used to turn a fetus from a breech position or transverse position into a **vertex position before labor begins**. It is done to bring the favorable cephalic pole in the lower pole of the uterus to **avoid complications of vaginal breech delivery and also to avoid lower segment cesarean section (LSCS)**.

The **ACOG recommends** that efforts should be made to reduce breech presentation by ECV whenever possible.

The success rate for external cephalic version ranges from **35–85%, with an average of about 60%**.

When to perform:
ECV should be performed at **36/37 weeks of gestation** for the following reasons:
- ❖ In case the version results in fetal distress and need for immediate LSCS, iatrogenic prematurity is avoided.
- ❖ The likelihood of spontaneous version is low.
- ❖ Although earlier attempts at version are more likely to be successful, they also are more likely to be associated with spontaneous reversion to breech.

PROCEDURE

- ❖ It should be attempted at 36/37 weeks in labor-delivery complex.
- ❖ Tocolytic drug should be given.
- ❖ USG should be done to confirm the diagnosis and amniotic fluid index (AFI).
- ❖ A **reactive nonstress test (NST) pre-procedure** should be ensured.

- After emptying her bladder, the patient should be made to lie supine with her shoulders slightly raised and thighs slightly flexed.
- **Forward roll movement:** The breech is mobilized with both hands to one iliac fossa toward which the fetal back lies. The podalic pole is grasped by the right hand like that of Pawliks grip and the left hand grasps the head. A firm intermittent unforceful pressure is exerted to the head and breech in opposite directions to keep the trunk well-flexed which facilitates the version and pushes the head toward the pelvis and breech toward the fundus till the lie becomes transverse. **The fetal heart surveillance (FHS) should be checked**. The hand should be changed one after the other so as to hold the fetal poles without crossing over of hands. The intermittent pressure is exerted till the head is brought to the lower pole of the uterus.
- **Postprocedure, a reactive NST should be obtained**. There may be transient bradycardia due to head compression which should settle within 10 minutes. If it persists, possibility of cord entanglement should be considered and reversion should be done.
- The patient should be observed for 30 minutes for FHS monitoring and to assess for vaginal bleeding in case prelabor rupture of membranes (PROM) has occurred.
- Rh negative nonimmunized women should be given anti-D gamma globulin.

■ CONTRAINDICATIONS OF ECV

- Multiple pregnancy.
- Previous LSCS (risk of scar rupture).
- Severe pre-eclampsia (risk of abruption).
- Oligo/polyhydramnios.
- Placenta previa/contracted pelvis **(version should not be attempted if there is a contraindication to vaginal delivery as in such cases delivery will be by LSCS).**
- Bad obstetric history (BOH)/precious pregnancy (LSCS safer in such cases)
- Intrauterine growth restriction (IUGR), intrauterine fetal death (IUFD), large fetus, major congenital anomalies.
- PROM
- Active labor.

■ COMPLICATIONS OF ECV

- Fetal distress
- IUFD
- Preterm labor, PROM
- Abruption
- Cord entanglement, true knot
- Amniotic fluid embolism
- Fetomaternal hemorrhage
- Rupture uterus.

■ FACTORS WHICH INCREASE THE SUCCESS OF ECV

- Complete breech
- Nonengaged breech

- ❖ Sacroanterior position
- ❖ Adequate liquor
- ❖ Nonobese patient.

CAUSES OF FAILED ECV

- ❖ Frank breech: Early engagement and difficulty in flexion due to splinting action of the fetal limbs
- ❖ Scanty liquor or big baby
- ❖ Mechanical: Obesity, irritable uterus, increased tone of abdominal muscles
- ❖ Short cord
- ❖ Uterine malformations: Septate/bicornuate.

INDICATIONS FOR CESAREAN SECTION IN BREECH PRESENTATION

Because of complications of vaginal breech delivery, LSCS in breech presentation is done mainly for a good fetal outcome.

Compared with vaginal birth, **planned cesarean section reduces perinatal or neonatal death** or serious neonatal morbidity. Hence, in following cases LSCS is done:

- ❖ Primi with breech: In modern day obstetrics primigravida with breech presentation should be delivered by LSCS.
- ❖ **Footling breech (very high risk of cord prolapse)**.
- ❖ **Twins with first baby in breech** (risk of interlocking of twins and risk of cord prolapse).
- ❖ Previous LSCS with breech (risk of scar rupture).
- ❖ **Preterm breech** (risk of intraventricular hemorrhage increases with vaginal delivery).
- ❖ **Stargazing/flying fetus:** In about 5% of term breech presentations, the fetal head may be in extreme hyperextension. This presentation is referred to as the flying fetus or stargazer fetus. With such hyperextension, vaginal delivery may result in injury to the cervical spinal cord.
- ❖ Big baby (fetal weight >3.5 kg) or contracted pelvis.
- ❖ Precious pregnancy (like BOH, previous stillbirths, previous complications during vaginal breech delivery, IVF conception, etc.).

Q. Etiology of transverse lie.

DEFINITION

When the long axis of fetus lies perpendicular to the maternal spine or centralized uterine axis, it is called transverse lie. In transverse lie **shoulder is the presenting part**.

The dorsoanterior position is most common (60%).

- ❖ In dorsoposterior, the chance of fetal extension is common with increased risk of arm prolapse and cord prolapse.

ETIOLOGY

- ❖ Multiparity: Lax abdomen and imperfect uterine tone
- ❖ Prematurity

Chapter 14: Malpresentations and Malposition

- Multiple pregnancies: More common for the second baby
- Polyhydramnios
- Uterine anomalies
- Placenta previa
- Pelvic tumors (fibroids/ovarian cysts)
- CPD/contracted pelvis.

There is no mechanism of labor in transverse lie. Delivery is by LSCS.

Vaginal delivery with **conduplicato corpore** is possible. If the fetus is nonviable (extremely preterm) and very small (usually < 800 g) and the pelvis is large, spontaneous delivery is possible in transverse lie. The fetus is compressed with the head forced against the abdomen. A portion of the thoracic wall below the shoulder becomes the most dependent part, appearing at the vulva. The head and thorax then pass through the pelvic cavity at the same time, and the fetus, which is doubled upon it, is expelled—this is referred to as conduplicato corpore.

Q. Clinical diagnosis and mechanism of labor in occipitoposterior (OP) position.

Q. Management of OP position.

Q. Various outcomes in OP position.

■ DEFINITION

In a vertex presentation when the occiput is placed directly over the sacrum or sacroiliac joint, it is called an **occipitoposterior (OP) position**.

■ INCIDENCE

- 10% of all vertex positions
- **Right OP position is 5 times more common** than left OP (LOP) since dextrorotation of the uterus and presence of the sigmoid colon on the left disfavor LOP.

■ CAUSES

- Pelvic inlet: Usually associated with anthropoid or android pelvis.
- Fetal head deflexion due to:
  - High pelvic inclination
  - Anterior placentation
  - Primary brachycephaly
- Abnormal uterine contraction.

■ DIAGNOSIS

Abdominal Examination

Umbilical Grip

- Fetal limbs are felt more easily on either side of the midline
- Fetal back is felt in the flank away from the midline
- Anterior shoulder away from the midline.

Pelvic Grip
- Head is not engaged
- The cephalic prominence (sinciput) is not as prominent as it is in OA.

Auscultation
Maximum intensity of **FHS is on the flank** and often difficult to locate in LOP position. **In direct OP position, the FHS is noted directly in the midline.**

Per Vaginum (P/V)
- Elongated bag of membranes
- Sagittal suture occupies any oblique diameters of the pelvis
- Posterior fontanelle is felt near the sacroiliac joint
- **Anterior fontanelle is felt more easily** and at a lower level than the posterior one.
- In late labor, caput obliterates the sutures and fontanelles. For diagnosis, **the unfolded pinna points towards the occiput.**

MECHANISM OF LABOR

The mechanism of labor has been described in **Flowchart 14.1**.

COURSE OF LABOR

Both first and second stages of labor are longer.

First stage

Increased duration due to:
- **Delayed engagement** due to persistent deflexion of the head thereby increasing the diameter of engagement (occipitofrontal = 11.5 cm). The driving force transmitted through the fetal axis is not in alignment with the axis of the inlet.
- Membrane status: Deflexed head becomes ovoid and this cannot fit well in the spherical lower segment → loss of ball valve action during uterine contraction → early rupture of membranes and drainage of liquor.
- Uterine contractions may be abnormal with slow cervical dilatation due to ill-fitting of the deflexed head to the lower uterine segment. The occiput presses on the rectum causing premature desire to bear down in the first stage.

Second Stage

It is often delayed due to **long internal rotation or malrotation, with arrest** of the head at times.

Third Stage

Increased incidence of PPH and trauma to the genital tract.

Chapter 14: Malpresentations and Malposition

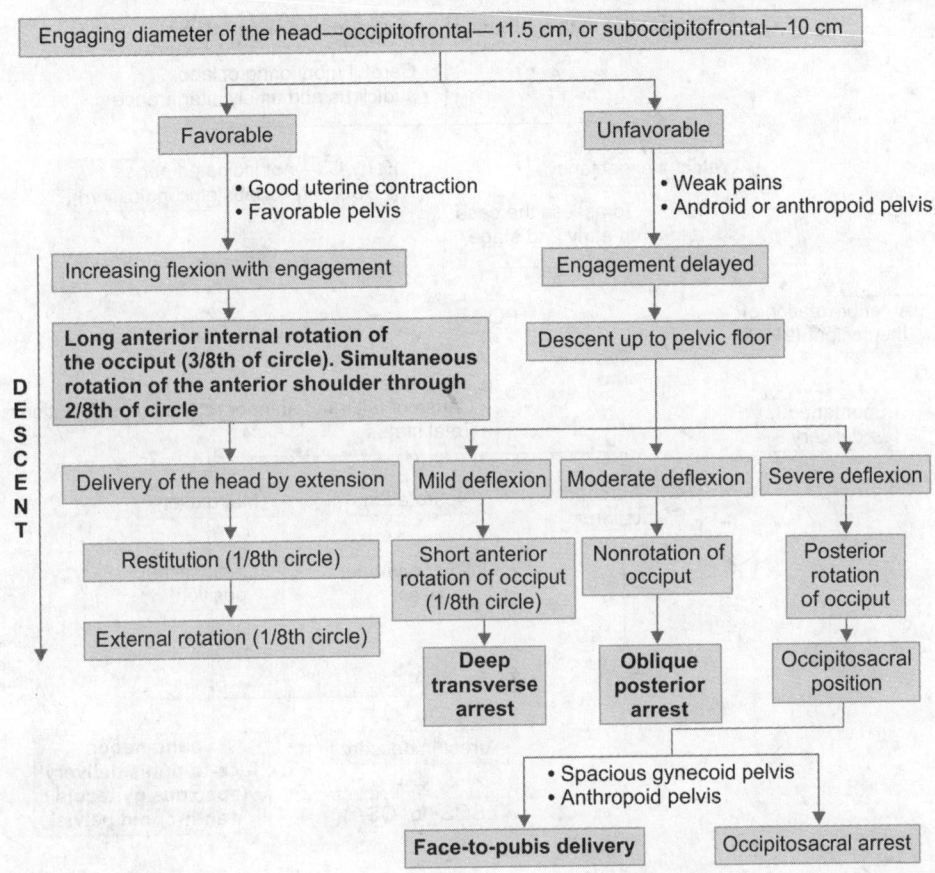

Flowchart 14.1: Scheme of mechanism of labor in occipitoposterior position.

■ MODE OF DELIVERY

- ❖ Long anterior rotation of occiput (OP becomes OA): Spontaneous or assisted vaginal delivery happens (90%).
- ❖ Short posterior rotation: Spontaneous or assisted vaginal delivery may happen as **face to pubis** leading to increased risk of perineal injuries or there may be occipitosacral arrest (OSA).

  Reason for perineal injury: BPD (9.5 cm) stretches the perineum and occipitofrontal diameter (11.5 cm) emerges out of the introitus.
- ❖ Nonrotation or short anterior rotation: Spontaneous vaginal delivery is very rare. LSCS is done, else it may lead to prolonged/obstructed labor.

■ MANAGEMENT OF LABOR (FLOWCHART 14.2)

The principles are:
- ❖ Early diagnosis
- ❖ Strict vigilance and watchful expectancy
- ❖ Judicious and timely interference.

Flowchart 14.2: Scheme of management of occipitoposterior position.

```
Scheme of management of occipitoposterior position
            • Careful monitoring of labor
            • Judicious and timely interference
     ┌──────────────┴──────────────┐
Watchful expectancy          Early CS—not indicated per se
To assess the case           (LSCS only for obstetric indication)
in early 2nd stage
     ┌────────────┴────────────┐
Anterior rotation of         POP
the occiput (90%)            Assess
     │                       • The pelvis
Spontaneous                  • Cause of failure of anterior rotation or malrotation
delivery                     • Fetal status
         ┌───────────────┬───────────────┐
   Partial anterior   Nonrotation     Malrotation
      rotation           │                │
        │          Oblique posterior  Occipitosacral
       DTA            arrest            position
        │                │                │
      LSCS             LSCS         Spontaneous
                        │           face-to-pubis delivery
                 Arrest in descent  (spacious gynecoid
                        │           or anthropoid pelvis)
                 LSCS (for OSA)
```

OP position is per say not an indication for LSCS.
- Labor is allowed to proceed like normal labor.
- IV line, RL infusion started.
- Blood to be cross-matched and kept ready (LSCS may be needed and more risk of PPH).

Indications for LSCS in cases of OP position:
- DTA.
- Oblique posterior arrest.
- Occipitosacral arrest (OSA).

Q. Deep transverse arrest (DTA).

■ DEFINITION

The head is **deep into the cavity**, sagittal suture is in the **transverse bispinous diameter, at station "0"** and there is no progress in descent of the head even after ½–1 hour of full cervical dilatation.

So, it can be defined as a failure of both rotation and descent of the head from a transverse position at or just above the level of the spines, provided that the cervix is fully dilated and the uterine contractions are adequate.

Chapter 14: Malpresentations and Malposition

This arrest may be due to nonrotation of primary occipitotransverse position or incomplete anterior rotation (1/8th of a circle) of oblique OP position.

■ CAUSES

- Pelvic architecture: Prominent ischial spines, android pelvis, convergent walls
- Deflexed head
- Weak uterine contractions.

■ DIAGNOSIS

- The head is engaged
- Sagittal suture is in the transverse bispinous diameter
- PV examination: most of the times, station is at "0" or just above 0
- Anterior fontanelle is palpable.

■ MANAGEMENT

- If vaginal delivery is unsafe due to big baby or inadequate pelvis → LSCS.
- If vaginal delivery is safe and the obstetrician is skilled, operative vaginal delivery can be attempted. Methods are:
  - Ventouse.
  - Manual rotation and forceps application.
  - Forceps rotation and delivery with Kiellands forceps.

  However in modern day obstetrics, manual rotation and Kielland forceps are not done and LSCS is always to be done and preferred.

■ COMPLICATIONS

- Prolonged labor.
- Obstructed labor with higher incidence of rupture uterus.
- Increased incidence of:
  - Operative delivery
  - Trauma to the genital tract
  - PPH and puerperal infection
  - Perinatal morbidity and mortality.

CHAPTER 15

Abortions/Miscarriages

Q. Define spontaneous abortion. Discuss the etiologies of abortion in first and second trimester.

DEFINITIONS

Abortion is defined as expulsion/extraction, from its mother, of an embryo or fetus weighing **500 g or less** when it is not capable of independent survival.

Abortion occurring without **medical or mechanical means** to empty the uterus is referred to as spontaneous. **Spontaneous miscarriage** is typically defined as a clinically recognized (i.e., by blood test, urine test, or ultrasonography) pregnancy loss before 20 weeks of gestation.

Approximately **5–15%** of diagnosed pregnancies result in spontaneous miscarriage.

About 75% of abortions happen before 16 weeks and out of these around 75% happen before 8 weeks of gestation.

ETIOLOGY

The causes of spontaneous abortions in first trimester are different from those in the second trimester (**Flowchart 15.1**).

Common Causes of Abortion

First Trimester

- **Genetic factors (50%):**
  - More than 80% of abortions occur in the first 12 weeks of pregnancy, and at least half result from chromosomal anomalies. After the first trimester, both the abortion rate and the incidence of chromosomal anomalies decrease. **Advanced maternal age** is contributory factor.
  - **Trisomy 16 is the most common abnormal karyotype found in the abortus**
  - **Monosomy X (45,X), the second most frequent** chromosomal abnormality (after trisomy), usually results in abortion and much less frequently in live born female infants (Turner syndrome)
  - Advanced maternal and paternal ages do not increase the incidence of triploidy

Flowchart 15.1: Main causes of abortion in first and second trimester.

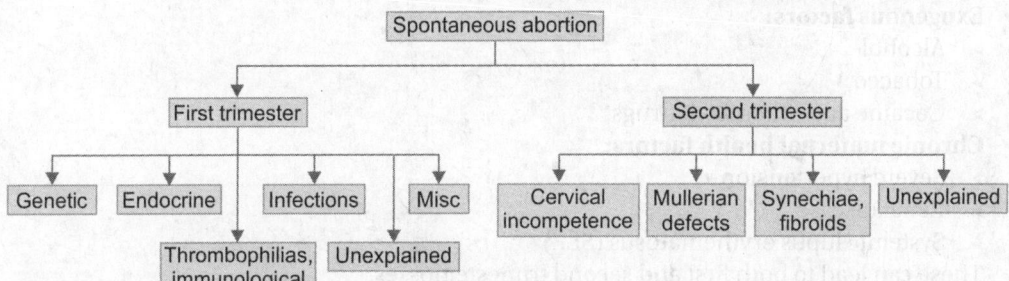

- Euploid abortion: Euploid fetuses tend to abort later in gestation than aneuploid ones. Three-fourths of aneuploid abortions occur before 8 weeks; euploid abortions peak at about 13 weeks. The incidence of euploid abortions increases dramatically after maternal age exceeds 35 years.
- **Endocrine disorders (10–15%):**
  - **Luteal phase defect**/progesterone deficiency would always result in early first trimester abortions **(mainly before 8 weeks)**. After around 10 weeks the placenta completely secretes progesterone
  - **Thyroid disorders** both hypo and hyperthyroidism can lead to recurrent first trimester abortion
  - **Overt diabetes mellitus** would also lead to congenital anomalies and recurrent first trimester abortions.
- **Thrombophilias and immunological disorders (autoimmune and alloimmune)—10%:**
  - **Autoimmune factors:** Antinuclear antibodies (ANA) and anti-DNA antibodies and antiphospholipid antibodies
  - Antiphospholipid antibodies are a family of autoantibodies that bind to negatively charged phospholipids, phospholipid-binding proteins, or a combination of the two. Two of these are **lupus anticoagulant and anticardiolipin antibody,** and have been implicated in spontaneous abortion
  - The mechanism of pregnancy loss in women with these antibodies involves **placental thrombosis and infarction**
  - In one postulated mechanism, antibodies may inhibit the release of prostacyclin, a potent vasodilator and inhibitor of platelet aggregation. In contrast, platelets produce thromboxane A2, a vasoconstrictor and platelet aggregator. They have also been shown to inhibit protein C activation, resulting in coagulation and fibrin formation
  - **Alloimmune disease:** Normally there are blocking antibodies which prevent the maternal immune cells from recognizing the fetus as foreign and prevent abortion
  - Lack of production of these antibodies can lead to abortion
  - **Inherited thrombophilias (protein C and S deficiency, factor V Leiden mutation, and hyperhomocysteinemia)** can lead to early and late miscarriages due to intravascular coagulation.
- **Infection:** For example, rubella, cytomegalovirus, mycoplasmal, ureaplasmal, listerial, and toxoplasmal infections.
- **Unexplained:** In many cases exact cause is not found. However, it is certain that risk of abortion increases with increased maternal age
- **Trauma/severe emotional shock.**
- **Septate uterus or "T" shaped uterus**

Other factors that may contribute to miscarriage:
- **Exogenous factors:**
  - Alcohol
  - Tobacco
  - Cocaine and other illicit drugs.
- **Chronic maternal health factors:**
  - Severe hypertension
  - Renal disease
  - Systemic lupus erythematosus (SLE)

  These can lead to both first and second trimester losses.

Second Trimester

- **Anatomic abnormalities:**
  - **Cervical incompetence** (congenital or acquired) (details in the next answer)
  - **Müllerian fusion defects** (bicornuate uterus and unicornuate)
  - **Uterine synechiae:** Asherman syndrome, characterized by uterine synechiae, usually results from destruction of large areas of endometrium by overzealous curettage. The risk is maximum if curettage is done in the postpartum period.

    If pregnancy follows, the amount of remaining endometrium may be insufficient to support the pregnancy, and abortion may ensue. A hysterosalpingogram that shows characteristic multiple filling defects may indicate Asherman syndrome, but hysteroscopy most accurately and directly identifies this condition.
- Uterine fibroid.
- **Maternal medical illness:** Chronic maternal health factors—severe hypertension, renal disease, and systemic lupus erythematosus (SLE) can lead to both first and second trimester losses.
- Unexplained.

Q. What are the causes and management of cervical incompetence?

Q. Cervical encerclage.

Q. OS tightening.

DEFINITION

Mechanical or functional defect in the cervix which leads to inability of cervix to hold pregnancy is known as **cervical incompetence**.

ETIOLOGY

- Although the cause of cervical incompetence is obscure, previous **trauma** to the cervix—especially in the course of dilatation and curettage, **conization**, cauterization, or **amputation**—appears to be a factor in some cases
- In other instances, abnormal cervical development, including that following exposure to diethylstilbestrol in utero, may play a role
- It is also **associated with uterine anomalies** like bicornuate and unicornuate uterus
- Multiple pregnancy, past history.

CLINICAL FEATURES

Symptoms

Classically, it is characterized by **painless** cervical dilatation in the **second trimester**, with prolapse and ballooning of membranes into the vagina, preterm premature rupture of membranes **(PPROM)**, followed by expulsion of an immature fetus. Unless effectively treated, this sequence may **repeat in future pregnancies**.

Examination

Internal examination in interconceptional may reveal cervical tear (unilateral or bilateral) and gaping of cervix.

INVESTIGATIONS

The diagnosis is generally made on the **classical history. In the interconceptional period:**
- Passage of no. 6–8 Hegar's dilator without pain and absence of snap on withdrawal
- Premenstrual hysterocervicography shows a **funnel-shaped shadow** (the cervix is supposed to be closed due to progesterone).

During pregnancy:
- **Cervical length (TVS preferred) less than 2.5 cm** is considered as short cervix
- Funneling—ballooning of the membranes into a dilated internal os >1 cm but with a closed external OS may also be seen
- Closed cervix (competent os) on USG appears like the **letter T**. Incompetent os on USG shows the following features: Before opening, the cervix shortens and then funneling can take place, which on USG looks like **the letter Y** (indicating incompetent os) that can progress to look like the **letter V** (cervix is just about to open). When the os is open the membranes can herniate, giving the appearance of **letter U**.
- Per speculum (PS): Dilatation of cervix and herniation of membranes may be seen.

TREATMENT

- The treatment of classical cervical incompetence is **cerclage (os tightening)**.
- The operation is performed to surgically reinforce the weak cervix by some type of purse-string suturing.
- Cerclage procedure: Two types of vaginal operations are commonly used during pregnancy. One is **McDonald (Figs. 15.1A and B)** and the other is **Shirodkar**. Success rates of these operations are **80–90%.**

Timing of Operation

- Emergency cerclage is done when there is **cervical dilatation** and bulging membranes or detection of **short cervix (<2.5 cm) on USG**
- Prophylactic cerclage is done 2 weeks prior to the previous second trimester abortion.

Anesthesia

Regional (spinal or caudal block) or short general anesthesia (TIVA).

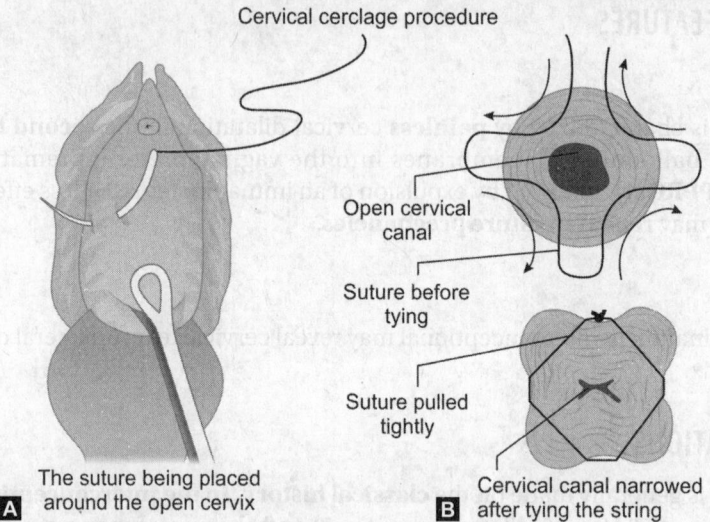

Figs. 15.1A and B: McDonald cerclage operation.

McDonald's Cerclage

- The McDonald's cerclage is performed using a permanent suture
- The bladder emptied and the cervix is exposed
- A purse-string suture of **nonabsorbable material** like Mersilene or Mersilk on a Mayo needle is inserted around the exocervix as high as possible to approximate to the level of the internal os. This is at the junction of the rugose vagina and smooth cervix
- Five or six bites with the needle are made
- The stitch is pulled tight enough to close the internal os, the knot being made in **front of the cervix**.

Shirodkar's Cerclage

- The cervix is pulled down, a transverse incision is made above the cervix and the bladder is pushed well up above the internal os
- A vertical incision is made posteriorly on cervicovaginal junction
- The **nonabsorbable suture** material (Mersilene) is passed **submucously** through the right and left corner of the anterior incision with an aneurysm needle so as to bring it out of the posterior incision
- The ends of the tape tied **posteriorly**
- The anterior and posterior incisions are closed with chromic catgut no. 0.

Postoperative Care

- **Bedrest** for 2–3 days
- **Uterine relaxants** (tocolytics like isoxsuprine, ritodrine, etc.) to be given (injectables followed by oral) for few days.

Advise on Discharge

- Avoid intercourse

Chapter 15: Abortions/Miscarriages

- Routine antenatal care
- To report if bleeding, leaking PV or pain in abdomen.

Contraindications

- Vaginal bleeding
- Uterine contractions
- Ruptured membranes
- Intrauterine infections
- Intrauterine fetal death/severe congenital anomalies
- Dilation >4 cm.

Removal of Stitch

The knot is usually cut at **37 weeks** or any time **before, if the patient goes in labor**. If the knot is not cut, then during labor there can be cervical tears or rupture uterus.

Complications

While cerclage is generally a safe procedure, there are a number of potential complications that may arise during or after surgery. These include the two types of complications as described here.

Immediate

- Risks associated with regional or general anesthesia
- Premature labor
- Premature rupture of membranes
- Chorioamnionitis
- Injury to the cervix or bladder
- Bleeding.

Delayed

- Cervical dystocia with failure to dilate requiring cesarean section
- Cervical tear/uterine rupture (may occur if the stitch is not removed before onset of labor).

Benson and Durfee Cerclage

- It is an **abdominal encerclage** operation reserved in cases when previously vaginal operations have failed (abortion has occurred in spite of vaginal cerclage).
- Similar surgery can be done **laparoscopically during the nonpregnant state**.

Q. Missed abortion.

DEFINITION

A **missed miscarriage** is when the embryo or fetus has died and is retained inside the uterus (so miscarriage/abortion process has not yet occurred). It is also referred to as delayed miscarriage, silent miscarriage, or **missed abortion**.

Carneous mole (blood mole, fleshy mole) is the pathological variant of missed abortion affecting the fetus before 12 weeks. Small repeated hemorrhage in the choriodecidual space disrupts the villi from its attachments. The clotted blood with the contained embryo is known as a blood mole. The embryo becomes dead and is either completely aborted or remains as a rudimentary structure. Gradually the fluid portion of the blood surrounding the embryo gets absorbed and the wall becomes fleshy, hence the term fleshy or carneous mole.

The whole mass can be expelled out as a decidual cast.

CLINICAL FEATURES

- Amenorrhea for a variable period of 2–3 months
- Bleeding PV: Slight bleeding, brownish vaginal discharge/spotting, absence of pain/discomfort
- Subsidence of pregnancy symptoms, uterus stops growing and retrogression of breast changes
- Fetal heart sounds cannot be heard even with Doppler ultrasound.

COMPLICATIONS

- DIC (rare): If retained inside for 4 or more weeks, risk of DIC in the patient, however the risk is less compared to IUFD
- Psychological upset
- Infection.

MANAGEMENT

Diagnosis

- Transvaginal ultrasound is the mainstay in the diagnosis
- USG features: Gestation sac diameter is ≥25 mm with no obvious yolk sac or a fetal pole with a crown rump length of ≥7 mm without evidence of fetal cardiac activity.

Treatment

Once the diagnosis is done, the patient can then be offered different types of management depending on their clinical status and patient's choice:

- **Expectant management (rarely done)** is possible, with a "wait and watch" approach. Women may expel the conceptus spontaneously.
- **Medical management:** Misoprostol (PGE1) is the drug of choice. 400 microgram orally/sublingual or 800 microgram vaginally is given. Expulsion occurs within 12–24 hours.
- **Surgical management:** Suction evacuation/dilatation and evacuation.

Indications of surgical management:
- Hemodynamically unstable patient (IV fluids and blood transfusions may be required)
- Persistent excessive bleeding
- Evidence of infected retained tissue
- Failure of expectant or medical management
- Recurrent miscarriage, to assess for cytogenetics of products of conception
- Patient choice.

Q. Inevitable abortion.

■ DEFINITION

Inevitable abortion is the clinical type of abortion where the changes have progressed to a state from where continuation of pregnancy is not possible. The abortion has not occurred but it is bound to happen and nothing can be done to avoid this.

It is usually preceded by threatened abortion. Essentially, a threatened miscarriage progresses to an inevitable miscarriage if cervical dilatation occurs. Once some tissue has passed through the cervical os, this will then be termed an **incomplete miscarriage**.

■ CLINICAL FEATURES

- **Amenorrhea:** There is history of amenorrhea, usually of 2–3 months. Other early pregnancy symptoms are also seen in most of the patients, like morning sickness, breast enlargement, and discomfort.
- **Bleeding per vagina:** The bleeding per vagina in the beginning is bright red and scanty in amount, later becomes heavy, with passage of clots.
- **Pain:** Pain is a characteristic feature of inevitable abortion. It is characterized by lower abdominal cramps/colicky pain (because of painful uterine contractions).
- **Size of the uterus:** In inevitable abortion, the uterus size corresponds to the duration of gestation as the products of conception are still in place in the uterine cavity.
- **Dilatation of cervix**: A **pathogenic sign of inevitable abortion**. Dilation of the internal os of the cervix indicates inevitable abortion. The products of conception may be felt through the dilated cervix. **In threatened abortion, the internal os is closed**.

■ DIFFERENTIAL DIAGNOSIS

- Cervical ectopic pregnancy is a rare but potentially catastrophic differential that should be excluded by means of a repeat ultrasound and serial beta-hCG.
- If cervical ectopic is not considered as a differential for a gestational sac in the endocervix, curettage of a presumed incomplete miscarriage may result in unexpected severe hemorrhage.

■ MANAGEMENT

The principles are:
1. To accelerate the process of expulsion.
2. To maintain strict asepsis.

General Measures

Excessive bleeding should be controlled by administering **methergine** 0.2 mg if the cervix is dilated and the size of the uterus is less than 12 weeks. The shock if present is corrected by IV fluid therapy and blood transfusion.

Active Treatment (to Evacuate the Uterus)

- **Before 12 weeks:** Dilatation and evacuation/suction evacuation

- Medical management with **misoprostol** (as in missed abortion) can also be tried in stable patients
- **After 12 weeks:** The uterine contraction is accelerated by oxytocin drip (10–20 units in 500 mL of normal saline) 40–60 drops per minute. If the fetus is expelled and the placenta is retained, it is removed by ovum forceps (check curettage).

Q. Threatened abortion.

DEFINITION

Threatened abortion is a clinical entity where the process of abortion has started but has not progressed to a state from which recovery is impossible.

Threatened abortion is the earliest stage of most spontaneous abortions. There is bleeding from the genital tract, but the cervix (internal os) is closed and there is no discharge of products of conception.

CLINICAL FEATURES

- Vaginal bleeding—the bleeding is usually slight, as faint brown discharge or red discharge. The bleeding can stop spontaneously.
- There is generally no pain although there may be a dull ache or discomfort due to congestion of the pelvic organs
- PS: Bleeding from the os may be seen
- PV: To be performed very gently and generally avoided if USG is available
- Uterus corresponds to period of amenorrhea
- **Cervix (internal os) is closed**, but, the **external os of a multigravida can normally admit a fingertip**.

INVESTIGATIONS

Routine investigations:
- Blood for hemoglobin estimation, ABO and rh grouping.
- Blood transfusion may be required urgently if abortion becomes incomplete and there is profuse bleeding/shock.

Special investigation:
- TVS should be performed.
  - A well-formed gestational sac (double decidual sign) with the live embryo indicating healthy fetus
  - Observation of fetal cardiac motion. With this there is 98% chance of continuation of pregnancy
  - Subchorionic bleeding (hematoma) may be seen
  - Irregular sac, smaller mean gestational sac diameter, and absent fetal pole or absent fetal cardiac movements are all ominous signs.
- Serum progesterone of 25 ng/mL or more generally indicates a viable pregnancy and rules out ectopic pregnancy.
- Serial beta-hCG level is useful to assess fetal wellbeing and rule out ectopic pregnancy.

MANAGEMENT

- **Bed rest/pelvic rest:** The patient should be in bed for few days until bleeding stops. Prolonged restriction of activity has got no value. Coitus to be avoided.
- Anti-D gamma globulin has to be given in Rh-negative nonimmunized women.
- Progesterone supplementation is to be given in patients of luteal phase defect. It also helps in decreasing the cramping pain.
- **Dydrogesterone (10 mg bd to qds) has additional immunomodulatory effect and is associated with approximately two-fold significant reduction in the miscarriage rate in threatened miscarriages.**
- There is no evidence that hCG is of any help in the treatment of threatened abortion, hence not recommended.
- The patient is advised to preserve the vulval pads and anything expelled out per vaginam, for inspection.

ADVICE ON DISCHARGE

- To report if bleeding and/or pain increases
- The patient should limit her activity for at least 2 weeks and avoid heavy work and coitus
- Ultrasound should be repeated after 1–2 weeks.

PROGNOSIS

- The prognosis is very unpredictable. In approximately 65–75% cases, pregnancies continue. In rest, it leads to inevitable or missed abortion.
- If the pregnancy continues, watch for intrauterine growth restriction (IUGR) and preterm labor.

CHAPTER 16

Ectopic Pregnancy

Q. Discuss etiology of ectopic pregnancy.

Q. Signs and symptoms and management of acute/ruptured ectopic pregnancy.

Q. Signs and symptoms and management of unruptured ectopic pregnancy.

■ DEFINITION

The term ectopic is derived from the Greek word **ektopos, meaning out of place**.

In ectopic pregnancy, the fertilized ovum is implanted (and develops) **outside the normal endometrial cavity**. The gestation grows and draws its blood supply from the site of abnormal implantation.

Most common site is the Fallopian tube. In tubal pregnancy, most common site is ampulla followed by isthmus.

■ INCIDENCE

It is around **1 in 150–300 deliveries**. It is increasing due to increase in pelvic inflammatory disease, tuboplasty surgeries and IVF.

■ ETIOLOGY

Pelvic Inflammatory Disease (PID)

- The most common cause of PID is an infection caused by *Chlamydia trachomatis*. Other organisms such as *Neisseria gonorrhoeae*, also increase the risk of ectopic pregnancy, and a history of salpingitis **increases the risk of ectopic pregnancy 4–10 fold**.
- Genital tuberculosis also increases the risk of ectopic pregnancy.
- Loss of cilia, narrowing of lumen and intra and peritubal adhesions contribute.

Contraception Failure

- All contraceptive methods lead to an overall lower risk of pregnancy and, therefore, to an **overall lower risk** of ectopic pregnancy. However, **contraceptive failure increases the risk of ectopic pregnancy**.

- Intrauterine copper device (IUCD): The modern copper intrauterine device (IUD) does not increase the risk of ectopic pregnancy. However, there is a **relative increase in tubal pregnancy** (7 times more) should pregnancy occur with IUCD in situ.
- Only progestasert has a rate of ectopic pregnancy higher than that for women not using any form of contraception (as it decreases tubal motility).
- **Sterilization: There is 15–50% chance of ectopic pregnancy if pregnancy occurs (sterilization failure). The risk is the highest with bipolar coagulation.**

Tubal Surgery
Previous tubal surgery can increase the risk of developing ectopic pregnancy. Surgeries carrying higher risk of subsequent ectopic pregnancy include salpingostomy, neosalpingostomy, fimbrioplasty, tubal reanastomosis, and lysis of peritubal or periovarian adhesions.

History of Previous Ectopic Pregnancy
After one ectopic pregnancy, a patient has a 7–13 fold increase in the likelihood of another ectopic pregnancy. A patient with a previous ectopic pregnancy has a **10–25% chance of a future tubal pregnancy**.

Assisted Reproductive Technology (ART)
- Ovulation induction with clomiphene citrate or gonadotropin therapy has been linked to a 4-fold increase in the risk of ectopic pregnancy.
- The risk of ectopic pregnancy and heterotopic pregnancy dramatically increases when a patient has used assisted reproductive techniques—such as in vitro fertilization (IVF) or gamete intrafallopian transfer (GIFT)—to conceive. **The risk of ectopic is 5–7%.**
- Studies have demonstrated that up to 1% of pregnancies achieved through IVF or GIFT can result in a heterotopic gestation, compared with an incidence of 1 in 30,000 pregnancies for spontaneous conceptions.

Pelvic Adhesions
Due to previous pelvic or abdominal surgery.

Increasing Age
The highest rate of ectopic pregnancy occurs in women aged 35–44 years. A 3–4 fold increase in the risk of developing an ectopic pregnancy exists compared with women aged 15–24 years.

Smoking
Cigarette smoking has been shown to be a risk factor for ectopic pregnancy development. Studies have demonstrated an elevated risk ranging from **1.6 to 3.5 times** that of nonsmokers.

■ TYPES OF PRESENTATION
- Acute (ruptured)

- Unruptured
- Subacute (chronic)

CLINICAL FEATURES

Acute (Ruptured) Ectopic Pregnancy

Symptoms

- Ampullary pregnancy generally ruptures at 8 weeks and isthmic at 6 weeks. Implantation within the tubal segment that penetrates the uterine wall results in an interstitial pregnancy which generally ruptures at 16 weeks.
- It is associated with tubal rupture or tubal abortion and massive intraperitoneal hemorrhage.
- Only 50% of patients with an ectopic pregnancy present with the **classic triad of abdominal pain, amenorrhea and vaginal bleeding**.
- **Abdominal pain:** It is the **most constant** feature (seen in almost 100% patients). It is acute, agonizing or colicky, in lower abdomen unilateral, bilateral or generalized. Shoulder tip pain (due to diaphragmatic irritation from hemoperitoneum) is seen in around 25% patients.
- **Amenorrhea:** There is generally short period (5-8 weeks) of amenorrhea (in around 75% patients) or it may even be absent.
- **Bleeding per vaginum:** May be spotting or slight continuous bleeding (in around 70%). This is due to shedding of endometrium (due to decreased progesterone as there is insufficient HCG). There may also be expulsion of endometrial cast. Very rarely, the bleeding maybe due to tubal abortion through uterine ostium in interstitial pregnancy.
- **Syncopal attack** and vomiting due to peritoneal irritation.

Signs

- Pallor present
- Tachycardia, feeble pulse
- Hypotension
- Cold clammy extremities
- Lower abdomen is **tense and tender, no mass felt** and shifting dullness is present.
- Abdominal rigidity and severe tenderness, as well as evidence of hypovolemic shock such as orthostatic blood pressure changes and tachycardia, should alert the clinician to a surgical emergency.

Per Vaginum (PV)

- Vaginal mucosa is blanched.
- Uterus: Slightly bulky or normal size and **floats as if in water.**
- Cervical motion tenderness.
- Unilateral or bilateral tenderness on fornix palpation—usually much worse on the affected side.
- **No mass felt through the fornix usually.**

The presence of uterine contents in the vagina, which can be caused by shedding of endometrial lining stimulated by an ectopic pregnancy, may lead to a misdiagnosis of an incomplete or complete abortion and, therefore, a delayed or missed diagnosis of ectopic pregnancy.

Unruptured Tubal Pregnancy

The physician should be **ectopic minded** and include ectopic pregnancy in differential diagnosis when a sexually active female has abnormal bleeding, more so in patients with risk factors.

Symptoms

- Presence of delayed periods/spotting with **features of early pregnancy.**
- Flank pain, mild, colicky or continuous.

Signs: Bimanual Examination

The palpation should be **gentle to avoid iatrogenic rupture.**
- Uterus is soft, normal or just bulky.
- A well circumscribed, **pulsatile, tender mass felt through one of the fornices, separate from the uterus**.

Subacute/Chronic/Old Ectopic Pregnancy

Symptoms

- Short period of amenorrhea, 6–8 weeks.
- *Lower abdominal pain:* Starts as acute and gradually becomes dull or colicky.
- *Vaginal bleeding:* Scanty, dark and continuous. There could be expulsion of endometrial cast.
- Bladder symptoms like dysuria, frequency or retention may be present.
- Rectal tenesmus if infected hematocele.

Signs

- Patient looks ill with varying degree of pallor.
- Tachycardia, even at rest.
- **Features of shock are absent.**
- Temperature: May be mildly elevated.

Abdominal Examination

- Tenderness and guarding in lower abdomen on the affected side.
- Irregular and tender mass may be felt in lower abdomen.
- **Cullen's sign:** Dark bluish discoloration around umbilicus, suggestive of intraperitoneal hemorrhage.

Bimanual Examination

- Vaginal mucosa-pale
- Uterus normal size or bulky and may be pushed to one side
- Cervical movement tenderness ++
- **Ill defined, tender, boggy mass** felt through the posterolateral fornix, which may push the uterus to opposite side.

■ DIFFERENTIAL DIAGNOSIS

Acute Ectopic Pregnancy

- ❖ Acute appendicitis
- ❖ Ruptured corpus luteum
- ❖ Ruptured chocolate cyst
- ❖ Ovarian torsion
- ❖ Perforated peptic ulcer.

Pregnancy test would be negative in all of the above.

Chronic Ectopic Pregnancy

- ❖ Incomplete abortion
- ❖ Appendicitis
- ❖ Salpingitis
- ❖ Ruptured corpus luteum
- ❖ Ruptured chocolate cyst
- ❖ Ovarian torsion.

■ MANAGEMENT

Acute Ectopic Pregnancy

Shock in early pregnancy should be thought to be due to ruptured ectopic unless proven otherwise.

Investigations

As it is an **emergency situation**, only hemoglobin and blood group and cross match should be done.

Treatment

- ❖ The principle is **resuscitation and laparotomy**
- ❖ Two wide bore IV lines
- ❖ IV fluids: RL (crystalloid) and colloids (haemaccel)
- ❖ Blood transfusion
- ❖ Exploratory laparotomy **(quick in, quick out)**
- ❖ **Linear salpingectomy** is the gold standard surgery. The tube is sent for histopathology
- ❖ The blood supply to the ovary is preserved, and oophorectomy is not to be done.

Chronic Ectopic Pregnancy

Investigations

- ❖ **Blood:**
  - ▷ CBC (hemoglobin and total WBC count).
  - ▷ Blood grouping and cross match.

- ❖ **Serial beta hCG monitoring:**
  - ▷ Beta hCG is positive. A single value is not important as it diagnoses pregnancy but not its location. However, a lower level than weeks of gestation would raise suspicion.
  - ▷ Beta hCG would not double after 48 hours.
  - ▷ As per the **Kadar's rule, there would be <66% increase** in beta hCG in cases of ectopic pregnancy.
- ❖ **USG:** TVS is the most important.
  - ▷ Uterus is empty. **Pseudo sac** maybe seen.
  - ▷ Echogenic fluid in pouch of Douglas.
  - ▷ Adnexal mass, separate from ovary.
  - ▷ On **color Doppler, ring of fire appearance** around the mass.
- ❖ **Laparoscopy:** If the patient is hemodynamically stable, laparoscopy is preferred as it is not only diagnostic but also therapeutic. The blood in the POD is aspirated and salpingectomy can be done.
- ❖ **Serum progesterone:** >25 ng/mL is suggestive of viable intrauterine pregnancy and <5 ng/mL suggest an ectopic or abnormal intrauterine pregnancy.
- ❖ **Culdocentesis:** Very rarely done today. In absence of TVS or laparoscopy, it can be done through 18 G lumbar puncture needle, posterior fornix is punctured.
  However, a **negative culdocentesis does not rule out an ectopic, neither a positive result is specific.**
- ❖ **Dilatation and curettage (D&C):** Very rarely needed. Chorionic villi float in normal saline is diagnostic of intrauterine pregnancy.

Treatment

If patient is unstable or if facilities for laparoscopy are not available:
- ❖ Exploratory laparotomy (quick in, quick out).
- ❖ Linear salpingectomy is the gold standard. The tube is sent for histopathology.
- ❖ The blood supply to the ovary is preserved, and oophorectomy is not to be done.
- ❖ If the patient is hemodynamically stable, **laparoscopy is preferred** as it is not only diagnostic but also therapeutic. The blood in the POD is aspirated and salpingectomy can be done.

Unruptured Ectopic Pregnancy

Investigations

- ❖ **Serial beta hCG monitoring:**
  - ▷ Beta hCG is positive. A single value is not important as it diagnoses pregnancy but not its location. However, a lower level than weeks of gestation would raise suspicion.
  - ▷ Beta hCG would not double after 48 hours.
  - ▷ As per the **Kadar's rule, there would be less than 66%** increase in beta hCG in cases of ectopic pregnancy.
- ❖ **TVS:**
  - ▷ USG (especially TVS) is probably the most important tool for diagnosing an extrauterine pregnancy, although, it is more frequently used to confirm an intrauterine pregnancy.
  - ▷ **Presumed ectopic pregnancy: An empty uterus on TVS in patients with a serum β-hCG levels greater than the discriminatory cut-off value** is an ectopic pregnancy until proven otherwise. The endometrium may be thick and/or there could be presence of a pseudo sac.

- **Definite ectopic pregnancy:** Presence of a **thick, brightly echogenic, ring-like** structure is located outside the uterus, with a gestational sac containing an obvious fetal pole, a yolk sac or both. The endometrium could be thick or shows pseudo sac.
- The presence of a tender adnexal mass on USG suggests an ectopic pregnancy.
- **Laparoscopy:** It can be both **diagnostic as well as therapeutic**.

Management

Medical

Medical management (methotrexate) is the treatment of choice for an ectopic pregnancy whenever the required criteria are fulfilled.

The following criteria should be fulfilled for medical management of ectopic pregnancy:
- Patient should be **hemodynamically stable (unruptured tubal ectopic pregnancy)**.
- Fetal cardiac activity absent. Presence of cardiac activity is a relative contraindication.
- β-hCG levels <5,000 μIU/mL (levels more than 5,000 μIU/mL is a relative contraindication).
- Gestational sac diameter **<4 cm**.
- Free fluid in POD less than 100 mL: According to ACOG, contraindications for methotrexate include: breastfeeding, alcoholism, immunodeficiency, liver or renal disease, blood dyscrasias, active pulmonary disease and peptic ulcer.

Candidates for methotrexate therapy must be hemodynamically stable. They are instructed that:
- Medical therapy fails in at least **5–10% of cases**.
- If tubal rupture occurs (5–10% chance), emergency surgery is necessary.
- If the woman is treated as an outpatient, rapid transportation must be reliably available.
- Signs and symptoms of tubal rupture such as vaginal bleeding, abdominal and pleuritic pain, weakness, dizziness, or syncope must be reported promptly.
- Until the ectopic pregnancy is resolved, sexual intercourse is prohibited, alcohol should be avoided, and folic acid supplements including prenatal vitamins should not be taken.

Methotrexate therapy for primary treatment of ectopic pregnancy.

Regimen	Follow-up
Single dose: Methotrexate, 50 mg/m^2	• Measure β-hCG at days 4 and 7 • If difference is ≥15%, repeat weekly until undetectable • If difference is <15%, repeat methotrexate dose and begin new day 1 If fetal cardiac activity present at day 7, repeat methotrexate dose, begin new day • Surgical treatment if β-hCG levels not decreasing or fetal cardiac activity persists after three doses of methotrexate
Variable dose: Methotrexate, 1 mg/kg IM, days 1, 3, 5, and 7 plus leucovorin, 0.1 mg/kg IM, days 2, 4, 6, and 8	Continue alternate day injection until β-hCG levels decreases to >15% in 48 hours, or four does methotrexate given. Then, weekly β-hCG until undetectable

Surgical

- Laparoscopy is preferred. If facilities are not available then laparotomy maybe done. **Salpingectomy is preferred**.
- Conservative surgeries: **Not routinely recommended because of high-risk of recurrence on the same side.**

Various conservative surgeries include:
- **Linear salpingostomy:** Linear incision on tube, remove the products, incision kept open.
- **Linear salpingotomy:** Like above, but the incision is closed.
- **Segmental resection.**
- **Fimbrial expression:** In cases of distal pregnancy.

Anti-D Injection

- In all Rh negative patients (and if Rh positive partner) injection **anti D** is to be given **50 µg (<12 weeks of gestation)** or **300 µg (>12 weeks of gestation)** in all cases of ectopic pregnancy (ruptured, chronic, unruptured).
- In future pregnancy, TVS should be done early as there is a risk of recurrence.

CHAPTER 17

Preeclampsia/Eclampsia

Q. Classify hypertensive disorders of pregnancy.

Diagnosis of hypertensive disorders complicating pregnancy.

■ GESTATIONAL HYPERTENSION

- ❖ BP ≥140/90 mm Hg for first time during pregnancy.
- ❖ No proteinuria.
- ❖ BP returns to normal within 12 weeks of postpartum.
- ❖ Final diagnosis made only postpartum.

■ PREECLAMPSIA

Minimum Criteria (Hypertension and Proteinuria or Signs of End-Organ Damage)

- ❖ BP ≥140/90 mm Hg after 20 weeks of gestation (twice on measurements taken **four or more hours apart**)
  If severe hypertension: Systolic blood pressure of 160 mm Hg or more or diastolic blood pressure of 110 mm Hg or more (then do not wait for 4 hours) can be confirmed within a short interval (minutes) to facilitate timely antihypertensive therapy

  AND
- ❖ **Proteinuria ≥300 mg per 24 hours** or ≥2 + dipstick.
  As per the **new definition:** In absence of proteinuria signs of end-organ damage, such as thrombocytopenia, impaired liver function, severe persistent right upper quadrant or epigastric pain, excluding all other alternative diagnoses, new-onset headache unresponsive to all forms of management, pulmonary edema, or renal insufficiency with abnormal lab values.

Increased Certainty of Preeclampsia

- ❖ BP ≥160/100 mm Hg.
- ❖ Proteinuria 2.0 g per 24 hours or ≥2 + dipstick.
- ❖ Serum creatinine >1.2 mg/dL unless known to be previously elevated.
- ❖ Platelets <100,000/mm^3.

- Microangiopathic hemolysis (increased LDH).
- Elevated SGOT or SGPT.
- Persistent headache or other cerebral or visual disturbances.
- Persistent epigastric pain.

Hypertension is diagnosed when the resting blood pressure is 140/90 mm Hg or greater; Korotkoff phase V is used to define diastolic pressure. In the past, it had been recommended that an incremental increase of 30 mm Hg systolic or 15 mm Hg diastolic pressure be used as diagnostic criteria, even when absolute values were below 140/90 mm Hg. These criteria are **no longer recommended** because evidence shows that these women are not likely to suffer increased adverse pregnancy outcomes.

Edema has also been abandoned as a diagnostic criterion because it occurs in too many normal pregnant women.

ECLAMPSIA

Seizures that cannot be attributed to other causes in a woman with preeclampsia.

SUPERIMPOSED PREECLAMPSIA (ON CHRONIC HYPERTENSION)

New-onset proteinuria ≥300 mg per 24 hours in hypertensive women but no proteinuria before 20 weeks of gestation.

OR

A sudden increase in proteinuria or blood pressure or platelet count <1,00,000/mm³ in women with hypertension and proteinuria before 20 weeks of gestation.

CHRONIC HYPERTENSION

BP ≥140/90 mm Hg before pregnancy or diagnosed before 20 weeks of gestation.

OR

Hypertension is first diagnosed after 20 weeks of gestation and **persistent after 12 weeks postpartum.**

Q. Risk factors and etiopathology of preeclampsia.

DEFINITION

Preeclampsia is a **pregnancy specific syndrome** of reduced organ perfusion secondary to vasospasm and endothelial activation characterized by BP more than or equal to 140/90 mm Hg after 20 weeks of gestation and proteinuria more than or equal to 300 mg per 24 hours or signs of end organ failure, after 20th week in a previously normotensive and nonproteinuric patient.

RISK FACTORS FOR PREECLAMPSIA

- Patient younger than 20 or older than 35 years of age.
- Young primigravida (exposed to chorionic villi for the first time).
- Vesicular mole, multiple pregnancies (exposed to a superabundance of chorionic villi).

Flowchart 17.1: Pathogenesis of preeclampsia.

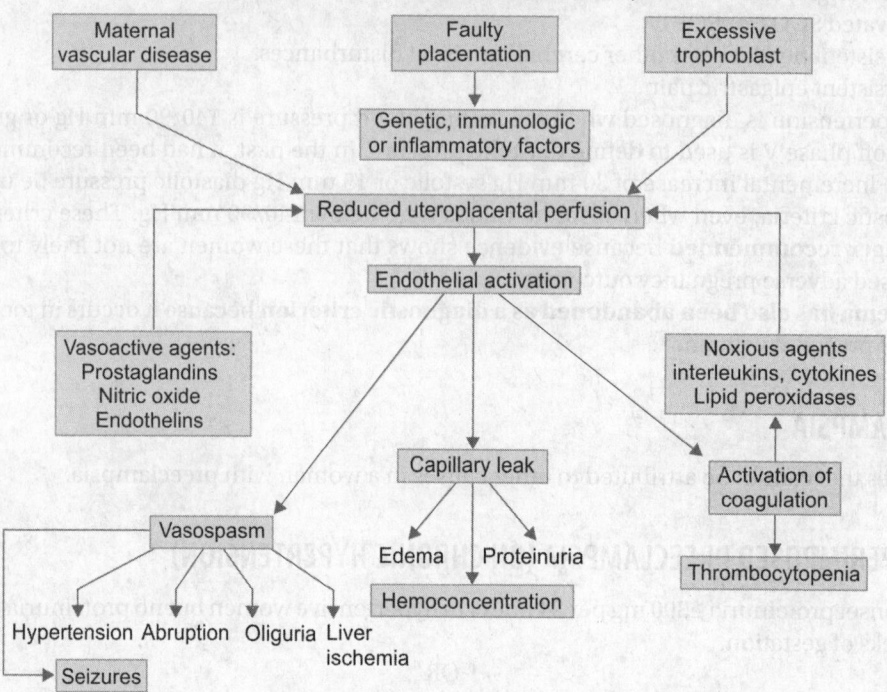

- Maternal obesity (pre-pregnancy body mass index greater than 30) insulin resistance, pre-existing DM, and pre-existing hypertension/renal/vascular disease.
- Past history: There is 25% chance of recurrence in subsequent pregnancy.
- Family history of preeclampsia.
- Gestational diabetes
- Systemic lupus erythematosus
- Thrombophilias (APLA syndrome, protein C, S deficiency, factor V Leiden).
- New paternity.
- Fetal hydrops.
- Assisted reproductive technology.
- Obstructive sleep apnea.
- Smoking is protective for preeclampsia.
- Placenta previa has also been reported to reduce the risk of hypertensive disorders in pregnancy.

According to Sibai, currently plausible potential causes include the following:
- Abnormal trophoblastic invasion of uterine vessels.
- Immunological intolerance between maternal and fetoplacental tissues (decrease in Th1 and increase in Th2 helper T-cells).
- Maternal maladaptation to cardiovascular or inflammatory changes of normal pregnancy [imbalance between vasoconstrictors and vasodilators, increase in TXA2, endothelin-1, and increase sensitivity to angiotensin II, whereas prostacyclin and nitric oxide (NO) decreases].
- Dietary deficiencies.
- Genetic influences (HLA-Dr4).

Abnormal trophoblastic invasion: In normal implantation, the **uterine spiral arteries** undergo extensive remodeling as they are invaded by endovascular trophoblasts (so high resistance, low flow system gets converted to a low resistance and high flow system). In preeclampsia, however, there is **incomplete trophoblastic invasion.** In preeclampsia, only the decidual vessels, but not myometrial vessels, become lined with endovascular trophoblasts (so high resistance persists in uterine arteries).

■ PATHOGENESIS

See **Flowchart 17.1**.

Q. Differences between mild and severe preeclampsia.

Abnormality	Mild	Severe
Diastolic blood pressure	<100 mm Hg	110 mm Hg or higher
Proteinuria	Trace to 1+	Persistent 2+ or more
Headache	Absent	Present
Visual disturbances	Absent	Present
Upper abdominal pain	Absent	Present
Oliguria	Absent	Present
Convulsion	Absent	Present (eclampsia)
Serum creatinine	Normal	Elevated
Thrombocytopenia	Absent	Present
Liver enzyme elevation	Minimal	Marked
Fetal growth restriction	Absent	Obvious
Pulmonary edema	Absent	Present

Q. HELLP syndrome.

■ INTRODUCTION

- ❖ **HELLP syndrome** is an acronym for hemolysis, elevated liver enzymes and low platelets.
- ❖ This is rare complication of preeclampsia (10–15% cases).

■ CRITERIA FOR THE DIAGNOSIS OF HELLP SYNDROME

Hemolysis (H)

- ❖ Schistocytes in the blood smear
- ❖ Bilirubin more than 1.2 mg/dL
- ❖ Absent plasma haptoglobin.

Elevated Liver Enzymes (EL)

- ❖ SGOT more than 72 IU/l.
- ❖ LDH more than 600 IU/l.

Low Platelet Count (LP)

Platelets less than $100 \times 10^3/mm^3$.

■ COMPLICATIONS

Maternal

- Eclampsia.
- Abruption.
- Disseminated intravascular coagulation (DIC).
- Pulmonary edema, respiratory failure.
- Pulmonary embolism, acute respiratory distress syndrome (ARDS).
- Stroke, cerebral edema.
- Central venous thrombosis, seizures, retinal detachment.
- Acute renal failure, chronic renal failure.
- Hepatic (usually subcapsular) hematoma with possible rupture, ascites, nephrogenic diabetes insipidus.
- Infection, sepsis.
- Death.
- Recurrence risk of HELLP syndrome: 3–19%.

Fetal/Neonatal

- Prematurity, respiratory distress syndrome (RDS).
- Intrauterine growth retardation.
- Thrombocytopenia.

■ INVESTIGATIONS

Laboratory evaluation should include the following:
- Blood group and cross matching.
- **Complete blood cell (CBC) count with platelets:** Anemia and thrombocytopenia.
- **Coagulation studies:** BT, CT, PT, aPTT, fibrinogen, D-dimer.
- **Peripheral smear: Schistocytes, helmet cells, and burr cells** secondary to microangiopathic hemolytic anemia.
- **LFT:** Bilirubin, SGOT, SGPT, LDH.
- **RFT:** BUN, creatinine.
- **Haptoglobin level:** Decreased secondary to hemolysis.

■ TREATMENT

Multidisciplinary Team Approach

This comprises the obstetrician, neonatologist, hematologist, intensivist and ICU facilities.
- **Delivery is the definitive treatment**
- Although controversial, **corticosteroids** can be given as a treatment regimen for patients with HELLP.

- Steroids are theorized to alter the degree of intravascular endothelial injury and prevent further hepatocyte death and platelet activation.
- There is improved platelet counts, liver function, blood pressure, and urine output with the use of high-dose dexamethasone. **Intravenous glucocorticoids** appear superior to intramuscular steroids and are dose-dependent.
- Steroids are also believed to improve fetal morbidity by reducing the incidence of rDS and intraventricular hemorrhage, as well as maternal morbidity.
- Dosing for high-risk patients with severe disease (platelet count less than 20,000 or CNS dysfunction): 20 mg IV dexamethasone every 6 hours for up to 4 doses.
- Dosing for all other patients with HELLP syndrome: 10 mg IV dexamethasone every 6 hours for 2 doses then 6 mg IV dexamethasone every 6 hours for 2 doses.
- Antihypertensive to control the high BP.
- **Prophylactic $MgSO_4$ should be started if impending eclampsia or actual eclampsia.**
- Platelet transfusion and FFP may be needed.
- **Labor should be induced irrespective of weeks of gestation.**
- LSCS for obstetric indication.
- The route of delivery should be selected on obstetric indications including cervical status, obstetric history, the maternal and the fetal condition. If the cervix is unfavorable for induction of labor, cervical ripening should be the first step.

Q. Complications, investigations and management of preeclampsia.

DEFINITION

As above.

COMPLICATIONS

Maternal

Antenatal

- Eclampsia.
- Abruption.
- Preterm labor.
- HELLP syndrome.
- DIC.
- Blindness.
- Cerebral hemorrhage.
- ARDS.
- Renal failure (oliguria, anuria).
- Increase risk of operative delivery.
- Death.

Intrapartum

Eclampsia.

Postpartum

- Postpartum hemorrhage (PPH).

- ❖ Eclampsia.
- ❖ Shock.
- ❖ Sepsis.
- ❖ Death.

Remote

- ❖ Residual hypertension may be present in about 50% cases even after 6 months of delivery.
- ❖ Recurrence risk: There is 25% chance of recurrence in subsequent pregnancy.

Fetal

- ❖ IUGR.
- ❖ IUFD.
- ❖ Prematurity.
- ❖ Oligohydramnios.
- ❖ Asphyxia.

MANAGEMENT

Investigations

- ❖ **Urine for proteins**/albumin 24 hours urine protein.
- ❖ **CBC:** There is hemoconcentration so Hb values are false elevated. Low platelets indicate HELLP syndrome.
- ❖ **Serum uric acid:** It is a **biochemical marker** of preeclampsia raised levels (>4.5 mg/dL) indicate renal involvement and also correlate with severity of preeclampsia, volume contraction and fetal jeopardy.
- ❖ LFT: SGOT, SGPT, bilirubin.
- ❖ RFT: Serum creatinine.
- ❖ **Coagulation profile** may be required in severe cases:
  - ▷ BT
  - ▷ CT
  - ▷ PT, APTT
  - ▷ Fibrinogen levels
  - ▷ FDP
- ❖ **Fundoscopy:** Papilledema in severe cases, constriction of arterioles, and alteration in a normal ratio of vein: Arteriole diameter from 3:2 to 3:1.
- ❖ **Tests for fetal well-being:**
  - ▷ Fetal kick count.
  - ▷ NST weekly or biweekly.
  - ▷ BPP.
  - ▷ USG: For fetal growth and AFI.
  - ▷ Color Doppler.

TREATMENT

- ❖ Admit the patient

Chapter 17: Preeclampsia/Eclampsia

- Bedrest
- Diet: Diet to contain adequate protein about 100 mg/day. Salt and fluid restriction not needed
- BP charting 4 times/day
- Daily weight record
- Antihypertensives in pregnancy
  - Alpha methyldopa: 250–500 mg tds to qds
  - Nifedipine (always oral, never sublingual): 5–10 mg bd to qds
  - Hydralazine 10–25 mg bds
  - Labetalol 100 mg bds to qds
  - ACE inhibitors are contraindicated.
- **As per the latest guidelines, DOC for hypertension in pregnancy = labetalol followed by alpha methyldopa.**
- **DOC for hypertensive crisis in pregnancy = labetalol followed by hydralazine.**
- Diuretics: Not routinely recommended except in cases of cardiac failure or pulmonary edema or massive edema not relieved by rest and causing discomfort to the patient.

■ MANAGEMENT (FLOWCHART 17.2)

- On antihypertensives, if the BP is under control and there are no premonitory symptoms, then the pregnancy is allowed to continue **till 37 weeks** (keeping a close watch on maternal and fetal well-being).

Flowchart 17.2: Management of preeclampsia.

```
                      Preeclampsia
                           │
                     Hospitalization
      ┌─────────┬───────────┬──────────────┬──────────────┐
   Bedrest      BP      Antihypertensives  Investigations  Tests for
              charting                         CBC       fetal well-being
                                               LFT
                                               RFT
                                            Uric acid
                                             24 hours
                                           Urine proteins

      ┌──────────────┐                  Persistently      Premonitory
      │ BP controlled│                   elevated BP       symptoms
      └──────┬───────┘                        or       (Impending eclampsia)
     ┌───────┴────────┐                HELLP syndrome         │
  Pregnancy >37    Pregnancy <37              │          Prophylactic
    weeks             weeks                   │             MgSO₄
      │                │                      │               │
   Delivery      Discharge + continue         └──────→    Delivery
                 maternal and fetal                   (Irrespective of weeks
                    surveillance                          of gestation)
                         │
                 Delivery at ≥37 weeks
```

- ❖ **Thereafter, the patient should be delivered even if the BP is under control**, as the risks of continuation of pregnancy far outweigh the benefits (as this is a pregnancy-induced condition and delivery is the ultimate or definitive treatment for pregnancy-induced hypertension).
- ❖ **It is not advisable to wait beyond 37 weeks** because the BP can rise and there can be complications (eclampsia, HELLP syndrome, IUFD, abruption, DIC, etc.) and there are no added benefits of continuing pregnancy beyond 37 weeks.

Impending Eclampsia

The dangerous symptoms **(premonitory symptoms)** that indicate impending eclampsia in case of preeclampsia are:
- ❖ Headache
- ❖ Oliguria
- ❖ Epigastric pain
- ❖ Nausea, vomiting
- ❖ Blurring of vision.

Whenever the above symptoms develop in a case of severe preeclampsia, the patient is at a risk of eclampsia; the patient should be given anticonvulsant ($MgSO_4$) and antihypertensive medication, and the patient to be **delivered irrespective of the weeks of gestation.**

Magnesium sulfate is the drug of choice for eclampsia and also for **impending eclampsia**. Prophylactic magnesium sulfate decreases the risk of convulsion, abruption, and maternal mortality in this scenario **(Magpie Trial).**

The indications for termination of pregnancy **irrespective of the weeks of gestation** in a case of preeclampsia are:
- ❖ Severe preeclampsia, with impending eclampsia.
- ❖ Eclampsia (give $MgSO_4$ first, followed by induction of labor).
- ❖ HELLP syndrome.

Methods of Delivery

- ❖ The route of delivery should be selected on obstetric indications including cervical status, obstetric history, the maternal and the fetal condition. If the cervix is unfavorable for induction of labor, cervical ripening with PGs gel or inserts should be the first step.
- ❖ If cervix favorable: Oxytocin infusion, ARM.
- ❖ LSCS for obstetric indications or in cases of severe preeclampsia and unripe, closed cervix where there would be prolonged induction-delivery interval.

During Labor

- ❖ BP and urine output charting.
- ❖ Strict monitoring of fetal heart sounds (continuous EFM preferred).
- ❖ **Avoid methergin** after baby delivery as it can raise the BP.

■ PREVENTION OF HYPERTENSION IN FUTURE PREGNANCY

- ❖ **Low-dose aspirin** (75–150 mg/day till 34 weeks).
- ❖ Antioxidants (vitamin E, A, C, and **lycopene**).

- Calcium (2 g/day).
- Omega 3 fatty acids.

Q. Management of eclampsia.

DEFINITION

Preeclampsia when complicated by convulsion and/or coma is called eclampsia.

MANAGEMENT (FLOWCHART 17.3)

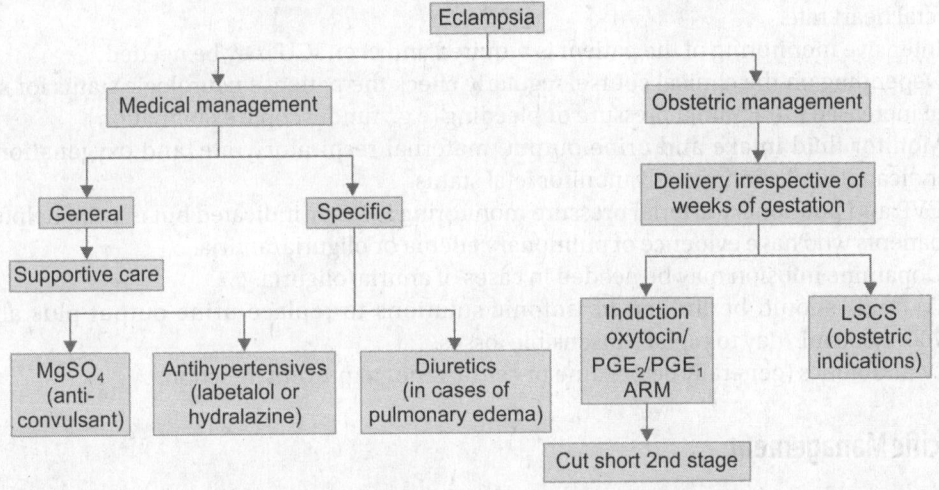

Flowchart 17.3: Management of eclampsia.

Medical

- Eclamptic convulsions are life-threatening emergencies and require the proper treatment to decrease maternal morbidity and mortality.
- **Delivery is the only definitive treatment for eclampsia.**

Team Approach

The patient should be shifted urgently to a *tertiary care center* for further management.

An experienced obstetrician, a pediatrician or neonatologist, anesthetist, intensivist and ICU and NICU backup are essential.

General Management

Supportive Care

- To prevent maternal **injury** and **fall**.
- To prevent aspiration.
- Maintain airway.
- Place the patient in the left lateral position. This positioning decreases the risk of aspiration and will help to improve uterine blood flow.

- Protect the patient against injury during the seizure by padding and raising guardrails, using a padded tongue blade between the teeth.
- **Suctioning** the oral secretions.
- Oxygenation by face mask (8–10 L/min). Monitor the oxygen saturation.
- Sodium bicarbonate may be given if acidosis.
- Secure an intravenous (IV) line with a large-bore catheter for drawing specimens and administering fluids and medications.
- **Catheterization** to monitor the urine output and collect urine for proteins (proteinuria).
- Detailed history to be taken from relatives.
- **Examination:** Quick but thorough general, abdominal and vaginal examination to be done.
- **Monitor:** Pulse, respiratory rate, BP half hourly. Also monitor the progress of labor and fetal heart rate.
- Intensive monitoring of the patient is required and even ICU may be needed.
- Depending on the clinical course, regularly check the patient's neurologic status for signs of increased intracranial pressure or bleeding (e.g., funduscopic examination).
- Monitor fluid intake and urine output, maternal respiratory rate, and oxygenation, as indicated, and continuously monitor fetal status.
- CVP and pulmonary arterial pressure monitoring is rarely indicated but may be helpful in patients who have evidence of pulmonary edema or oliguria/anuria.
- Dopamine infusion may be needed in cases of anuria/oliguria.
- IV fluids should be limited to isotonic solutions to replace urine output plus about 700–1,000 mL/day to replace insensible losses.
- IV antibiotics (generally cefotaxime or ceftriaxone) to prevent infection.

Specific Management

- Anticonvulsant therapy (magnesium sulfate).
- Blood pressure (BP) control.
- Diuretics are used only in the setting of pulmonary edema.

Anticonvulsant Therapy

Magnesium sulfate is the DOC for eclampsia. It can be given by various protocols:
- Pritchard.
- Sibai.
- Zuspan.
- Sardesai.

Pritchard Protocol

Loading dose: 14 g
4 g (20 mL of 20%) IV over 4 min immediately followed by 10 g (20 mL of 50%) IM—5 g in each buttock.
  If convulsions persist after 15 min, IV 2 g (10 mL of 20%) over 2 min (if the woman is large—4 g).

Maintenance dose:
- 5 g (10 mL of 50%) IM every 4 h—alternate sides.

Sibai Protocol

Loading dose:
- 6 g IV over 20 min

Maintenance dose:
- 2–3 g/h IV

$MgSO_4$ is continued till 24 hours postdelivery or 24 hours after the last convulsion whichever is later.

Monitoring of $MgSO_4$ Therapy

- Patellar reflexes
- Respiratory rate (>14/min)
- Urine output (100 cc in 4 hours or 30 cc/h)
- **Therapeutic range of magnesium is 4–7 mEq/L**
- When plasma levels rise above 10 mEq/L, respiratory depression develops, and at 12 mEq/L or more, respiratory paralysis and arrest follow
- Calcium gluconate, 1 g intravenously, is the drug of choice for $MgSO_4$ toxicity, along with withholding further magnesium sulfate.

Status Eclampticus

- For the rare patient who continues to have seizure activity while receiving adequate magnesium therapy, seizures may be treated with sodium amobarbital, 250 mg IV over 3–5 minutes or thiopentone sodium 0.5 g IV slowly. The procedure to be monitored by expert anesthetist.
- If this fails complete anesthesia with muscle relaxant and assisted ventilation may be required.
- In unresponsive cases an emergency LSCS may be lifesaving.

Antihypertensives

- Control of hypertension is essential to prevent further morbidity or possible mortality. The most commonly used antihypertensive agents are hydralazine, labetalol, and nifedipine.
- As per the latest guidelines, DOC for hypertensive crisis in pregnancy = Labetalol followed by hydralazine.
- The goal is to maintain systolic BP between 140 and 160 mm Hg and diastolic BP between 90 and 110 mm Hg.
- An IV bolus of hydralazine (5–10 mg every 20 min) or labetalol (20–40 mg every 15 min) is recommended. Other potent antihypertensive medications, such as sodium nitroprusside or nitroglycerin can be used but are rarely required.
- Care must be taken not to decrease the BP too drastically; an excessive decrease can cause inadequate uteroplacental perfusion and fetal compromise.
- Diuretics are used *only in the setting of pulmonary edema*. Frusemide 40 mg IV followed by 20 g mannitol IV reduces pulmonary edema and also prevents ARDS.

Obstetric Management

Delivery

- **Delivery is the only definitive treatment for eclampsia.**
- Induction of labor must be initiated **(irrespective of weeks of gestation)** after MgSO$_4$ and antihypertensives.
- A dose of antenatal steroids may be administered when gestational age is less than 34 weeks. Betamethasone (12 mg IM q24h × 2 doses) or dexamethasone (6 mg IM q12h × 4 doses) is recommended.
- The mode of delivery should be based on obstetric indications but should be chosen with an awareness that *vaginal delivery is preferable from a maternal point of view.*
- In the absence of fetal malpresentation or fetal distress, oxytocin or prostaglandins may be initiated to induce labor.
- Fetal heart rate and uterine contractions should be continuously monitored. Fetal bradycardia is common following the eclamptic seizure. Typically, emergency LSCS is not indicated for this postseizure transient bradycardia as it spontaneously resolves.
- Prophylactic forceps or ventouse to be used to cut short second stage of labor.
- LSCS is indicated in cases of:
  - Uncontrolled fits in spite of therapy.
  - Unconscious patients and if prospects of vaginal delivery are remote.
  - Worsening of maternal neurological, hepatic or renal condition and when anticipated delivery time is remote.
  - Obstetric indications like fetal distress, abruption, malpresentations.
  - It may also be considered in patients with an unfavorable cervix and a gestational age of 30 weeks or less (as induction under these circumstances may result in a prolonged intrapartum course and intrapartum complications).
- When emergent cesarean delivery is indicated, coagulopathy if present should be corrected before the procedure.
- **Watch for PPH after delivery and methergine to be avoided.**

Anesthesia

- For nonemergency cesarean delivery, epidural or combined techniques of regional anesthesia are preferred.
- Regional anesthesia is contraindicated in the presence of coagulopathy or severe thrombocytopenia (<50,000 platelets/µL).
- General anesthesia in women with eclampsia increases the risk of aspiration, and airway edema may make intubation difficult. It can also produce significant increases in systemic and cerebral pressures during intubation and extubation.
- The use of spinal anesthesia requires caution because of the possibility of total sympathetic blockade, resulting in maternal hypotension and uteroplacental insufficiency.

CHAPTER 18

Antepartum Hemorrhage and Postpartum Hemorrhage

Q. Etiology, signs, symptoms, and management of abruption.

Q. What are the types of abruption, management, and complications?

ABRUPTIO PLACENTAE/ABRUPTION

Definition

It is a form of APH where the bleeding occurs due to premature separation of **normally implanted** placenta. It is the **most common cause of APH**, followed by placenta previa.

Risk Factors for Abruptio Placentae

- Increased age and parity
- Preeclampsia and chronic hypertension. This is the **most important predisposing factor**. The vasospasm in uteroplacental bed leads to anoxic endothelial damage and rupture of vessels or extravasation of blood
- Cigarette smoking and cocaine use (vasospasm and transient hypertension)
- Thrombophilia: Hereditary or acquired [antiphospholipid antibody (APLA) syndrome]
- Prior abruption (risk of recurrence is **17% for patients with one abruption and 25% for patients with more than one abruption)**
- Uterine leiomyoma: If the placenta is implanted over a fibroid
- Sudden decompression of uterus as in cases of multifetal gestation (after delivery of first baby) or in cases of premature rupture of membranes (PROM) and polyhydramnios (sudden escape of liquor)
- External trauma or trauma during external cephalic version (ECV)
- Short cord
- Folic acid deficiency is also thought to play a role.

Clinical Features

The signs and symptoms of abruptio placentae with frequency are:

Signs and symptoms	Frequency (%)
Vaginal bleeding	78
Uterine tenderness or back pain	66
Fetal distress	60
High-frequency contractions	17
Hypertonus	17
Idiopathic preterm labor	22
Dead fetus	15

Types/Varieties of Abruption (Fig. 18.1)

❖ *Revealed:* The blood insinuates between membranes and decidua and comes out of the external os.

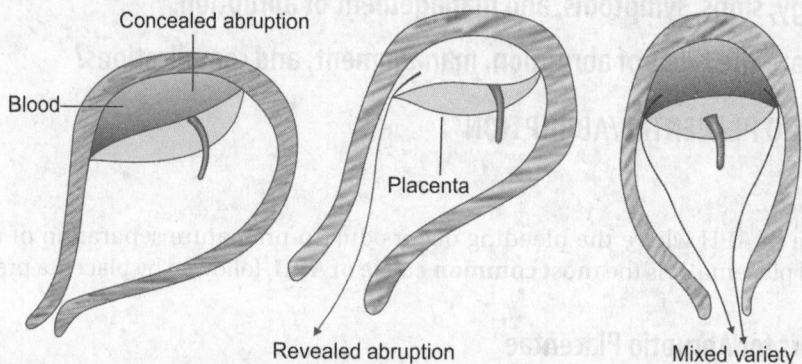

Fig. 18.1: Types of abruption.

❖ *Concealed:* The blood collects behind the placenta or the membrane and the decidua and does not come out of cervix.
❖ *Mixed:* Combination of above 2 types.

Clinical features depend on:
❖ Degree of placental separation
❖ Speed at which the separation occurs
❖ Variety of abruption (concealed or revealed).

Differences between Revealed and Concealed Variety

Revealed	Concealed
External bleeding (bleeding PV) present	Absent
Generally, condition and pallor is proportional to the amount of blood loss	Shock and pallor out of proportion to the blood loss
Uterine height corresponds to period of gestation	More than period of gestation
Uterine feel normal with localized tenderness	Uterus tense, tender, and tonically contracted
Fetal parts can be identified easily	Difficult to make out
Hb: Low, proportional to the amount of blood loss	Markedly low and out of proportion to the blood loss

Couvelaire Uterus

This is condition associated with **severe variety of concealed abruption.** This condition is diagnosed only laparotomy **[on operation table, if the delivery is by lower segment cesarean section (LSCS)]**.

There is widespread extravasation of blood into the uterine musculature and beneath the uterine serosa. This uteroplacental apoplexy, was first described by Couvelaire in the early 1900s, is now frequently called Couvelaire uterus.

The uterus looks **dark port wine in color** which may be patchy or diffuse. Such effusions of blood are also occasionally seen beneath the tubal serosa, in the connective tissue of the broad ligaments, and in the substance of the ovaries, as well as free in the peritoneal cavity. These myometrial hemorrhages rarely interfere with uterine contractions to produce severe PPH and are not an indication for hysterectomy.

Complications

Maternal

- Hemorrhage and hypovolemic shock
- Disseminated intravascular coagulation (DIC)
- PPH (remember APH predisposes to PPH)
- Renal failure [hypovolemia and acute tubular necrosis (ATN)], oliguria and anuria
- Sheehan's syndrome (postpartum pituitary necrosis)
- Increased risk of operative delivery (LSCS)
- Death.

Fetal

- Fetal distress/hypoxia
- Intrauterine fetal death (IUFD) (with IUFD the placental detachment is usually greater than 50%)
- Prematurity
- Anemia in the newborn.

Management

Emergency and Definitive

Emergency:
- Two wide bore intravenous (IV) lines
- IV fluids (crystalloids and colloids)
- **Blood transfusion** (in cases of hemodynamic instability in the patient) and fresh frozen plasma (FFP) and platelets transfusion in cases of DIC
- Close monitoring of maternal and fetal condition.
  Pritchard's rule for management of abruption: Keep **hematocrit (HCT) at least 30% and maintain urine output of at least 30 mL/hour.**
- **Collect blood for:**
  - Complete blood count (CBC) and platelet count
  - Grouping and cross-matching
  - DIC profile
  - Bleeding time, clotting time

Flowchart 18.1: Management of abruption.

```
                    Abruptio placentae
                    /              \
            FHS present         FHS absent (IUFD)
            /         \          /           \
    Fetal distress  No fetal    DIC present   DIC absent
         |         distress         |              |
       LSCS          |          Correct DIC        |
                  Oxytocin          |              |
                 augmentation       ↓              |
                     |          Vaginal delivery ←─┤
                  Normal              
                  delivery    
                         ┌──────────────┴──────────────┐
                      Possible                     Not possible
              Oxytocin augmentation ↓        (e.g., transverse lie/prev 2 LSCS)
                   Vaginal delivery                   |
                                                     LSCS
```

(DIC: disseminated intravascular coagulation; FHS: fetal heart sound; IUFD: intrauterine fetal death; LSCS: lower segment cesarean section)

- Prothrombin time (PT), activated partial thromboplastin time (APTT)
- Serum fibrinogen
- Fibrin degradation product (FDP).

Ultrasonography:
- Helps in placental localization. In abruption, it is in the upper segment as compared to previa in which the placenta is in the lower segment.
- Retroplacental collection can be seen.
- Early hemorrhage is hyperechoic or isoechoic.
- Negative findings do not rule out abruption.

Definitive Management:
- **Definitive management = immediate delivery** as abruption is progressive and the bleeding will only stop, once the placenta is delivered and the uterus contracts.
- If the fetus is alive and there is **no fetal distress** [reassuring fetal heart rate (FHR) tracing] and **there is a possibility that delivery can happen soon, then labor should be augmented** by artificial rupture of membranes (ARM) and oxytocin drip, keeping a close watch on FHR **(Flowchart 18.1).**

Q. What are the types of placenta previa?

Q. Clinical features and management of placenta previa.

PLACENTA PREVIA

Definition

Previa in Latin means 'in front of'. In placenta previa, the placenta is in front of presenting part, and implanted over and adjacent to the internal cervical os.

Variants include complete implantation over the os (complete placenta previa), a placental edge partially covering the os (partial placenta previa) or the placenta approaching the border of the os (marginal placenta previa).

Four degrees of placenta previa have been recognized **(Fig. 18.2)**.
1. *Total placenta previa:* The internal cervical os is covered completely by placenta.
2. *Partial placenta previa:* The internal os is partially covered by placenta.
3. *Marginal placenta previa:* The edge of the placenta is at the margin of the internal os.
4. *Low-lying placenta:* The placenta is implanted in the lower uterine segment such that the placenta edge actually does not reach the internal os but is in close proximity to it.

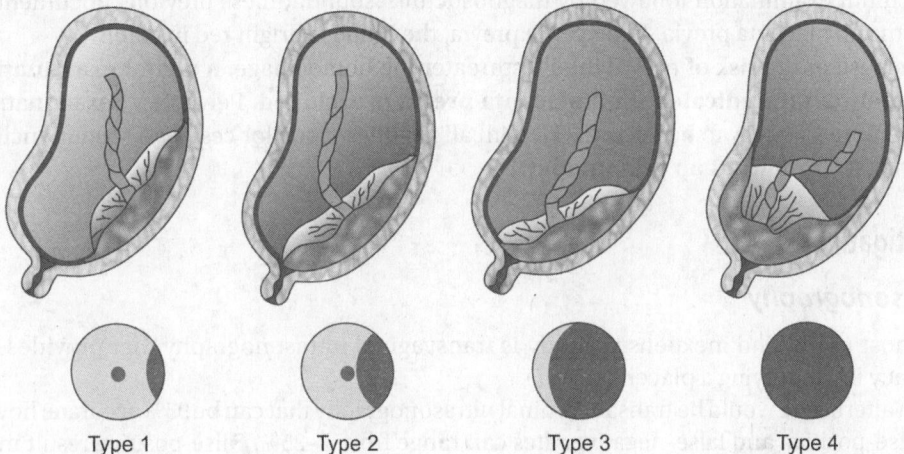

Fig. 18.2: Degree of placenta previa with findings on ultrasound examination.

Risk Factors

- Increasing age and increasing parity
- **Past history** (12 times risk of another placenta previa)
- Previous LSCS (probability of previa is four times greater than in patients without any uterine scar)
- Multiple pregnancy
- Prematurity
- Smoking.

Clinical Features

Symptoms

- Remember **4P's:** Painless, profuse, periodic and purposeless (causeless)
- The classic presentation of placenta previa is **painless vaginal bleeding**
- Nearly two-thirds of symptomatic patients present before 36 weeks' gestation, with half of these patients presenting before 30 weeks' gestation.

Signs

- *General condition and anemia:* Proportional to visible blood loss

- *Features of preeclampsia:* Unrelated/absent
- *Height of uterus:* Proportionate to the period of gestation
- *Feel of uterus:* Soft and relaxed without any localized tenderness
- **Malpresentation:** Malpresentation is common (breech, transverse lie or unstable lie)
- The head is **high floating (unengaged)**
- *Stallworthy's sign:* Slowing of fetal heart rate on pressing the head down into the pelvis and prompt recovery on release of pressure is termed Stallworthy's sign. This sign is suggestive of posterior placenta previa.

Any pregnant patient beyond the first trimester who presents with vaginal bleeding requires a speculum examination followed by diagnostic ultrasound, unless previous documentation confirms no placenta previa. In placenta previa, the blood is bright red in color.

Because of the risk of provoking life-threatening hemorrhage, **a digital examination is absolutely contraindicated until placenta previa is excluded.** Pelvic (PV) examination (if at all required) is only to be done in OT, with all facilities ready for cesarean section including anesthetist **(Double set up examination)**.

Investigations

Ultrasonography

The most useful and inexpensive study is transvaginal ultrasonography that provides 100% accuracy in identifying a placenta previa.

An alternative would be transabdominal ultrasonography that can be 95% accurate; however, the false-positive and false-negative rates can range from 2–25%. False-positive result may be due to full bladder.

Transperineal sonography is another alternative.

Color Doppler

Prominent venous flow in hypoechoic areas near cervix is consistent with the diagnosis of placenta previa.

Magnetic Resonance Imaging (MRI)

Very accurate, safe and without the risk of ionizing radiation. But expensive and not routinely done.

Management

Emergency

- Two wide bore IV lines
- IV fluids (crystalloids and colloids)
- **Collect blood for:**
  - CBC and platelet count
  - Grouping and cross-matching.
- **Blood transfusion** (in cases of hemodynamic instability in the patient and FFP and platelets transfusion in cases of DIC)
- Close monitoring of maternal and fetal condition

- ❖ Abdominal examination to rule out tenderness and vulval inspection for presence of bleeding
- ❖ Confirm the diagnosis with ultrasonography.

McAfee and Johnson Regimen (Conservative/Expectant Management in Placenta Previa)

This consists of complete bed rest, tocolysis, and close observation of patient. Steroids are generally given to enhance lung maturity.

To undertake this regimen (to wait and watch), **all the three criteria should be fulfilled:**
1. Mother should be hemodynamically stable.
2. There should be no fetal distress.
3. Pregnancy should be <36 weeks of gestation.
   If any one of these criteria is not met, then the patient should be **delivered by LSCS**.
   The expectant management is continued till 37 weeks. Then the patient is to be delivered by cesarean section, as now there is no point of further waiting.

Active Management (Delivery)

In cases of placenta previa, the delivery is by cesarean section.

Vaginal delivery is only possible in cases where the placental edge is **>3 cm away from internal os on USG (low-lying placenta).**

Immediate delivery (irrespective of weeks of gestation) is to be done in following cases:
- ❖ Patient is in shock/hemodynamic instability (resuscitation followed by LSCS)
- ❖ Fetal distress or IUFD or severe congenital malformation in fetus
- ❖ Pregnancy >37 weeks.

Q. Differentiate between placenta previa and abruption.

Distinguishing features of placenta previa and abruptio placentae are:

Clinical features	Placenta previa	Abruptio placentae
Nature of bleeding	• Painless, profuse • Bleeding is always revealed • Periodic	• Painful • Revealed, concealed, or usually mixed • Progressive
General condition and anemia	Proportional to visible blood loss	Out of proportion to the visible blood loss in concealed or mixed variety
Features of preeclampsia	Unrelated (absent)	Very likely to be present
Height of uterus	Proportionate height	May be disproportionately enlarged in concealed type
Feel of uterus	Soft and relaxed	Tonically contracted uterus
Malpresentation	Malpresentation is common (breech, transverse lie). The head is high floating	Unrelated the head may be engaged
Placentography	Placenta in lower segment	Placenta in upper segment
Tocolysis	Can be given	Never
Wait and watch	Can be done	Never
Delivery	LSCS	LSCS or vaginal delivery
DIC	Less common	More common

Q. Define PPH. What are the causes of PPH?
Q. Management of atonic PPH.

POSTPARTUM HEMORRHAGE (PPH)

Introduction
Hemorrhage is the most common direct cause of maternal mortality in India and developing countries. Majority of these cases are due to PPH.

Definitions
- Blood loss of 500 mL or more following a vaginal delivery or more than 1000 mL following cesarean delivery
- **Decrease in HCT by 10%** or more, after delivery **(ACOG)**.
- Any amount of blood loss requiring 1 unit or more blood transfusion in the postpartum period.
- **Any amount of bleeding** from or into the genital tract following the birth of the baby up to the end of puerperium which causes **hemodynamic instability** in the patient.

There are two types of PPH. **Primary** PPH occurs **within the first 24 hours** after delivery. **Secondary** PPH occurs **after 24 hours to 12 weeks postpartum**.

Predisposing Factors and Causes of Immediate Postpartum Hemorrhage

Bleeding from Placental Implantation Site
- **Hypotonic myometrium:** Uterine atony (most common) 80% cases
- **Hypertensive disorders:** Preeclampsia, eclampsia
- **Antepartum hemorrhage:** Abruption (remember: APH predisposes to PPH)
- **Over distended uterus** (e.g., large fetus, twins, and hydramnios): Imperfect retraction
- Following prolonged/obstructed labor: Poor retraction and amnionitis
- Following precipitate labor
- Following oxytocin-induced or augmented labor
- **High parity:** Inadequate retraction, and increased risk of adherent placenta and anemia all contribute
- Uterine **atony in previous pregnancy**
- Chorioamnionitis
- Drugs—tocolytic agents, halothane
- Retained placental tissue, avulsed cotyledon and succenturiate lobe
- Abnormally adherent—accreta, increta, and percreta
- Fibroids: Mechanically cause imperfect retraction.

Trauma to the Genital Tract (20%)
- Large episiotomy, including extensions
- Lacerations of perineum, vagina or cervix in cases of instrumental deliveries
- Ruptured uterus.

Coagulation Defects like DIC, HELLP Syndrome
Intensify all of the above.

Management

- Call for extra help
- Put two wide bore IV cannulas
- Send blood for grouping and cross-matching
- IV fluids (crystalloids and colloids) infuse normal saline 2 liters rapidly and plasma expanders like haemaccel
- Injection tranexamic acid 1 g IV
- Catheterize (Foley catheter) the patient and monitor the urine output
- To monitor the vitals like pulse, BP, and CVP, if needed
- Give oxygen by mask
- Blood transfusion.

Specific

- Palpate the abdomen for the feel of the uterus
- If the uterus is flabby its atonic PPH
- If the uterus is well-contracted and firm, the bleeding is due to trauma.

Atonic PPH

Medical Management

- Massage the uterus
- *Use of utero tonic drugs:*
  - Injection **oxytocin drip** (10–20 units in 500 mL of saline) @ 40–60 drops/minute. **As per the ACOG guidelines, oxytocin is the first line drug of choice for atonic PPH.**
  - Injection methergine 0.2 mg IV.
- The 15-methyl derivative of prostaglandin F2 (carboprost tromethamine). The initial recommended dose is 250 µg (0.25 mg) given intramuscularly, and this is repeated if necessary at 15–90 minutes intervals up to a maximum of eight doses.
- Misoprostol (800-1000 µg, can be used oral, sublingual, buccal, or per rectal), a synthetic prostaglandin E1 analog, is also effective for the treatment of uterine atony. WHO recommends that misoprostol (800 µg) be given per rectally.

Recent Advances

Carbetocin is a newer drug used for prevention and treatment of PPH.
- It is stable at room temperature (unlike oxytocin) and hence does not require refrigeration.
- It can be administered **intravenously or intramuscularly**. The recommended dose is **100 µg, administered slowly over a minute**. Contractile effects of the uterus are apparent within two minutes and can be observed for approximately one hour.

Intrauterine Packing

If the uterine atonicity persists: Intrauterine packing is done.
- **Shivkar's pack:** Condom inflated with saline acts as tamponade. Bakri balloon or Sengstaken–Blakemore tube can also be used. This can avoid a hysterectomy in around 80% patients **(Fig. 18.3)**.

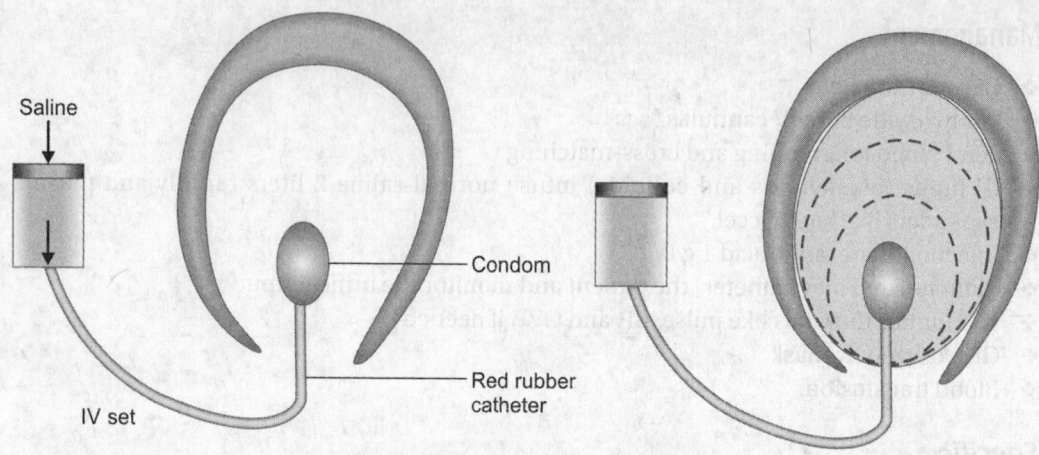

Fig. 18.3: Shivkar's pack.

Recent Advances

PPH suction canula is a vacuum suction hemostatic device for treating postpartum hemorrhage. Negative pressure created within the uterine cavity results in cessation of bleeding from the postpartum uterus including atonic postpartum hemorrhage.

Surgical Management

If all these medical methods fail to control the bleeding, then surgical methods are required.
Stepwise devascularization of the uterus:
- Uterine artery ligation **(Fig. 18.4)**
- **Internal iliac artery ligation:**
  - Ligation of the internal iliac arteries **(anterior division)** at times reduces the hemorrhage appreciably.
  - The most important mechanism of action with internal iliac artery ligation is an 85% reduction in pulse pressure in those arteries distal to the ligation.
  - This converts an arterial pressure system into one with pressures approaching those in the venous circulation and more amenable to hemostasis via simple clot formation. Bilateral ligation of these arteries does not appear to interfere with subsequent reproduction.

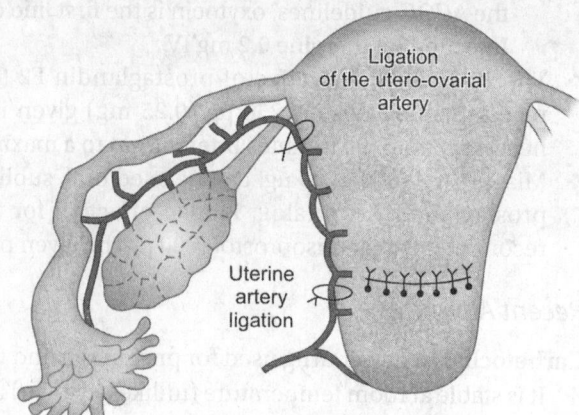

Fig. 18.4: Ligation of the utero-ovarian artery.

- **Uterine compression sutures:**
  - In 1997, **B-Lynch** described a surgical technique for severe postpartum hemorrhage in which a pair of vertical brace chromic sutures were secured around the uterus, giving the appearance of suspenders, to compress together the anterior and posterior walls (tamponade effect) success rate is about 80% **(Fig. 18.5)**.

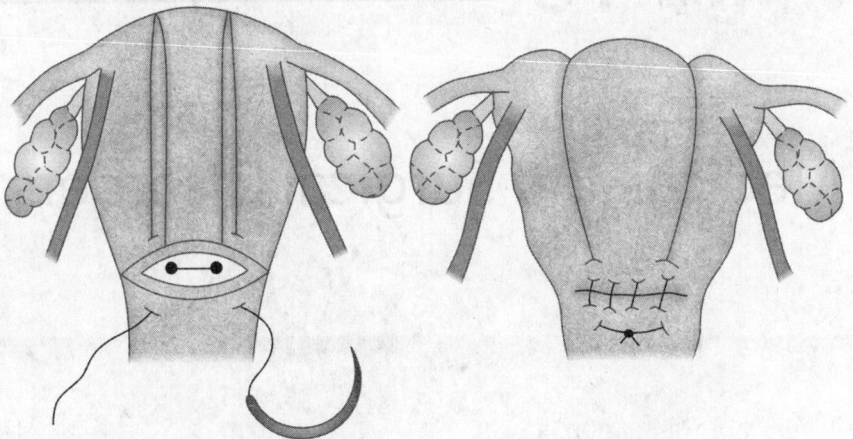

Fig. 18.5: B-Lynch brace suture for control of atonic PPH.

- Hayman sutures.
- Cho square sutures.
- Gunshella sutures.

❖ **Uterine artery embolization** under fluoroscopic guidance can be tried.
❖ **Obstetric hysterectomy** is used as the last resort.
Hysterectomy performed at or following delivery may be lifesaving if there is severe obstetrical hemorrhage. It can be carried out in conjunction with cesarean delivery or following vaginal delivery.

CHAPTER 19

Medical and Surgical Disorders

Q. Signs and symptoms suggestive of heart disease in pregnancy.

■ METCALFE'S CRITERIA FOR HEART DISEASE IN PREGNANCY

The following findings are suggestive of heart disease in pregnancy:

Symptoms:
- Progressive dyspnea or orthopnea
- Nocturnal cough
- Hemoptysis
- Syncope
- Chest pain.

Clinical findings:
- Cyanosis
- Clubbing of fingers
- Persistent neck vein distention
- Systolic murmur grade 3/6 or greater
- Diastolic murmur
- Cardiomegaly
- Persistent split-second sound
- Criteria for pulmonary hypertension
- Persistent arrhythmias.

Q. Intrapartum management of cardiac patient.

■ INTRODUCTION

Mitral stenosis is the most common valvular disease in pregnancy. The patient with heart disease belongs to a **high-risk category** and there is increased risk of mortality during pregnancy and especially during labor.

■ TEAM APPROACH

Obstetrician, cardiologist, anesthetist, neonatologist, and intensive care unit (ICU) facilities.

Chapter 19: Medical and Surgical Disorders

■ GENERAL MEASURES FOR THE CARDIAC PATIENT IN LABOR

First Stage

- Labor and delivery in **lateral decubitus position or propped up position**
- Adequate pain relief **(epidural analgesia is the best)**. Pain can cause tachycardia, which in turn can precipitate failure
- **Restrict intravenous (IV) fluids** to 75 mL/hour (except in aortic stenosis) to prevent congestive cardiac failure (CCF)
- **Oxygen** by breathing mask at the rate of 5–6 L/minute
- Careful monitoring of the vital parameters. Cardiac monitoring and pulse oximeter monitoring. Central venous pressure (CVP) monitoring in selected cases. If pulse rate exceeds 110/minute in between contractions, rapid digitalization is done by IV digoxin 0.5 mg
- Antibiotics (infective endocarditis prophylaxis = ampicillin and gentamicin). Ampicillin 2 g and gentamicin 1.5 mg/kg at the onset of labor followed by repeat doses at 8 hourly interval.

Second Stage

Avoid maternal pushing efforts and so to **cut short II stage of labor by use of prophylactic forceps or vacuum**.

Third Stage

- Prevention of postpartum pulmonary edema by giving **IV furosemide after placental delivery**
- **Methergine is absolutely contraindicated** and not to be given. To prevent excessive blood loss oxytocin infusion can be used.

■ PLACE FOR LOWER SEGMENT CESAREAN SECTION (LSCS)

- In heart disease patients, LSCS should be done for obstetric indications only
- Heart disease in which **elective LSCS should be done is Marfan syndrome with aortic root dilatation is >4 cm. Coarctation of aorta is a relative indication for elective LSCS.**

Q. Short note: red degeneration.

■ INTRODUCTION

- Fibroids are the most common benign tumors of the uterus. They are also the most common pelvic tumors in females.
- Fibroids can undergo various types of degeneration. One of it is called red degeneration which occurs **exclusively during pregnancy**.

■ RED DEGENERATION

- **Also known as carneous degeneration**
- Occurs because fibroid overgrows its blood supply **(micronecrothrombosis)**

- Most commonly occurs in **second trimester of pregnancy** followed by in the **puerperium** period
- *Cut section:* Raw beefy appearance, fishy odor.

CLINICAL FEATURES

Patient presents with:
- Acute abdomen
- Vomiting
- Fever.

There is presence of leukocytosis.

DIFFERENTIAL DIAGNOSIS

- Acute appendicitis
- Pyelonephritis
- Abruption.

MANAGEMENT

- Always conservative management (never surgery)
- Hospitalization
- Bed rest
- Analgesics
- IV fluids
- IV antibiotics (SOS).

Q. Complications of anemia in pregnancy.
Q. Investigations for case of anemia in pregnancy.
Q. Management of iron deficiency anemia in pregnancy.

INTRODUCTION

Anemia is the most common hematological disorder to occur in pregnancy. Dimorphic anemia is the most common type of anemia.

It is the **most common indirect cause of maternal mortality**.

COMPLICATIONS MATERNAL ANTENATAL

- **Infections:** Anemia and malnutrition decreases resistance to infections
- **Cardiac failure** at 30–32 weeks
- Preterm labor
- Abruption (folic acid deficiency).

Intrapartum

Cardiac failure: Due to increased cardiac output.

Postpartum

- **PPH: Patients may not tolerate even minimal blood loss**
- **Maternal mortality**
- Puerperal sepsis
- Subinvolution
- Poor lactation
- Poor wound healing
- Puerperal venous and pulmonary embolism.

Fetal

- The baby does not have anemia at birth, but the iron stores may be less
- Intrauterine growth restriction (IUGR)
- Increased in perinatal loss.

CRITERIA OF PHYSIOLOGICAL ANEMIA

- Hemoglobin (Hb): 10 g%
- Red blood cells (RBC): 3.2 million/mm^3
- Packed cell volume (PCV): 32%
- Peripheral smear: **Normocytic and normochromic**
- Mean corpuscular hemoglobin concentration remains unchanged in pregnancy.

INVESTIGATIONS

For the Degree of Anemia

- Hemoglobin
- Hematocrit (PCV).

Type of Anemia

- **Peripheral blood smear** (stained with **Leishman stain**) is the most important
- RBC morphology gives the idea about the type of anemia.

Iron Deficiency

- Hypochromic, microcytic
- Anisocytosis
- Poikilocytosis
- Increased in reticulocyte count.

Megaloblastic Anemia

Vitamin B$_{12}$ and folic acid deficiency:
- Macrocytes
- Hypersegmented neutrophils
- Howell-Jolly bodies
- Giant polymorphs.

Hematological Indices

Indices	Iron deficiency anemia	Megaloblastic anemia
MCV	Decreased (<75 u^3)	Increased (>100 u^3)
MCH	Decreased (< than 25 pg)	Increased (>33 pg)
MCHC	Decreased (< than 30%)	Normal

(MCH: mean corpuscular hemoglobin; MCHC: mean cell hemoglobin concentration; MCV: mean corpuscular volume)

Other Blood Investigations

In Iron Deficiency

- Serum iron below 30 mg/dL
- Total iron binding capacity test (TIBC) increased (>400 mg/dL)
- Percentage saturation decreased (10% or less)
- As per Centers for Disease Control and Prevention (CDC), **serum ferritin <15 µg/L** confirms iron deficiency anemia.

In Megaloblastic Anemia

- Serum iron, normal or high
- Serum folate <3 ng/mL
- Serum B_{12} <90 pg/mL
- Associated leukopenia and thrombocytopenia.

To Find the Cause of Anemia

- Stool examination to detect helminthic infestation
- Clean catch midstream, urine sample for pus cells, protein, and sugars
- Other appropriate investigations as per history and clinical examination
- Hemoglobin electrophoresis to rule out thalassemia especially in cases of refractory anemia
- *In specific cases:* Chest X-ray to rule out tuberculosis (TB), fractional test meal analysis of gastric juice for achlorhydria in pernicious anemia.

■ TREATMENT

Curative

General and specific.

General

- **Diet:** A balanced diet rich in iron and protein
    - The best source of iron is red meat, especially beef and liver. Chicken, turkey, pork, fish, and shellfish also are good sources of iron.
    - Vegetarian sources include:
        - Iron-fortified breads and cereals
        - Peas; lentils; white, red, and baked beans; soybeans; and chickpeas
        - Tofu, jaggery

- Dried fruits, such as prunes, raisins, and apricots
- Spinach and other dark green leafy vegetables
  ▸ Iron utensils should be used for cooking.
- **Vitamin C:** Vitamin C helps the body absorb iron. Good sources of vitamin C are vegetables and fruits, especially citrus fruits.
- To cure the diseases contributing to anemia
- To eradicate any focus of infection
- **Anthelmintics** to eradicate worm infestation.

Factors that inhibit iron absorption	Factors that enhance iron absorption
Foods rich in calcium	Heme iron
Tannins in tea	Ferrous iron (Fe^{2+})
Phytates in cereals	Ascorbic acid

Specific Therapy

- Oral and parenteral forms are available.
- Blood transfusion

1. Oral Iron

- Once women become iron deficient in pregnancy, it is not possible to ensure repletion through diet alone and at least oral supplementation is needed
- Oral iron is an effective, cheap, and safe way to replace iron. Ferrous salts (sulfate, gluconate, fumarate, succinate) show only marginal differences between one another in efficiency of absorption of iron
- Ferric salts are much less well-absorbed
- Generally, a 200 mg tablet contains 60 mg elemental iron. One tablet is to be given three times a day (180 mg) to a max of six tablets. Higher doses should not be given, as absorption is saturated and side effects increased
- Oral iron supplementation should be taken on an empty stomach, as absorption is reduced or promoted by the same factors that affect absorption of dietary nonheme iron.
- Folic acid and vitamin B_{12} and C supplementation should also be given along with iron.

Side effects:
- Epigastric pain
- Nausea, vomiting
- Diarrhea or constipation
  ▸ Patients need to be informed that **stools would black in color**
  ▸ The side effects can be minimized by starting with a small dose or change of preparation
  ▸ With oral treatment, the absorption of iron is an issue as it is effected by various factors
  ▸ The serum iron maybe restored but there is difficulty in replenishing the stores.

Response is evident by:
- Sense of well-being
- Increased appetite
- Rise in hemoglobin and hematocrit which is preceded by reticulocytosis.

Causes of failure of oral treatment:
- Improper typing of anemia: Wrong diagnosis, thalassemia
- Defective absorption

- Noncompliant patient
- Nontolerance
- Concurrent blood loss like piles or hookworm infestation.

2. Parenteral Iron

- **Intravenous:** Iron sucrose, iron dextran
- **Intramuscular:** Iron dextran and iron sorbitol citric acid complex.

Indications for parenteral iron:
- Noncompliant patient
- Nontolerance to oral iron
- **Malabsorption syndrome**
  - Parenteral iron is not given for rapid rise of Hb as the rise in Hb is the same with oral, IM and IV iron.
  - It is about **0.7–1 g/dL per week**
  - **Fastest rise of Hb is with blood transfusion.**

The main advantages of parenteral iron are:
- Surety or certainty of administration
- Helps in replenishing the iron stores faster.

Different formulae for calculations of dose of parenteral iron:
- Formula 1 = (Normal Hb in g – patient's Hb in g) × Weight (in kg) × 2.21 + 1,000 (for stores) = mg of iron needed
- Formula 2 = 250 mg of iron is required for each gram of Hb below normal
- Formula 3 = 0.3 × weight (in pounds) × (100 – Hb%) = mg of iron needed. Add 50% of this for stores.

For IV iron test dose is to be given by IV route and for IM iron test dose is to be given IM. However for the newer preparation, **iron sucrose, test dose is not needed**.

Intramuscular injections are to be given by **Z technique** to prevent staining of the skin and to minimize the pain.

Side effects:
- Pain
- Abscess formation, skin discoloration
- *Reactions:* Fever, headache, lymphadenopathy, nausea, vomiting and rarely allergic reactions.

3. Blood Transfusion

Packed cells are preferred over whole blood (to avoid the risk of CCF). To be given when rapid rise of hemoglobin is required:
- Severe anemia with advanced pregnancy (>36 weeks)
- Severe anemia in early labor
- Anytime, if the patient has CCF due to severe anemia (under the cover of diuretics).

Advantages of blood transfusion:
- Increase in oxygen carrying capacity of blood
- Hb from lysed red cells may be utilized for formation of new RBCs
- Stimulates erythropoiesis
- Improvement expected in 3 days.

Chapter 19: Medical and Surgical Disorders

Precautions:
- Properly typed and cross matched blood to be used
- Patient needs to be admitted
- Blood to be given under the cover of diuretics (frusemide)
- To monitor vitals and watch for crepitations in the base of lungs
- Emergency resuscitation trolley ready to manage anaphylaxis reaction.

Management during Labor

Blood to be collected for grouping and **cross matching and be kept ready**.

First Stage
- Patient should be in bed (lateral or propped-up position preferred)
- Oxygen inhalation
- Strict asepsis
- To avoid fluid overload.

Second Stage
- Strict asepsis
- **Cut short second stage of labor** by use of prophylactic forceps or vacuum.

Third Stage
- **Active management of third stage of labor** (oxytocin or methergine following delivery of anterior shoulder) should be done to prevent PPH
- Blood loss to be replenished with blood transfusion, if required
- To avoid fluid overload and watch for CCF.

Management during Puerperium
- Prophylactic antibiotics to prevent infection
- Hematinics to be continued for at least 3 months postpartum
- **Contraceptive advice:** Patient to be counseled and explained the importance of birth spacing
- Depot medroxyprogesterone acetate (DMPA) and progestogen-only pills (POP) are suitable. Intrauterine contraceptive devices (IUCDs) preferably to be avoided
- Patient to be warned of danger of recurrence in subsequent pregnancies.

Q. Complications of diabetes in pregnancy.

INTRODUCTION

About 1–14% of all pregnancies are complicated by diabetes mellitus (DM). Diabetes in pregnancy could be:
- **Overt DM:** Pre-existing diabetes which is detected before pregnancy or detected for first time during pregnancy.
- **Gestational diabetes (GDM):** It is defined as **carbohydrate intolerance** resulting in hyperglycemia of variable severity with onset or first recognition during pregnancy, whether or not insulin is used for treatment and whether or not the condition persists

after pregnancy. It generally develops at 26–28 weeks of gestation **as insulin resistance in pregnancy is maximum at 28 weeks of gestation**.

Pregnancy is a diabetogenic state because of:
- Insulin resistance
  - Production of HPL
  - Increased production of cortisol, estrogen, and progesterone
  - Increased destruction of insulin by kidneys and placenta
- Increased lipolysis
- Altered gluconeogenesis.

COMPLICATIONS

Effects of Pregnancy on Diabetes

- Increased insulin requirement
- Progression of diabetic retinopathy
- Worsening of diabetic nephropathy
- Worsening of diabetic cardiomyopathy.

Effects of Diabetes on Pregnancy

Diabetes causes maternal, fetal and neonatal complications.

Maternal Complications

During Pregnancy

- *Abortion:* **Recurrent first trimester abortions** with uncontrolled diabetes
- Increased risk of preeclampsia (25%)
- *Polyhydramnios (25–50%):* Fetal hyperglycemia leading to polyuria, large baby and large placenta are responsible for polyhydramnios
- *Preterm labor (20%):* Due to overdistended uterus (polyhydramnios, macrosomia), infections and preeclampsia
- *Higher risk of infection:* Urinary tract infection (UTI) and vulvovaginitis
- *Maternal distress:* Due to polyhydramnios and macrosomia
- Ketoacidosis.

During Labor

- Prolonged labor, obstructed labor
- *Shoulder dystocia:* Six times more risk compared to nondiabetics. With birth weight remaining same, the babies of diabetic mothers are more prone to develop shoulder dystocia compared to babies of nondiabetic mothers.
- *PPH:* Due to overdistended uterus (polyhydramnios, macrosomia) and preeclampsia
- *Pelvic floor trauma:* More risk of 3rd and 4th degree perineal tears
- *Operative delivery:* LSCS rates vary from 25% to 80%.

Puerperium

- Puerperal sepsis
- Lactational failure.

Late

Nearly 50% women with gestational DM (GDM) will become overt DM over a period of 5–20 years.

Fetal Complications

- **Congenital anomalies (3–10%):** It is related to severity of diabetes during organogenesis. It has been found that **higher the HbA1c, higher is the risk of anomalies**.
- **Most common anomaly:** Cardiac anomalies (VSD) followed by neural tube defects (NTD) (anencephaly/spina bifida)
- **Most specific anomaly:** Caudal regression syndrome/sacral agenesis.

Central Nervous System

- Anencephaly and spina bifida
- Encephalocele
- Meningomyelocele and holoprosencephaly
- Microcephaly.

Cardiovascular

- Transposition of the great vessels (most specific cardiac anomaly)
- Ventricular septal defect (VSD) and atrial septal defect (ASD)
- Hypoplastic left ventricle
- Hypertrophic obstructive cardiomyopathy (HOCM).

Note: VSD is the most common cardiac anomaly; transposition of the great vessels (TGV) is the most specific cardiac anomaly in infants of diabetic mothers.

Skeletal

Caudal regression syndrome (sacral agenesis).

Genitourinary

- Absent kidneys
- Polycystic kidneys
- Double ureter.

Gastrointestinal

- Tracheoesophageal fistula
- Bowel atresia
- Imperforate anus.

Macrosomia (30–40%)

- The American College of Obstetricians and Gynecologists (ACOG) definition: Birth weight >4.5 kg
- **Pedersen's hypothesis:** Maternal hyperglycemia causes fetal hyperglycemia, which in turn causes fetal hyperinsulinemia and also increases insulin-like growth factor (IGF) I and II which leads to fetal macrosomia.

Others

- Elevation of maternal free fatty acids lead to its increased transfer to the fetus.
- **Birth injuries:** Brachial plexus injury. Shoulder dystocia and prolonged labor are responsible for this injury.
- **IUGR:** *Only in cases of long standing diabetes* **associated with maternal vasculopathy.**
- **Sudden IUFD at term:** Exact reason is not known but final event is hypoxia and acidosis. There is increase in fetal oxygen demand and glycosylated HB binds more avidly to oxygen and releases less oxygen.
- *Gestational diabetes mostly develops at around 24-28 weeks, and hence, there is no risk of first trimester abortions and congenital anomalies in the fetus as sugars would be normal in the first trimester*
- **So remember that the 2 'A's: 'Anomalies' and 'abortions' are seen only in overt diabetes and not in GDM.**

Neonatal Complications

- Hyaline membrane disease or respiratory distress syndrome
- Hyperviscosity syndrome
- Genetic transmission (infants of mothers with type I diabetes have 4–5% risk of acquiring diabetes; infants of mothers with type II diabetes have 25–50% risk of diabetes)
- Hypoglycemia
- Hypocalcemia
- Hypomagnesemia
- Hyperbilirubinemia
- Polycythemia
- Cardiomyopathy
- Increase in perinatal mortality (PNM) (2-3 times).

Q. Thrombophilias/APLA syndrome in pregnancy (short note).

INTRODUCTION

- Thrombophilia is an abnormality of blood coagulation that increases the risk of thrombosis
- The most common conditions associated with thrombophilia are deep vein thrombosis (DVT) and pulmonary embolism (PE).

Types of Thromobophilias

Thrombophilias can be congenital (hereditary thrombophilia) or acquired (APLA syndrome = antiphospholipid antibody syndrome).

Congenital

- Factor V Leiden mutation
- Prothrombin G20210A mutation
- Antithrombin deficiency
- Protein C deficiency
- Protein S deficiency
- Hyperhomocysteinemia

All these are **autosomal dominant** inheritance except **hyperhomocysteinemia** which is **autosomal recessive**.

Acquired

APLA syndrome, is an autoimmune, hypercoagulable state caused by antiphospholipid antibodies. It provokes thrombosis in both arteries and veins as well as pregnancy-related complications such as miscarriage, stillbirth, preterm delivery, and severe preeclampsia. The diagnostic criteria require one clinical event (i.e., thrombosis or pregnancy complication) and two positive blood test results spaced at least three months apart that detect **lupus anticoagulant (LA), anti-apolipoprotein antibodies, or anti-cardiolipin antibodies (ACL).**

The anticardiolipin antibodies and the lupus anticoagulant bind to "annexin V" and "beta-2 microglobulin," which are naturally occurring anticoagulants present in our body. This leads to decrease in levels of free "annexin V" and "beta-2 microglobulin," leading to thrombosis.

Obstetric Complications of Thrombophilias (Congenital and Acquired)

- Recurrent abortions
- Severe preeclampsia
- IUGR
- Sudden unexplained IUFD
- Abruption

Treatment of Thrombophilias (Acquired and Congenital)

Anticoagulation prevents pregnancy complications

- Warfarin prevents coagulation but as **warfarin is a teratogenic drug, heparin is the drug of choice during pregnancy**
- Treatment includes low-dose aspirin (75–150 mg) and injection heparin 5,000 IU SC twice daily. LMWH preferred, as less side effects. Treatment is started as soon as the pregnancy is confirmed. Aspirin is to be omitted at 34 weeks and heparin is stopped 24 hours before planned delivery (induction) or LSCS
- Postpartum, warfarin can be used or heparin can be continued to prevent DVT.

CHAPTER 20

Preterm, Intrauterine Growth Restriction and Postdatism

Q. Etiology of preterm labor.
Q. Management of threatened preterm labor.
Q. Management of preterm labor.

DEFINITION

Onset of labor before 37 completed weeks of gestation is called preterm labor.

INCIDENCE

Varies in the range of 5–10%.

RISK FACTORS/ETIOLOGY (FLOWCHART 20.1)

- **Most common cause: Idiopathic.** In about 50% cases the cause is not known.
- *Infections:* Urinary tract, dental caries, genital tract infections such as bacterial vaginosis, *Chlamydia, Mycoplasma*, etc.
- *Over distended uterus:* Multiple gestation, polyhydramnios, uterine anomalies like unicornuate, bicornuate uterus, macrosomia, etc.

Flowchart 20.1: Etiopathogenesis of preterm labor.

Choriodecidual bacterial colonization ↑ TNF, ↑ IL → Chorion, amnion and decidua → ↑ PGE_2, $F_{2\alpha}$, ↑ TXA_2, Leukotrienes, ↑ Proteases, ↑ Collagenase → ↑ Myometrial contraction, ↑ Cervical ripening → Preterm labor and delivery

Pathologic uterine enlargement (Polyhydramnios, multiple pregnancy) ↑ Mechanical stretch, ↑ IL, ↑ Gap junction, ↑ PG synthetase

(IL: interleukin; PGE: prostaglandin E2; TNF: tumor necrosis factor; TXA_2: thromboxane A_2)

Chapter 20: Preterm, Intrauterine Growth Restriction and Postdatism

- *Prior preterm delivery:* 16% risk of recurrence of birth before 34 weeks, if prior one delivery is before 34 weeks and 41% risk of recurrence, if prior two birth before 34 weeks.
- Pregnancy complications like preeclampsia, premature rupture of membranes (PROM), antepartum hemorrhage (APH), intrauterine fetal death (IUFD).
- *Medical and surgical illness:* Acute fever, acute pyelonephritis (APN), acute appendicitis, any abdominal surgeries.
- Fibroids.
- Smoking, illicit drug use (especially cocaine).
- Low socioeconomic status.
- *Iatrogenic:* Indicated preterm delivery due to medical or obstetric complications like severe preeclampsia, eclampsia, uteroplacental insufficiency, etc.

MANAGEMENT

Investigations

- Complete blood count (CBC)
- Urine routine and culture and sensitivity
- High vaginal and cervical swab for culture
- Ultrasonography (USG) for fetal biometry, weight, well-being, cervical length, dilatation of os, placental localization.

Treatment

- *Bed rest:* Preferably in left lateral position
- Adequate hydration
- Antibiotics, if infection is present
- Two most important drugs used are **corticosteroids** and **tocolytic agents.**

Steroids

- Steroids (dexamethasone or betamethasone) are given to enhance **fetal lung maturity and they also decrease the incidence of intraventricular hemorrhage (IVH) and necrotizing enterocolitis (NEC). This is beneficial if the delivery is delayed beyond 48 hours of the first dose.**
  - **Betamethasone 12 mg IM 2 doses 24 hours apart or dexamethasone 6 mg IM every 12 hours for 4 doses.**
  - **Betamethasone is preferred over dexamethasone, as it also prevents periventricular leukomalacia.**
- **Chorioamnionitis** and active infection in mother (e.g., open pulmonary Koch) are the only contraindications for the use of steroids. They can be given to patients of hypertension and diabetes mellitus.
- Repeated doses of steroids (weekly) are **to be avoided** as they are a/w risk of necrotizing enterocolitis, intrauterine growth restriction (IUGR), pulmonary edema, and pregnancy-induced hypertension (PIH).

Tocolytic Agents

- Beta-2 agonist (e.g., isoxsuprine, ritodrine, terbutaline, etc.)
- Calcium channel blocker (nifedipine): **Orally, never sublingual**

- Indomethacin
- Magnesium sulfate
- Atosiban (oxytocin antagonist)
- Progesterone (can be used for **prevention** of preterm birth in patients with past history of preterm delivery. However, it is not effective once the contractions have started).

Tocolytics can be used for short-term use or long-term use. **Long-term use is generally avoided**. The objectives of short-term use are:
- To delay the delivery for **at least 48 hours** for steroids to act [to prevent respiratory distress syndrome (RDS) and IVH]
- **In utero transfer** of the patient to higher center with neonatal intensive care unit (NICU) facilities.

Potential Complications of Tocolytic Agents

- **Beta-adrenergic agents**
  - Hyperglycemia
  - Hypokalemia
  - Hypotension
  - Pulmonary edema
  - Cardiac insufficiency
  - Arrhythmias
  - Myocardial ischemia
  - Maternal death.
- **Magnesium sulfate**
  - Pulmonary edema
  - Respiratory depression
  - Cardiac arrest
  - Maternal tetany
  - Muscular paralysis.
- **Indomethacin**
  - Oligohydramnios
  - Premature closure of ductus arteriosus (DA)
  - Renal failure
  - Gastrointestinal bleeding.
- **Nifedipine**
  - Transient hypotension
  - Headache.

Contraindications to Tocolysis

Conditions where delivery is beneficial or needed are contraindications to tocolysis.
- Chorioamnionitis
- Severe preeclampsia or eclampsia
- Advanced labor
- Fetal distress
- Abruption
- Intrauterine fetal death (IUFD)
- Congenital anomalies not compatible with life
- Pregnancy >34 weeks.

Management of Preterm Labor

Multidisciplinary team approach: Obstetrician, anesthetist, neonatologist, and NICU facilities.
- Patient is put to bed to prevent early rupture of membranes
- Adequate pain relief (epidural analgesia)
- Oxygen by breathing mask
- To watch for fetal distress during labor (**preferably continuous EFM**)
- **Birth should be gentle and slow to prevent sudden decompression**
- **Episiotomy preferred to** prevent head compression
- Tendency to delay is curtailed by low or outlet forceps
- Early cord clamping was previously recommended to prevent hypervolemia and hyperbilirubinemia in the baby. However, given the benefits to most newborns the ACOG now recommends a **delay in umbilical cord clamping** in **vigorous term and preterm infants** for at least 30–60 seconds after birth.
- Neonatologist to be present and immediately shift the newborn to NICU.
- Lower segment cesarean section (LSCS) should be done for obstetric indications only.

RECENT ADVANCES

- Magnesium sulfate for fetal neuroprotection (BEAM study: Beneficial effects of antenatal magnesium sulfate)
- Magnesium sulfate reduces the severity and risk of cerebral palsy in surviving infants if administered to mother when birth is anticipated before 32 weeks of gestation.
- If a woman is at risk of preterm birth, she should receive $MgSO_4$ for 12–24 hours to reduce the risk of cerebral palsy.
- Fetal fibronectin (FFN) in cervical/vaginal secretions is a predictor of preterm labor. Increase in maternal salivary estriol is also a predictor.
- **The most sensitive antenatal predictor of preterm birth is cervical length (CL) assessment by TVS**, particularly at 24–28 weeks of gestation. TVS measured cervical length at 24 weeks highly correlates with the risk of preterm delivery. The risk of preterm delivery among women with a **cervix 25 mm or shorter** at 24 weeks is very high.
- Past history of preterm birth (PTB), and short CL are the most important predictive factors for preterm delivery.
- **Progesterone supplementation** (injections/oral/vaginal) in future pregnancies is one of the proven effective methods to prevent PTB in women with history of spontaneous PTB and in women with short CL.

Q. Complications of preterm neonate.

INTRODUCTION

- Baby born before 37 weeks of gestation is preterm. Preterm neonates can have various complications
- Developmental immaturity affects a wide range of organ systems
- The complex interplay of the mechanisms involved in preterm delivery, including inflammation and cytokine injury has been implicated in the pathogenesis of chronic lung disease, necrotizing enterocolitis, retinopathy of prematurity (ROP), and brain white matter injury.

LUNGS AND RESPIRATORY SYSTEM

- ❖ **Respiratory distress syndrome (RDS)**
  - ▷ RDS is associated with surfactant deficiency
  - ▷ The incidence of RDS increases with decreasing gestational age. Respiratory distress is less common in infants born at 33–36 weeks of gestation and is rare in full-term infants
  - ▷ Antenatal administration of glucocorticoids to women at risk for preterm delivery reduces the incidence and severity of RDS as well as the rate of mortality
  - ▷ Soon after birth, preterm infants with RDS develop rapid breathing, grunting, poor color, and crackling or diminished breath sounds breathing requires increased work. Respiratory failure because of fatigue, apnea, hypoxia, or an air leak (from alveolar injury) results from stiff lungs that need high pressures for ventilation.
- ❖ **Congenital pneumonia**
- ❖ **Bronchopulmonary dysplasia and chronic lung disease:** The chronic lung disease (CLD) that sometimes follows RDS in preterm infants is also called bronchopulmonary dysplasia (BPD). BPD/CLD is a chronic disorder that results from inflammation, injury, and scarring of the airways and the alveoli.
- ❖ **Apnea:** Another complication of preterm birth is apnea in which infants may stop breathing for 20 seconds or more, sometimes accompanied by bradycardia.

GASTROINTESTINAL SYSTEM

- ❖ **Necrotizing enterocolitis (NEC)**
  - ▷ It is an acute injury of the small or large intestines that causes inflammation and injury to the bowel lining and that primarily affects preterm infants.
  - ▷ NEC occurs in 3% of infants born before 33 weeks of gestation and in 7% of infants with birth weights less than 1,500 grams.
  - ▷ It typically occurs within 2 weeks of birth and presents as feeding difficulties, abdominal swelling, hypotension, and other signs of sepsis.
  - ▷ The exact cause of NEC is unknown. The preterm infant's intestinal lining is fragile, and stresses (infections and insufficient oxygen or blood flow) can injure it. Inflammation is important in terms of both the etiology and the outcomes.
  - ▷ Injury to the gastrointestinal (GI) tract lining can progress through the wall of the intestines, causing perforation and spilling of the intestinal contents into the abdomen, which causes peritonitis and sepsis.
- ❖ **Gastroesophageal reflux (GER)** is common in preterm infants, often presents as regurgitation, and may adversely affect growth and health. It may also be manifested by aspiration pneumonia, wheezing, or worsening of bronchopulmonary dysplasia (BPD) or chronic lung disease (CLD).

SKIN

- ❖ Skin plays an important role in fluid balance, temperature regulation, and the prevention of infection. The skin of infants born at the lower limit of viability is generally gelatinous, is easily injured when touched, allows tremendous loss of fluids, and does not provide an adequate barrier to infection.
- ❖ **Hypothermia** can develop as there is reduced subcutaneous and brown fat.

INFECTIONS AND THE IMMUNE SYSTEM

- Preterm infants have immature immune systems that are inefficient at fighting off the bacteria, viruses, and other organisms that can cause infections.
- The most serious manifestations of infections commonly seen in preterm infants include **pneumonia, sepsis, meningitis, and urinary tract infections.**
- As many as 65% of infants with birth weights of <1,000 grams have at least one infection during their initial hospitalization.
- Invasive fungal infections occur in 6-7% of infants in NICU, and the rates of such infections increase with decreasing gestational age and birth weight.

CARDIOVASCULAR SYSTEM

- **Patent ductus arteriosus (PDA):** This can lead to heart failure and reduced blood flow to vital body organs.
- **Hypotension** is a frequent concern in preterm infants. The administration of boluses of normal saline and pressors is used to support blood pressure.

HEMATOLOGIC SYSTEM

Anemia: Fetal blood loss, fetomaternal hemorrhage, and hemolysis can all result in congenital anemia, but the most common hematologic complication in preterm infants is anemia of prematurity. Anemia of prematurity is an exaggeration of the physiological anemia of infancy because of suppressed hematopoiesis for 6-12 weeks after birth and is earlier in onset and symptomatic.

AUDITORY SYSTEM

- **Hearing disorder** is attributed to infections, immaturity, asphyxia, ototoxic medications, and hyperbilirubinemia.
- Ventilated infants are at increased risk for **otitis media**.

OPHTHALMIC SYSTEM

- **Retinopathy of prematurity (ROP)** is the most common eye abnormality in preterm infants. It is a neovascular retinal disorder, and its incidence increases with decreasing gestational age and decreasing birth weight. It is multifactorial in etiology with the primary determinant being immaturity with an avascular retina. Environmental factors, including hypoxia, hyperoxia, variations in blood pressure, sepsis, and acidosis may injure the endothelium of the immature retinal blood vessels.
- Other ophthalmologic complications of prematurity include:
  - Refractive disorders (especially myopia)
  - Strabismus
  - Amblyopia
  - Optic nerve atrophy
  - Cataracts
  - Cortical visual impairment
  - Angle closure glaucoma
  - Retinal detachment.

CENTRAL NERVOUS SYSTEM

The most common signs of central nervous system (CNS) injury in preterm infants are:
- IVH
- Intraparenchymal hemorrhage
- White matter injury including periventricular leukomalacia
  - IVH generally begins with bleeding into the germinal matrix just below the lateral ventricles (i.e., a subependymal or germinal matrix hemorrhage).
  - The incidence and severity of IVH increase with decreasing gestational age and birth weight. Factors that contribute to IVH include hypotension, hypertension, fluctuating blood pressures, poor autoregulation of cerebral blood flow, disturbances in coagulation, hyperosmolarity, and injury to the vascular endothelium by oxygen free radicals.
  - Severe IVH can lead to ventricular dilation and posthemorrhagic hydrocephalus, if there is an obstruction to the flow of cerebrospinal fluid with increased intracranial pressure.
- White matter injury and periventricular leukomalacia
- Injury to the periventricular white matter is a sign of CNS injury and is a complication of preterm birth. White matter injury includes a spectrum of CNS injuries, from focal cystic necrotic lesions (also called PVL) to ventricular dilation with irregular ventricular edges or cerebral atrophy.

RENAL SYSTEM

Oliguria and anuria: The immature kidneys are unable to handle water, solute and acid loads.

Q. Types of IUGR.

Q. Etiology of IUGR.

DEFINITION

Birth weight is below the tenth percentile of average for the gestational age.

Comparison of symmetric and asymmetric IUGR fetuses:

Symmetric (20%)	Asymmetric (80%)
Symmetrically small	Head larger than abdomen
Normal ponderal index	Low ponderal index
Head/abdomen and femur/abdomen ratios = normal	Elevated head/abdomen and femur/abdomen ratios
Associated with genetic disease, infection	Placental vascular insufficiency
Total number of cells = less	Normal
Cell size = Normal	Smaller
Complicated neonatal course;	Usually uncomplicated neonatal course
Poor prognosis	Good prognosis
Insult is early in pregnancy	Fetus affected in later months
Brain sparing effect: Absent	Present

INCIDENCE
About 5–15%.

CAUSES OF IUGR

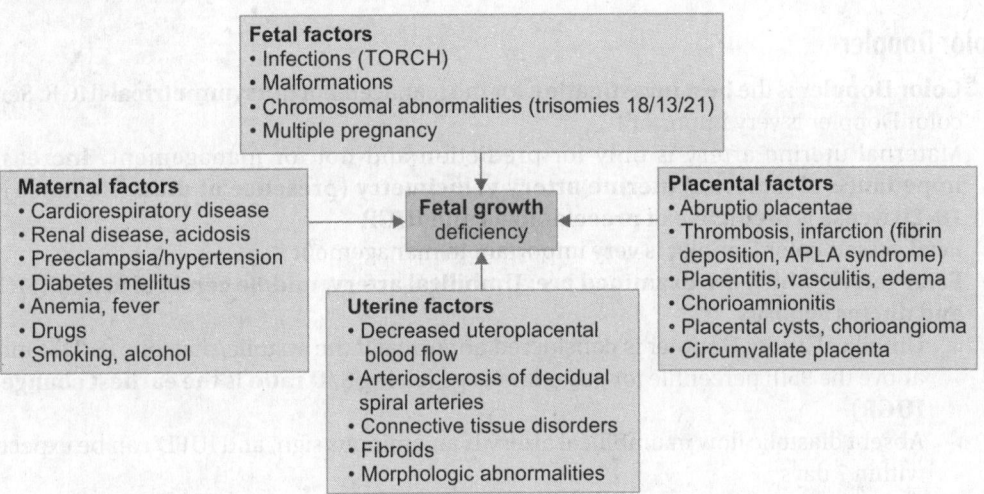

The cause remains unknown in about 40% cases.

DIAGNOSIS

Clinical
- Palpation of uterus for fundal height, approximate liquor volume, and fetal weight
- **Symphysis-fundal height (SFH)** correlates with gestational age. It would be less than what it should be. A lag of 4 cm or more suggests growth restriction. Serial measurement is important
- Abdominal girth will be less than expected
- Maternal weight gain remains stationary or can even decrease.

Ultrasonography (USG)
Ultrasonography helps to diagnose IUGR and also its type (symmetric or asymmetric). Also, it can detect associated oligohydramnios, the estimated birth weight (EBW) and any congenital anomalies in the fetus.

USG Markers for Asymmetric IUGR
- **Abdominal circumference (on USG) is the best marker** for IUGR followed by ponderal index (PI)
- PI = fetal weight divided by third power of femur length. Normal = 8.3
- PI less than 7 indicates IUGR
- FL/AC = 22% is normal, more than 23.5% suggests IUGR
- **Normally, after 34 weeks, HC/AC is less than one.** If it is more than one it suggests asymmetric IUGR

- Fetal glycogen stores from liver are depleted and there is redistribution of blood flow; therefore, AC is smaller than other parameters (BPD and femur length) on USG. FL is not affected by nutrition status
- **Amniotic fluid index (AFI):** In asymmetric IUGR, the liquor would be less because of brain sparing effect.

Color Doppler

- **Color Doppler** is the **best investigation** for the management of **asymmetrical** IUGR. Serial color Doppler is very important
- Maternal uterine artery is only for prediction and not for management: **Increased impedance of maternal uterine artery velocimetry (presence of diastolic notch) at 16–20 weeks is predictive of preeclampsia and IUGR**
- Fetal vessels color Doppler is very important in management
- **Fetal vessels which are examined are: Umbilical artery, middle cerebral artery (MCA) and ductus venosus**
  - Umbilical artery Doppler is considered abnormal if the systolic/diastolic (S/D) ratio is above the 95th percentile for gestational age **(rising S/D ratio is the earliest change in IUGR)**
  - Absent diastolic flow in umbilical artery is an ominous sign, and IUFD can be expected within 7 days
  - In extreme cases of growth restriction, end-diastolic flow in **umbilical artery and ductus venosus may become reversed** and IUFD will occur within 48 hours
  - As the S/D ratio begins to rise in fetus with asymmetric IUGR, **the blood flow in middle cerebral artery (MCA)** increases. There is redistribution of blood flow, and vital organs like brain continue to receive adequate blood at the expense of liver and kidney. This is called as **brain-sparing effect.**
  - **Absent and reversed diastolic flow in umbilical artery on color Doppler is an indication of immediate LSCS (as they indicate impending death).**

■ MANAGEMENT (FLOWCHART 20.2)

Symmetric IUGR

In cases of symmetric IUGR, congenital anomalies, infections, and chromosomal abnormalities should be ruled out. There is no effective treatment.

Asymmetric IUGR

- To monitor for fetal well-being very closely and
- Timely delivery to prevent IUFD.

General

There is **no proven definitive treatment**, but the following may help:
- Adequate bed rest in left lateral position
- **High protein diet**, 300 extra calories/day, hyperalimentation by amino acids especially arginine
- **Corticosteroids** to be given prophylactically to enhance the lung maturity, as early delivery may be necessary

Chapter 20: Preterm, Intrauterine Growth Restriction and Postdatism

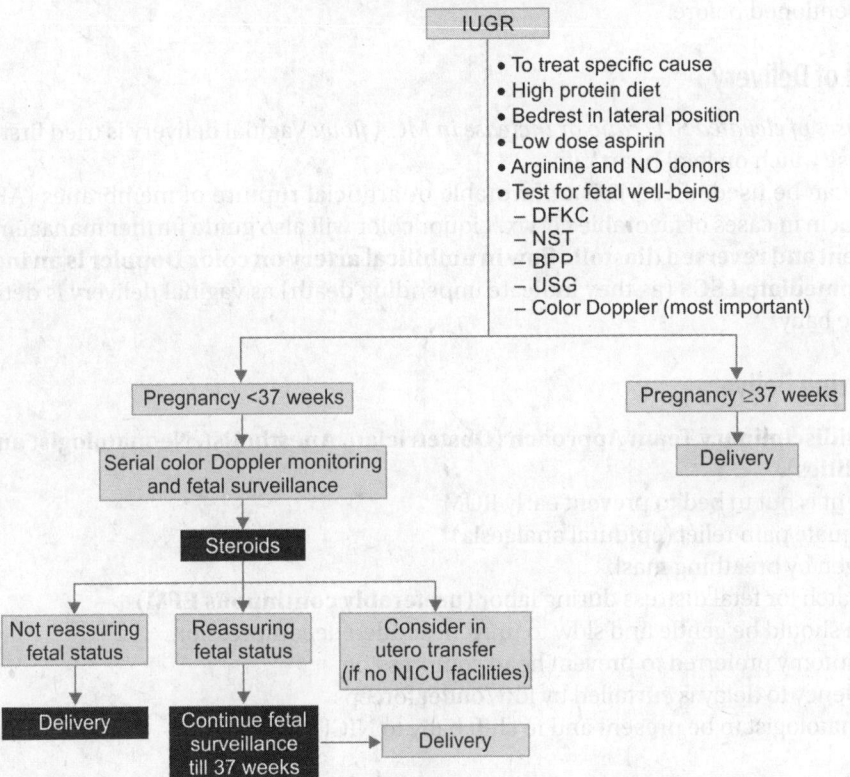

Flowchart 20.2: Management of IUGR.

(BPP: biophysical profile; DFKC: daily fetal kick counts; NICU: neonatal intensive care unit; NST: nonstress test; USG: ultrasonography)

- Avoiding smoking, nicotine, tobacco, and alcohol
- Control of hypertension, preeclampsia if present
- Maternal hyperoxygenation @2.5 liters/day
- Maternal volume expansion may help in improving placental perfusion
- **Low dose aspirin 75–150 mg** may be helpful in selected cases of pre-eclampsia, thrombophilias
- DHA supplementation may also help
- **Arginine and nitric oxide donors** are known to increase the placental blood flow and help in uteroplacental insufficiency
- NTG patches applied on the abdomen are also known to have similar effect
- **Sildenafil 25 mg two to three times** a day can be tried to improve placental blood flow and help in uteroplacental insufficiency.

Test for Fetal Well-being

- Daily fetal kick count (DFKC)
- Nonstress test (NST), weekly or biweekly
- Biophysical profile (BPP)
- USG for AFI, EBW, placental maturity. Serial USG 3–4 weeks interval may be needed

- ❖ Color Doppler is the most important and serial color Doppler helps in timing of the delivery as mentioned before.

Method of Delivery

- ❖ *In cases of elevated S/D ratio or increase in MCA flow:* Vaginal delivery is tried first keeping a close watch on fetal heart rate.
- ❖ PGs can be used, if cervix is unfavorable or artificial rupture of membranes (ARM) and oxytocin in cases of favorable cervix. Liquor color will also guide further management.
- ❖ **Absent and reversed diastolic flow in umbilical artery on color Doppler is an indication of immediate LSCS** (as they indicate impending death) as vaginal delivery is detrimental of the baby.

Care During Delivery

- ❖ **Multidisciplinary Team Approach (Obstetrician, Anesthetist, Neonatologist and NICU Facilities).**
- ❖ Patient is put to bed to prevent early ROM
- ❖ Adequate pain relief (epidural analgesia)
- ❖ Oxygen by breathing mask
- ❖ To watch for fetal distress during labor **(preferably continuous EFM)**
- ❖ Birth should be gentle and slow to prevent sudden decompression
- ❖ Episiotomy preferred to prevent head compression
- ❖ Tendency to delay is curtailed by low/outlet forceps
- ❖ Neonatologist to be present and to shift baby to NICU, if needed.

Q. Complications and management of postdatism.

■ DEFINITION

Postdatism is defined as pregnancy continuing beyond EDD or 40 weeks of gestation whereas post-term is pregnancy continuing more than 42 weeks.

■ ETIOLOGY/RISK FACTORS

- ❖ Idiopathic
- ❖ Past history/family history
- ❖ Anencephaly
- ❖ Fetal adrenal hypoplasia
- ❖ X-linked placental sulfatase deficiency
- ❖ Primiparity.

■ COMPLICATIONS

Fetal

Antenatal

Placental ageing leads to placental insufficiency leading to:
- ❖ **Oligohydramnios:** Liquor is 800 mL at 40 weeks and about 450 mL at 42 weeks

- ❖ Meconium stained amniotic fluid (MSAF)
- ❖ Fetal hypoxia, distress and **sudden IUFD**.

Intrapartum
- ❖ Meconium aspiration
- ❖ Cord compression
- ❖ Shoulder dystocia, birth trauma
- ❖ Uterine dysfunction
- ❖ Increased risk of operative delivery
- ❖ Fetal hypoxia, distress.

After Birth
- ❖ Meconium aspiration syndrome
- ❖ Hypoglycemia
- ❖ Polycythemia.

Maternal

Increased risk of induction of labor, instrumental delivery, and LSCS.

CLINICAL FEATURES

In cases of post-term pregnancy the following features may be seen:
- ❖ Stationary or falling weight
- ❖ Diminished abdominal girth due to decrease in liquor
- ❖ Uterus feels **'full of fetus' due to decrease in liquor**
- ❖ Hard skull bones on abdominal and vaginal examination.

MANAGEMENT (FLOWCHART 20.3)

To **confirm postdatism** and fetal maturity:
- ❖ **Menstrual history:** It is very useful to calculate the period of gestation, if the patient is sure of her dates and has previous regular cycles.
- ❖ But in cases of mistaken/wrong dates or if the patient has conceived in lactational amenorrhea then the following clinical criteria are needed to confirm a term gestation:
  - ▸ Fetal heart tones have been demonstrated for at least 20 completed weeks by stethoscope or at least 30 completed weeks by Doppler ultrasound
  - ▸ Appropriate uterine size was established by pelvic examination prior to 16 weeks.
- ❖ Ultrasound determinations needed to confirm a term gestation:
  - ▸ Gestational age based on the measurement of **crown-rump length obtained between 6–11 weeks of gestation (dating scan)**
  - ▸ To confirm postdatism USG in first trimester (dating scan) is most useful.
  - ▸ Very rarely amniocentesis and biochemical (L:S ratio) and cytological evaluation of amniotic fluid may be required. However in presence of USG this is rarely required.

Flowchart 20.3: Management of postdatism.

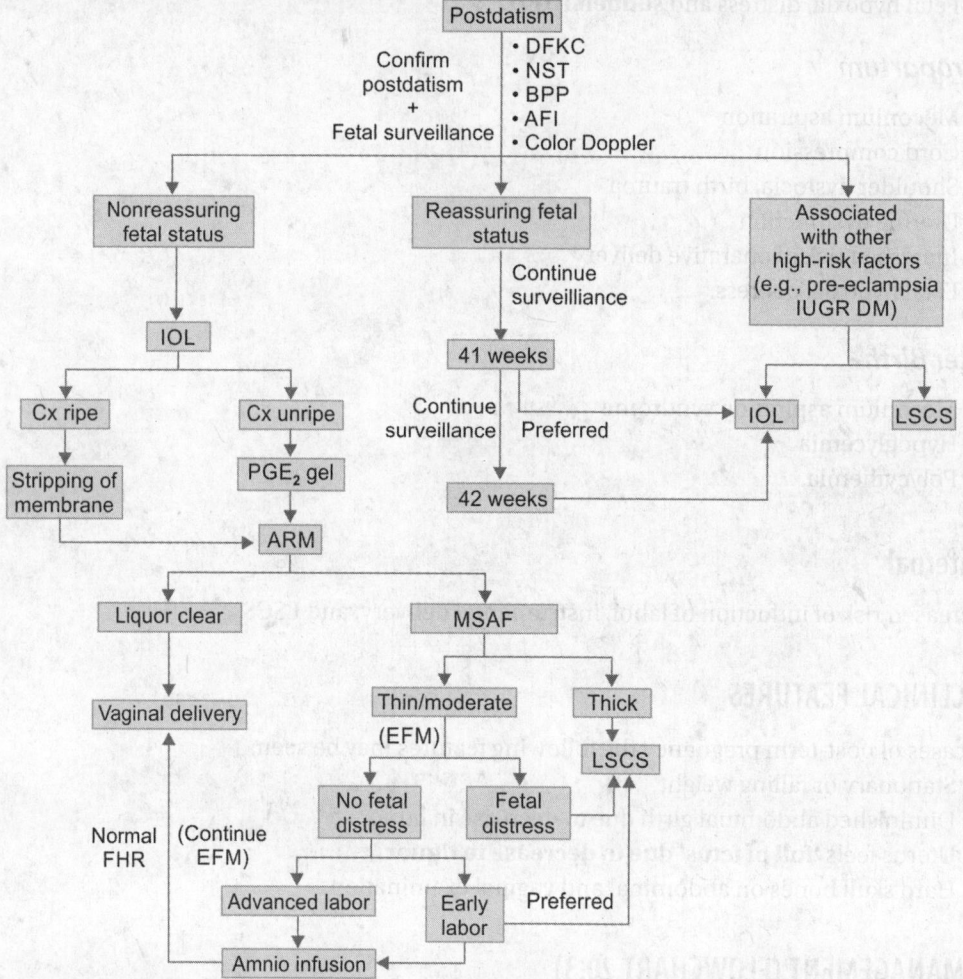

(AFI: amniotic fluid index; ARM: artificial rupture of membranes; BPP: biophysical profile; DFKC: daily fetal kick counts; DM: diabetes mellitus; EFM: electronic fetal monitoring; FHR: fetal heart rate; IOL: induction of labor; IUGR: intrauterine growth restriction; LSCS: lower segment cesarean section; MSAF: meconium-stained amniotic fluid; NICU: neonatal intensive care unit; NST: nonstress test; USG: ultrasonography; Cx: cervix)

- ❖ Assessment of fetal well-being to detect placental insufficiency:
  - ➢ **NST (biweekly)**
  - ➢ BPP and AFI
  - ➢ Color Doppler
  - ➢ Delivery should be done, if there is evidence of fetal compromise or oligohydramnios.
  - ➢ Prostaglandin can be used for cervical ripening and labor induction.

CHAPTER 21

Puerperal Sepsis

Q. Define puerperal pyrexia. Causes of puerperal pyrexia.

Q. Puerperal sepsis.

■ PUERPERAL PYREXIA

Definition

A rise in temperature reaching **100.4°F (38°C) or more** (measured orally) on **two** separate occasions at 24 hours apart **(excluding the first 24 hours) within the first 10 days** following delivery is called puerperal pyrexia.

Causes

- Puerperal sepsis
- Acute pyelonephritis, cystitis
- Breast engorgement, mastitis, breast abscess
- Wound infection [lower segment cesarean section (LSCS)/episiotomy]
- Septic pelvic thrombophlebitis
- Atelectasis and pneumonia
- Unknown origin
- A recrudescence of malaria, pulmonary tuberculosis (TB).

Puerperal Sepsis

Puerperal sepsis is infection of the genital tract which occurs as a complication of delivery. Postpartum uterine infection has been called by various names as endometritis, endomyometritis, and endoparametritis. As the infection actually involves not only the decidua but also the myometrium and parametrial tissues, the preferred term is metritis with pelvic cellulitis.

Route of Delivery

The **single most significant risk factor** for the development of uterine infection is the **route of delivery**.

Compared with cesarean delivery, metritis following vaginal delivery is relatively uncommon. Most pelvic infections are caused by bacteria indigenous to the genital tract.

Predisposing Factors of Puerperal Sepsis
Antepartum
- Malnutrition and anemia
- Preeclampsia
- Premature rupture of membranes (PROM)
- Immunocompromised status [human immunodeficiency virus (HIV)]
- Diabetes mellitus
- Obesity.

Intrapartum
- Multiple cervical examinations
- Internal fetal monitoring
- Chorioamnionitis
- Retained bits of placenta or membranes
- Antepartum hemorrhage (APH) and postpartum hemorrhage (PPH)
- Prolonged labor (dehydration, ketoacidosis), prolonged rupture of membranes (>18 hours)
- Operative delivery (LSCS)
- Meconium stained amniotic fluid (MSAF)
- Traumatic operative delivery
- Placenta previa (placental site is close to vagina).

Bacteria Commonly Responsible for Female Genital Infections
Aerobes
- Group A, B, D beta-hemolytic streptococci
- Enterococcus
- Gram-negative bacteria—*Escherichia coli, Klebsiella* and *Proteus* species
- *Staphylococcus aureus*, MRSA
- *Gardnerella vaginalis*.

Anaerobes
- *Peptococcus* species
- *Peptostreptococcus* species
- *Bacteroides* species
- *Clostridium* species
- *Fusobacterium* species
- *Mobiluncus* species.

Other
- *Mycoplasma* species
- *Chlamydia trachomatis*
- *Neisseria gonorrhoeae*.

Most of the infections are polymicrobial.
- Fever is the most important feature for the diagnosis of postpartum metritis. Temperature commonly exceeds 38–39°C. Chills may accompany fever and suggest bacteremia, which is documented in 10–20% of women with pelvic infection following cesarean delivery.

Flowchart 21.1: Pathogenesis of metritis following cesarean delivery.

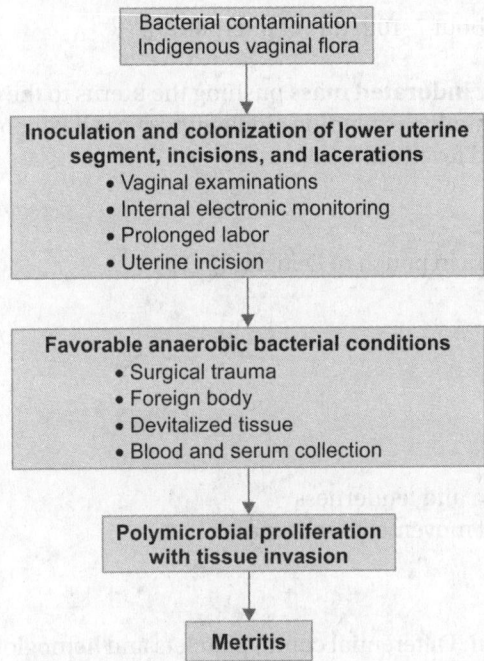

- Women have foul-smelling lochia. Other infections, notably those due to group A hemolytic streptococci, are frequently associated with scanty, odorless lochia.
- Leukocytosis may range from 15,000 cells/µL to 30,000 cells/µL.
- Complications of metritis that cause persistent fever despite appropriate therapy include a parametrial phlegmon or an area of intense cellulitis, a surgical incisional or pelvic abscess, and infected hematoma, and septic pelvic thrombophlebitis (**Flowchart 21.1**).

Clinical Features

Endometritis

- Fever with **chills and rigor**
- Tachycardia
- Lower abdominal tenderness on one or both sides of the abdomen
- Adnexal and parametrial tenderness
- **Foul-smelling lochia** without other evidence of infection
- Some infections, most notably caused by group A beta-hemolytic streptococci, are frequently associated with scanty, odorless lochia
- Uterus is tender and **subinvoluted**.

Wound Infections

Patients with wound infections, or episiotomy infections, have erythema, edema, tenderness out of proportion to expected postpartum pain, and discharge from the wound or episiotomy site. With severe infection there is fever with chills.

Parametritis

- The onset is usually about 7–10th day of puerperium
- Constant pelvic pain
- *PV*: **Unilateral tender indurated mass** pushing the uterus to the opposite side
- *PR*: Confirms the induration extending along uterosacral ligament
- Spiky temperature and fever with chills.

Pelvic Abscess

- Bulging, fluctuant mass in pouch of Douglas (POD)
- Swinging temperature
- Diarrhea.

Pelvic Peritonitis

- Pyrexia
- Tachycardia
- Lower abdominal pain and tenderness
- Forniceal and cervical movement tenderness.

Investigations

- *Complete blood count*: Differential count, platelets and hemoglobin (Hb)
- Electrolytes
- Thick blood film for malarial parasites
- Blood cultures, if sepsis is suspected
- "Clean catch" mid stream specimen for urinalysis, with cultures and sensitivity tests
- **High vaginal and endocervical swabs** for cultures (aerobic and anaerobic) and antibiotic sensitivity
- Wound cultures, if appropriate
- Coagulation studies, if pelvic thrombosis, deep vein thrombosis, pulmonary embolism, or invasive treatment (e.g., surgical procedure) is being considered
- Pelvic ultrasonography (USG) may be helpful in detecting retained products of conception, pelvic abscess, or infected hematoma. Color Doppler to detect venous thrombosis
- Contrast-enhanced computed tomography (CT) or magnetic resonance imaging (MRI) are useful in establishing the diagnosis of septic pelvic thrombosis
- Chest X-ray to detect pulmonary pathology like collapse and atelectasis and also in cases of pulmonary Kochs.

Treatment

- Patient isolation especially if hemolytic streptococci is obtained on culture
- Intravenous (IV) fluids
- To correct anemia with iron and blood transfusion in severe cases
- To maintain temperature, pulse, blood pressure (BP), urine output chart.

Antimicrobial Regimens for Pelvic Infection following Cesarean Delivery

- Clindamycin 900 mg + gentamicin 1.5 mg/kg, q8h intravenously gold standard, 90–97% efficacy, once-daily gentamicin dosing acceptable

- ❖ *Plus ampicillin:* Added to regimen with sepsis syndrome or suspected enterococcal infection
- ❖ *Clindamycin + aztreonam:* Gentamicin substitute in patients with renal insufficiency
- ❖ *Extended-spectrum penicillins:* Piperacillin, ampicillin/sulbactam can be used
- ❖ *Imipenem + cilastatin:* Reserved for special indications.

Surgical Treatment

- ❖ It has a limited role.
- ❖ **Wound infection or episiotomy infection**: Drainage, debridement, and irrigation may be required. After the infection is controlled secondary suturing may be required.
- ❖ **Retained products**: Surgical evacuation under antibiotic cover.
- ❖ **Pelvic abscess**: Drained by colpotomy under USG guidance.
- ❖ **Unresponsive peritonitis**: Laparotomy and drainage of pus.
- ❖ Hysterectomy only in cases of **rupture or perforation having multiple abscesses, gangrenous uterus or gas gangrene infection**. Ruptured tubo-ovarian abscess should be removed.

Q. Physiology of lactation.

LACTATION

Physiology

About 500–800 mL of milk is produced by a healthy mother per day which requires 700 kcal/day. Physiological basis consists of four phases:

1. **Mammogenesis:** Growth of both ductal and lobuloalveolar systems occur in pregnancy.
2. **Lactogenesis:** Colostrum secretion is noted during pregnancy and immediately postdelivery. Milk secretion starts around the third postpartum day. Despite high prolactin levels in pregnancy, milk is not secreted as the high levels of estrogen and progesterone make the breast tissue unresponsive. **With withdrawal of estrogen and progesterone levels postdelivery, prolactin acts on the breast tissue.** Growth hormone, thyroxine and insulin also increase secretory activity.
3. **Galactokinesis:** Milk is discharged due to the infant's suckling efforts and also a contractile mechanism which expresses milk from the alveoli into the ducts. **Oxytocin is a major galactokinetic hormone.**
4. **Galactopoiesis:** The most important hormone is **prolactin**. Suckling is essential for effective and continuous lactation. Periodic feeding is essential to relieve the pressure which then maintains the secretion.

Milk Ejection Reflex

Reflex by which milk is forced down into the ampulla of the lactiferous duct, where it can be sucked out by the baby. This reflex is inhibited by adverse psychic conditions, pain or breast engorgement **(Fig. 21.1)**.

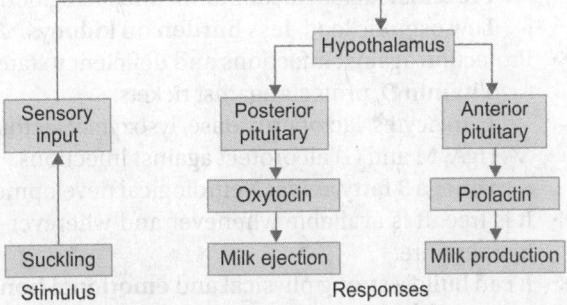

Fig. 21.1: Milk ejection reflex.

Stimulation of Lactation

Early motivation for breastfeeding. Early (within half an hour of delivery) and exclusive breastfeeding in the correct position should be encouraged.

Important steps are:
- To put the baby to breast every 2 hours
- Plenty of oral fluids
- To avoid breast engorgement.

Drugs that improve milk production (galactogogues): Metoclopramide 10 mg thrice daily increases prolactin levels. Oxytocin contracts myoepithelial cells and causes milk let down.

Lactation Suppression

Indications
- Intrauterine fetal death (IUFD), neonatal death
- Breastfeeding not possible due to personal or medical reasons
- Breastfeeding is contraindicated.

Methods
- To stop breastfeeding
- To avoid breast handling
- Tight breast support, compression bandage
- Icepacks
- Analgesics
- **Medical methods: Cabergoline, bromocriptine**, estrogen, androgen, pyridoxine.

Q. Advantages of breastfeeding.

BREASTFEEDING

Advantages

- Breast milk is the ideal and only natural food designed for baby. Its constituents are:
  - **Carbohydrates:** Mainly lactose, stimulates growth of intestinal flora and helps in vitamin B synthesis.
  - **Fat:** Smaller fat globules, easily digested.
  - **Proteins:** Rich in lactalbumin and lactoglobulin.
  - Low osmotic load, **less burden on kidneys**.
- Protection against infections and deficiency states:
  - **Vitamin D**, protects against rickets.
  - Leukocytes, lactoperoxidase, lysozyme, lactoferrin, **interferons and immunoglobulins** (IgA, M and G) all protect against infections.
  - **Omega 3 fatty acids:** Neurological development.
- It is free. It is available whenever and wherever the baby needs a feed and is at the right temperature.
- It can build a strong physical and **emotional bond** between mother and baby.
- Breastfed babies have:
  - Less chance of diarrhea and vomiting, fewer chest and ear infections.

- Less likelihood of becoming obese and therefore developing type 2 diabetes and other obesity-related illnesses later.
- Less chance of developing eczema.
- Decreased risk of developing chronic conditions, such as type I diabetes, celiac disease and Crohn's disease.
- Less chance of being constipated.
❖ Less risk of cancer: Breastfeeding can decrease baby's risk of some childhood cancers and **lowers mother's risk of premenopausal breast cancer and ovarian cancer.**
❖ Exclusive breastfeeding can also delay the return of periods and act as **natural contraception.**
❖ The oxytocin released when the baby nurses help uterus contract, reducing postdelivery blood loss. Breastfeeding also helps in involution of the uterus.

Q. Baby friendly hospital.

■ INTRODUCTION

The Baby Friendly Hospital Initiative (BFHI), also known as Baby Friendly Initiative (BFI), is a worldwide program of the **World Health Organization and UNICEF, launched in 1991** following the adoption of the Innocenti Declaration on breastfeeding promotion in 1990.

■ CRITERIA FOR ACCREDITATION

The criteria for a hospital's baby friendly accreditation include:
❖ Have a written breastfeeding policy that is routinely communicated to all healthcare staff.
❖ Train all healthcare staff in skills necessary to implement this policy.
❖ Inform all pregnant women about the benefits and management of breastfeeding.
❖ Help mothers initiate breastfeeding within one hour of birth.
❖ Show mothers how to breastfeed and maintain lactation, even if they should be separated from their infants.
❖ Give newborn infants no food or drink other than breast milk, not even sips of water, unless medically indicated.
❖ Practice rooming in, i.e., allow mothers and infants to remain together 24 hours a day.
❖ Encourage breastfeeding on demand.
❖ Give no artificial teats or pacifiers (also called dummies or soothers) to breastfeeding infants.
❖ Foster the establishment of breastfeeding support groups and refer mothers to them on discharge from the hospital or clinic.

CHAPTER 22

Obstructed Labor and Rupture Uterus

Q. Causes, clinical features, and management of obstructed labor.
Q. Bandl's ring.
Q. Difference between Schroeder's ring and Bandl's ring.

INTRODUCTION

Obstructed labor is one of the common preventable causes of maternal and perinatal morbidity and mortality in developing countries where there is no easy access to health facilities with the capability of carrying out operative deliveries.

DEFINITION

In spite of good/adequate uterine contractions, the progressive descent of presenting part is arrested due to mechanical obstruction (fault with passage and/or passenger).

The prevalence is 1-2% in developing countries.

CAUSES

There is no fault in power (remember the power is always normal or even more than normal in obstructed labor).

Fault in Passage

- **Cephalopelvic disproportion (CPD)**
- **Contracted pelvis** (undernutrition in childhood is common resulting in small pelvis in women)
- Cervical dystocia (prolapse or scarring)
- Cervical or broad ligament fibroid
- Impacted ovarian tumor or nongravid horn of bicornuate uterus below presenting part.

Fault in Passenger

- **Transverse lie**

- Brow/mentoposterior face presentation/compound presentation
- Occipitoposterior position
- **Hydrocephalus/fetal ascites**
- **Macrosomia**
- Locked twins.

EFFECTS/COMPLICATIONS

Maternal

Immediate

- Exhaustion
- Dehydration, **ketoacidosis** (increased muscular activity without fluids and accumulation of lactic acid and ketones)
- Genital sepsis, chorioamnionitis
- **Rupture uterus** (spontaneous or traumatic following instrumental delivery)
- **Postpartum hemorrhage (PPH)** and shock (atonic and traumatic)
- **Maternal morbidity and mortality** (death mainly due to rupture uterus, shock, and sepsis).

Late

- **Genitourinary fistula [vesicovaginal fistula (VVF) and rectovaginal fistula (RVF)]**
- Vaginal atresia
- **Sheehan's syndrome**
- Secondary amenorrhea (following hysterectomy in cases of rupture uterus).

Fetal

- Asphyxia (tonic uterine contractions or cord prolapse in transverse lie)
- Acidosis (fetal hypoxia and maternal acidosis)
- Intracranial hemorrhage (supermoulding, tentorial tear or traumatic delivery)
- Infections
- Intrauterine fetal death (IUFD)
- Perinatal mortality.

CLINICAL FEATURES

- Patient is in agony, discomfort, restless
- Exhaustion and ketoacidosis
- Other features of constriction and retraction ring are:

Features	Constriction ring (Schroeder's ring)	Retraction ring (Bandl's ring)
Nature	Due to localized incoordinate uterine contraction	It is an end result of tonic uterine contraction and retraction
Cause	Undue irritability of the uterus	Following obstructed labor
Position	Usually at the junction of upper and lower segment but may occur in other places. The position does not alter	Always situated at the junction of upper and lower segment. The position progressively moves upward

Contd...

Contd...

Features	Constriction ring (Schroeder's ring)	Retraction ring (Bandl's ring)
Lower segment	Upper segment contracts and retracts with relaxation in between, lower segment remains thick and loose	Upper segment is tonically contracted with no relaxation. The wall becomes thicker; lower segment becomes distended and thinned out
Abdominal examination	• Uterus feels normal and not tender • Fetal parts are easily felt • Ring is not felt • Round ligament is not felt • FHS is usually present	• Uterus is tense and tender • Not easily felt • Ring is felt as a groove placed obliquely • Taut and tender round ligaments are felt • FHS is usually absent (IUFD)
Vaginal examination	• The lower segment is not pressed by the presenting part • Ring is felt usually above the head • Features of obstructed labor are absent	• Lower segment is very much pressed by the forcibly driven presenting part • Ring cannot be felt vaginally • Features of obstructed labor are present
End result	• Exhaustion to the mother is a late feature • Fetal anoxia due to prolonged uterine hypertonic state may appear late • Chance of uterine rupture is absent	• Exhaustion and sepsis appear early • Fetal death is usually early due to tonic contraction and exaggerated retraction • Ruptured uterus more in multigravidas and uterine exhaustion and rupture in primigravidas are the common mode to terminations
Principle of treatment	To relax the ring followed by delivery of the baby. LSCS and cut the ring if needed	To relieve the obstruction by safe procedure (usually LSCS even in cases of IUFD) after excluding ruptured uterus

(FHS: fetal heart sound; IUFD: intrauterine fetal death; LSCS: lower segment cesarean section)

TREATMENT

The principles are **"never wait and watch and never use oxytocin"**
- To relieve the obstruction at the earliest by safe delivery
- To combat dehydration, ketoacidosis
- To control sepsis.

Preliminaries

- Two wide bore IV lines
- Send blood for cross matching and keep one pint ready
- Intravenous fluids [Ringer's lactate solution (RL)] at least 1 L in given in running drip. At least 3 L of fluid required
- Intravenous antibiotics cefotaxime or ceftriaxone 1 g and metronidazole.

Definitive Treatment

- Rupture uterus must be ruled out first.
- **"Never wait and watch and never use oxytocin"** as it increases the risk of rupture uterus.
- **There is no place for internal version and destructive operations in modern day obstetrics.**

- LSCS gives the best results and would be required in majority cases (will have to be done **even in cases of IUFD**).
- If the head is low down (station +2 or +3) and vaginal delivery is not risky the forceps extraction can be done.

■ PREVENTION

- **Antenatal** detection of factors likely to cause obstructed labor (macrosomia, CPD, short stature, malpresentations, etc).
- **Intranatal:** Use of **partograph**, strict vigilance and timely intervention and referral if needed.

Q. Causes of rupture uterus.
Q. Etiology, clinical features, and management of rupture uterus.

■ DEFINITION

Disruption in the continuity of all uterine layers—endometrium, myometrium and serosa anytime beyond 28 weeks of pregnancy is called rupture of uterus.

■ INCIDENCE

1 in 2,000 to 1 in 200 deliveries. Rupture uterus from obstructed labor is becoming less because of improved obstetric care, but prevalence of scar rupture is increased because of increase in LSCS rates.

■ ETIOLOGY

Rupture of previous LSCS scar during VBAC is one of the most common causes of rupture uterus today.
- Spontaneous (intact or unscarred uterus)
- Scar rupture
- Iatrogenic.

The rupture can happen during pregnancy or during labor **(Flowchart 22.1)**.
- **Spontaneous rupture** during pregnancy is **very rare** and is complete and involves the upper segment and occurs in later months of pregnancy
- Obstructive rupture (following obstructed labor) involves the lower segment and extends through one lateral wall to the upper segment
- Classical C section scar or hysterotomy scar generally gives way in **third trimester** of pregnancy
- **LSCS scar generally ruptures in labor (mainly in second stage** or toward end of first stage) and unlikely to rupture during pregnancy
- Iatrogenic rupture is mainly due to injudicious use of **oxytocin or prostaglandins** (for induction or augmentation of labor) and **very rarely due to internal podalic version and destructive operations as they are not performed in modern day obstetrics**.

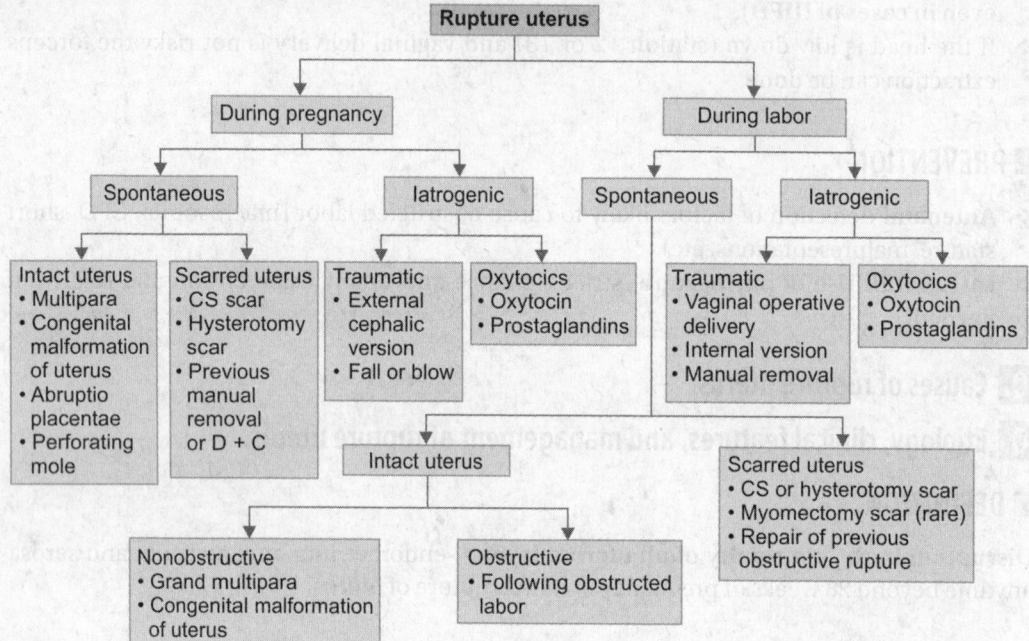

Flowchart 22.1: Scheme showing etiology of rupture uterus.

CLINICAL FEATURES

During Pregnancy

Classical or Hysterotomy Scar

- Dull abdominal pain over scar area
- Vaginal bleeding
- Tenderness on palpation
- Fetal distress/IUFD
- Something giving way, acute pain and collapse when the rupture is complete.

Following uterine ruptures the most common electronic fetal monitoring finding tends to be sudden, severe heart rate decelerations that may evolve into late decelerations, bradycardia, and undetectable fetal heart action (IUFD).

During Labor

Obstructive Rupture

Premonitory Phase

- Generally multipara in labor with features of obstruction
- Strong frequent uterine contractions followed by continuous pain in suprapubic area
- Dehydration, exhaustion, tachycardia, rise in temperature
- Distended lower segment, Bandl's ring
- Fetal distress/IUFD
- Presenting part jammed in pelvis, dry, edematous vagina.

Phase of Rupture

- **Something giving way** at height of contraction
- Cessation of contractions
- Shock and exhaustion
- **Superficial fetal parts**
- Absence of FHS
- A firm contracted uterus may at times be felt alongside the fetus
- **PV: Loss of station** (recession of presenting part)
- Bleeding PV.

With rupture and expulsion of the fetus into the peritoneal cavity, the chances for fetal survival are dismal and reported mortality rates range from 50–75%.

LSCS Scar Rupture

Impending scar rupture (scar dehiscence)	Scar rupture
Unexplained tachycardia	Weak thready fast pulse
Hypotension	Shock
Fetal tachycardia	Persistent fetal bradycardia/IUFD
Uterine scar tenderness	Hematuria
Bleeding PV	Bleeding PV
Hematuria	Recession of presenting part

(IUFD: Intrauterine fetal death)

Rupture following Instrumental or Manipulative Delivery

- Sudden deterioration of general condition of patient and vaginal bleeding following delivery
- Exploration of uterus to feel the rent confirms diagnosis
- Shock, broad ligament hematoma
- Shortening of cord immediately following a difficult vaginal delivery is pathognomonic.

■ TREATMENT

Resuscitation

- Two wide bore IV lines
- Send blood for cross matching
- **Intravenous fluids (Ringer's Lactate)** in running drip
- Intravenous antibiotics cefotaxime or ceftriaxone 1 g and metronidazole
- **Start blood transfusion**.

Laparotomy

Hysterectomy

- **Unless there is sufficient reason to preserve the uterus, quick subtotal hysterectomy** is needed in most of the cases, especially in multipara and obstructive rupture
- If condition permits and/or there is colporrhexis, total hysterectomy may be done.

Repair

- Mostly in cases of scar rupture, where margins are clean or in obstructive rupture and desirous of child
- Excision of fibrous/necrosed tissue followed by suturing the defect
- **Sterilization (tubal ligation) to be offered**.

PREVENTION

- Antenatal detection of factors likely to cause obstructed labor (macrosomia, CPD, short stature, malpresentations, etc.) and rupture uterus (previous cesarean section, hysterotomy, myomectomy) and **mandatory hospital delivery**
- Avoid undue force in external cephalic version (ECV)
- Judicious selection of cases for vaginal birth after one cesarean section (VBAC) and strict monitoring in labor
- Judicious use of oxytocin/prostaglandins (PGs) for induction/augmentation of labor and careful watch
- **Intranatal:** Use of partograph, strict vigilance and timely intervention and referral if needed
- Internal podalic version (IPV) and destructive operations not to be done in modern day obstetrics.

CHAPTER 23

Vesicular Mole and Liquor Disorders

Q. Mention the conditions in which uterus is more than weeks of gestation. Describe the clinical features of vesicular mole.

Q. Clinical features and complications of molar pregnancy.

Conditions in which uterus is **more than period of amenorrhea**:
- Wrong dates
- Twins, multiple pregnancy
- Polyhydramnios
- Macrosomia
- Ovarian tumors, fibroids
- Vesicular mole
- Concealed abruption.

DEFINITION

Gestational trophoblastic disease encompasses several disease processes that originate in the placenta. These include complete and partial moles, placental site trophoblastic tumors, choriocarcinomas, and invasive moles.

Vesicular mole is an abnormal condition of placenta where there is hydropic degeneration and proliferative changes in the young chorionic villi. It is a **benign condition with malignant potential**.

INCIDENCE OF MOLAR PREGNANCY

Incidence of molar pregnancy is highest in women aged **15 years or younger and those aged 45 years or older** (extremes of reproductive age). In the latter group, the relative frequency of the lesion is at least 10 times greater than that at ages 20–40 years.

CLINICAL FEATURES

Symptoms

- **Uterine bleeding** is almost universal and may vary from spotting to profuse hemorrhage. It is the most common presenting feature. The discharge has **"white currant in red currant juice"** appearance.

- *Lower abdominal pain*: The pain can be due to overstretching of the uterus, uterine contractions, infection, concealed hemorrhage and rarely perforation by invasive mole.
- *Constitutional symptoms*:
  - Excessive symptoms of pregnancy like nausea, vomiting and even hyperemesis [due to excessive human chorionic gonadotropin (hCG)]
  - Thyrotoxic features like tachycardia, tremors
- Passage of grapes-like vesicles is **pathognomonic**
- Fetal movements are not felt.

Signs

- Features suggestive of early pregnancy
- The patient looks ill
- Pallor is present and may be out of proportion to the visible loss (due to concealed hemorrhage)
- Feature of preeclampsia like hypertension, proteinuria edema are present in about 50% cases.

Per Abdomen

- The size of the uterus is **more than period of amenorrhea**
- Uterus feels firm elastic (doughy)
- The fetal parts cannot be felt and external ballottement cannot be elicited
- Fetal heart sounds cannot be heard or detected.

Per Vaginum (PV)

- Internal ballottement absent
- Bilateral or unilateral: Theca lutein cysts may be palpable in 25–50% cases
- **Finding of vesicles in the discharge is pathognomonic** and similarly if the os is open the vesicles may be felt.

INVESTIGATIONS

- Blood group.
- *Quantitative beta-hCG*: hCG levels greater than 1,00,000 mIU/mL indicate excessive trophoblastic growth and raise suspicion for a molar pregnancy. Serum hCG value more than 2 multiple of median (MOM) for the gestational age is of value. However, a molar pregnancy may have a normal hCG level. Pre-evacuation levels are very important for follow-up.
- *Complete blood cell count with platelets*: Anemia could be present and coagulopathy can occur.
- *Clotting function*: To exclude the development of a coagulopathy or to treat one if present.
- *Liver and renal function tests (LFT and RFT)*: Blood urea nitrogen (BUN) and serum creatinine.
- *Thyroxine*: Although women with molar pregnancies are usually clinically euthyroid, plasma thyroxine is usually elevated above the reference range for pregnancy. Patient may present with signs and symptoms of hyperthyroidism.

Chapter 23: Vesicular Mole and Liquor Disorders

- *USG*: Classical finding is the **snow storm appearance**.
  - **Theca lutein cysts:** These are ovarian cysts, may be greater than 6 cm in diameter and accompanying ovarian enlargement. These are identified by ultrasonography (USG). Patients may report pressure or pelvic pain. Because of the increased ovarian size, torsion is a risk. These cysts develop in response to high levels of beta-hCG. They spontaneously regress after the mole is evacuated, but it may take up to 12 weeks for complete regression.
- *Chest X-ray*: Once a molar pregnancy is diagnosed, a baseline chest radiograph should be taken. The lungs are a primary site of metastasis for malignant trophoblastic tumors and also to rule out pulmonary embolism.
- Definitive diagnosis is made by **histological examination** of the products.

COMPLICATIONS

- **Hemorrhage:** It could be due to separation of vesicles or rarely intraperitoneal hemorrhage due to perforating mole. Hemorrhage is a frequent complication during the evacuation of a molar pregnancy (atonic uterus and/or uterine injury). For this reason, intravenous oxytocin should be started at the initiation of the suctioning. Blood for possible transfusion should be readily available.
- **Perforation** of the uterus during suction and curettage sometimes occurs because the uterus is large and boggy. Rarely there may be a perforating mole.
- **Malignant trophoblastic disease** develops in 20% of molar pregnancies. For this reason, quantitative hCG should be serially monitored.
- **Disseminated intravascular coagulopathy (DIC):** Factors released by the molar tissue or trophoblastic pulmonary embolization could trigger the coagulation cascade. Patients should be monitored for DIC.
- **Acute pulmonary insufficiency**: Trophoblastic embolism could cause acute respiratory insufficiency. The greatest risk factor for this complication is a uterus larger than that expected for a gestational age of 16 weeks. The condition may be fatal.
- **Sepsis:** Absence of membranes, degenerated vesicles, old blood and operative interference all can contribute.
- **Preeclampsia and eclampsia** very rarely.

Q. Follow-up of a case of vesicular mole.

INTRODUCTION

Gestational trophoblastic disease encompasses several disease processes that originate in the placenta. These include complete and partial moles, placental site trophoblastic tumors, choriocarcinomas, and invasive moles.

Vesicular mole is an abnormal condition of placenta where there is hydropic degeneration and proliferative changes in the young chorionic villi. It is a benign condition with malignant potential.

AIM OF FOLLOW-UP

The prime objective is to diagnose persistent trophoblastic disease or choriocarcinoma.

PERIOD OF FOLLOW-UP

Routine follow-up is mandatory for all cases for at **least one year**. The reason is that the occurrence of choriocarcinoma is confined to this period.

INTERVAL OF FOLLOW-UP

- Serial quantitative serum beta-hCG levels should be determined.
- Serum hCG levels are obtained *weekly* until the levels are negative or within reference range.
- Levels should consistently drop and should never increase. **Normal levels are usually reached within 8–10 weeks after evacuation** of the hydatidiform mole. As long as the hCG levels are falling intervention is not needed.
- Once levels have reached the reference range for 3–4 weeks, check them *monthly for 6 months*. Then the follow-up is discontinued and pregnancy allowed.
- The patient should not become pregnant during the follow-up period. Effective contraception is recommended during the period of follow-up
- If the serum hCG levels plateau or rise, the patient is considered to have malignant disease (i.e., gestational trophoblastic neoplasia) and metastatic disease needs to be excluded.
- **Contraception:** Estrogen-progestin contraceptives or depot medroxyprogesterone is usually used to prevent a subsequent pregnancy during the period of surveillance. Intrauterine contraceptive device (IUCD) is avoided because of risk of perforation.

METHOD EMPLOYED AT EACH VISIT

History

Enquire about relevant symptoms like irregular vaginal bleeding, persistent cough, breathlessness or hemoptysis.

Abdominovaginal Examination to Note

- Uterine size and involution of the uterus
- Ovarian size for regression of the theca lutein cysts
- Malignant deposits **(bluish nodules)** in the anterior vaginal wall in the suburethral region.

Investigations

- Serum beta-hCG levels as mentioned above
- *Chest X-ray*: If the pre-evacuation X-ray shows metastasis, it should be repeated at 4 weeks interval until remission is confirmed
  - It is then repeated at 3 months interval during the follow-up period
  - When the pre-evacuation X-ray is normal, it is repeated only when beta-hCG plateaus or rises.

> **Q. Mention the conditions in which the uterus is more than weeks of gestation. Define polyhydramnios, and etiology, clinical features, complications, and management of polyhydramnios.**

Conditions in which uterus is more than period of amenorrhea:
- Wrong dates [mistaken date of last menstrual period (LMP)]
- Twins, multiple pregnancy

- Polyhydramnios
- Macrosomia
- Ovarian tumors, fibroids
- Vesicular mole
- Concealed abruption.

INTRODUCTION

Amniotic fluid index (AFI) is an estimate of the amount of amniotic fluid on USG. It is an index for fetal well-being and is a part of the biophysical profile.

AFI is the score (expressed in cm) given to the amount of amniotic fluid seen on USG.

To determine the AFI, the deepest, unobstructed, vertical length of each pocket of fluid is measured in each quadrant **(total 4 quadrants)** and then added up. **Single deepest pocket** can also be used to estimate the liquor volume.

DEFINITION OF POLYHYDRAMNIOS

More than 2 L of amniotic fluid is termed as polyhydramnios
OR
Amniotic fluid index more than or equal to 25 cm
OR
Single largest vertical pocket of liquor more than 8 cm (normal: 2–8 cm).

CLASSIFICATION

Single Largest Vertical Pocket (cm)

Mild	>8–11
Moderate	12–15
Severe	>15

INCIDENCE

1–2% of cases.

ETIOLOGY

- **Most common cause = Idiopathic**
- **Fetal anomalies:**
    - **Obstruction of fluid transit** through the gastrointestinal tract: Esophageal/duodenal atresia and diaphragmatic hernia
    - **Anencephaly:**
        - Transudation of fluid across the membranes
        - Absence of swallowing
        - Absent fetal pituitary [absence of antidiuretic hormone (ADH) implies that the baby passes more urine].
    - **Open spina bifida**
- Multiple pregnancy
- Hydrops fetalis (immune and nonimmune)

- Chromosomal abnormalities (e.g., trisomy 18)
- Twin-to-twin transfusion syndrome (the donor sac has oligohydramnios and recipient has polyhydramnios)
- Diabetes insipidus/Bartter's syndrome
- **Maternal: Diabetes mellitus** (leads to raised fetal blood sugars leads to fetal diuresis) and cardiac/renal disease (placental edema)
- **Placental:** Chorioangioma (associated with acute polyhydramnios).

CLINICAL FEATURES

Symptoms

- In majority cases, the liquor accumulation is gradual and patient may be asymptomatic
- Respiratory: Dyspnea
- Palpitations
- Edema feet
- Varicosities in legs, vulva and hemorrhoids
- Polyhydramnios associated with fetal hydrops may cause the **mirror syndrome**, where by the maternal condition mimics the fetus and mother develops edema, proteinuria, and pregnancy-induced hypertension (PIH).

On Examination

- The abdomen is markedly enlarged with fullness in flanks
- The skin is **tense, shiny**
- Height of the uterus is more than period of amenorrhea
- Abdominal girth will be more than normal
- **Fluid thrill present**
- Fetal parts **cannot be well palpated**. External ballottement can be elicited more easily
- Fetal heart sound (FHS) are difficult to hear and Doppler may be required
- PV: The cervix may be dilated and effaced and tense bulging membranes may be felt.

INVESTIGATIONS

- USG
  - To estimate AFI
  - To rule out multiple pregnancies and various fetal anomalies
- ABO and Rh blood group (Rh isoimmunization can cause immune hydrops)
- Fasting blood sugar (FBS) and post lunch blood sugar (PLBS) and if needed glucose tolerance test (GTT).

COMPLICATIONS

Maternal

Antenatal

- Preeclampsia
- **Preterm labor**
- Premature rupture of membrane (PROM)
- Malpresentation.

Intrapartum
- **Cord prolapse**
- Abruption (due to sudden decompression following sudden escape of large amount of liquor)
- Increased risk of operative delivery.

Postpartum
- **Postpartum hemorrhage (PPH; uterine atony)**
- Subinvolution of uterus.

Fetal
Increase in perinatal morbidity and mortality due to prematurity, cord prolapse, abruption, and anomalies.

TREATMENT
- Treatment is based on the underlying cause.
- Mild asymptomatic polyhydramnios is managed expectantly. For a woman with symptomatic polyhydramnios may need hospital admission. Antacids may be prescribed to relieve heartburn and nausea.
- No data to support dietary restriction of salt and fluid.
- **In severe cases:**
  - **Indomethacin (25 mg qds) and sulindac** are nonsteroidal anti-inflammatory drugs (NSAIDs) that decrease fetal urine production and are used in medical management of polyhydramnios in symptomatic patients.
  - A major concern for the use of indomethacin/sulindac is the risk of premature closure of the fetal ductus arteriosus. Hence, these drugs **should not be used beyond 34 weeks** of gestation.
- **In unresponsive cases with maternal distress:**
  - *Pregnancy <37 weeks*: **Amnioreduction (amniocentesis)** can be done. 1–1.5 liters of fluid should be removed slowly. The procedure may have to be repeated.
  - *If pregnancy is >37 weeks*: Induction of labor if normal presentation.
- **During labor:** Controlled artificial rupture of membrane (ARM) to be done **to prevent abruption and cord prolapse**.
- **Postpartum:** To watch for PPH and active management of the third stage of labor (**AMTSL**) should be done.

Q. Mention conditions in which uterus is smaller than period of amenorrhea. Define oligohydramnios. Give etiology of oligohydramnios.

Q. Oligohydramnios.

Conditions in which uterus is smaller than period of amenorrhea:
- Wrong dates (mistaken date of LMP)
- Intrauterine growth restriction (IUGR)
- Intrauterine fetal death (IUFD)
- Oligohydramnios.

INTRODUCTION

Amniotic fluid index (AFI) is an estimate of the amount of amniotic fluid and is an index for the fetal well-being. It is a part of the biophysical profile.

AFI is the score **(expressed in cm)** given to the amount of amniotic fluid seen on USG of a pregnant uterus. To determine the AFI, doctors may use a **four-quadrant technique**, when the deepest, unobstructed, vertical length of each pocket of fluid is measured in each quadrant and then added up to the others or the so-called **"single deepest pocket"** technique.

DEFINITION OF OLIGOHYDRAMNIOS

- Amniotic fluid index less than 5 cm is termed as oligohydramnios
  OR
- Amniotic fluid less than 100 mL
  OR
- Maximum vertical pocket less than 2 cm.

ETIOLOGY

Fetal

- Chromosomal abnormalities
- Congenital anomalies (e.g., **renal agenesis and posterior urethral valves**)
- IUGR
- **Postdatism/post-term pregnancy**
- PROM
- Twin-to-twin transfusion
- Intrauterine infections.

Maternal

- **Uteroplacental insufficiency**
- Hypertension
- Preeclampsia
- NSAIDs, angiotensin: Converting enzyme inhibitors
- Dehydration
- Idiopathic.

RENAL AGENESIS

This defect has an incidence of about 1 in 4,000 births. No kidneys are seen ultrasonographically. The adrenal glands typically enlarge and occupy the renal fossae, which is termed the **lying down adrenal sign. Without kidneys**, no urine is produced and the resulting severe oligohydramnios leads to **pulmonary hypoplasia, limb contractures**, a distinctive **compressed face**, and death from cord compression or pulmonary hypoplasia.

When this combination of abnormalities results from renal agenesis, it is called **Potter syndrome named after Dr Edith Potter** who described it in 1946. If these abnormalities result from scanty amniotic fluid of some other etiology, it is called **oligohydramnios sequence**.

- ❖ **Amnion nodosum** are tiny, light tan, creamy nodules in the amnion made up of vernix caseosa with hair, degenerated squames, and sebum. **They result from oligohydramnios** and are most commonly found in fetuses with renal agenesis and prolonged preterm ruptured membranes, or in the placenta of the donor fetus with twin-to-twin transfusion syndrome.
- ❖ Amniotic bands are caused when disruption of the amnion leads to formation of bands that entrap the fetus and impair growth and development of the involved structure. Fetal conditions due to this phenomenon include intrauterine amputations.

CLINICAL FEATURES

- ❖ Uterus size/height of the uterus is less than period of amenorrhea
- ❖ Abdominal girth will be less than normal
- ❖ The uterus is **"full of fetus" due to scanty liquor**
- ❖ Malpresentation (breech) is common
- ❖ Evidence of IUGR.

COMPLICATIONS

- ❖ Tetrad of early-onset oligohydramnios:
  - ▸ Facial clefts (cleft lip/palate)
  - ▸ IUGR
  - ▸ Limb reduction defects
  - ▸ Pulmonary hypoplasia
- ❖ Cord compression in labor
- ❖ Malpresentations
- ❖ Increase operative delivery
- ❖ High perinatal morbidity and mortality.

TREATMENT

- ❖ Rule out congenital anomalies in the fetus
- ❖ **Treatment of hypertension and IUGR** if present (refer to IUGR answer)
- ❖ Hydration therapy (oral or IV) may help to increase the liquor volumes
- ❖ Antenatal amnioinfusion is not recommended
- ❖ However **amnioinfusion can be done in labor to prevent cord compression and improve neonatal outcome**.

CHAPTER 24

Twins

Q. Complications of twins.

INTRODUCTION

Twins and higher order multiple pregnancies are at a risk of various complications as compared to singleton pregnancy **(Flowchart 24.1).**

COMPLICATIONS

Flowchart 24.1: Complications of twin pregnancy.

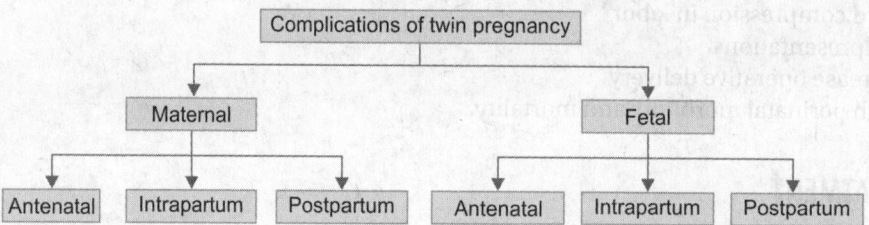

Maternal

Antenatal

There is increased risk of the following:

- **Anemia:** Due to increased requirements of iron, folic acid and vitamin B_{12} leading to dimorphic anemia
- **Hyperemesis, nausea:** Due to excessive hCG
- **Preeclampsia (25%):** Due to excessive chorionic villi. Multiple gestations are at increased risk for developing gestational hypertension and preeclampsia compared with singleton pregnancies. The incidence of preeclampsia is **2.6 times higher** in twin gestations than in singleton gestations
- **Polyhydramnios:** Due to increase in fetal renal perfusion. More common in monozygotic twins
- **Preterm labor (50%):** Over distention of the uterus, polyhydramnios and preeclampsia contribute

- **Gestational diabetes mellitus:** The incidence of gestational diabetes increases with each additional fetus in multiple gestations. Between 22–39% of triplet pregnancies and 3–6% of twin pregnancies are complicated by gestational diabetes
- **APH (placenta previa + abruption):** Large placenta which encroaches on the lower segment contributes to placenta previa. Abruption could be due to:
  - Preeclampsia
  - Sudden decompression of the uterus after the delivery of the first baby
  - Sudden escape of liquor from hydroamniotic sac
  - Folic acid deficiency
- **Malpresentations:** More common compared to single pregnancy. It is **more common in the second baby.** In 70% cases the first baby is vertex and in 50% cases both are vertex
- Mechanical distress such as palpitation, dyspnea, varicosities and hemorrhoids are increased compared to singleton pregnancy.

Intrapartum

- *Cord prolapse:* Around five times more common as compared to single term pregnancy and more common in second baby. Malpresentation and polyhydramnios contribute
- Cord entanglement and **interlocking of twins**
- *Operative delivery:* Increased risk of LSCS due to malpresentations, cord prolapse, preeclampsia, prematurity, etc.

Postpartum

- **PPH:** Uterine atony due to overdistension of the uterus, polyhydramnios, preeclampsia, placenta previa and APH all contribute
- Subinvolution of the uterus due to overdistension
- Infection due to anemia and operative interference
- Lactation failure due to more demand.

Fetal

- **Congenital anomalies:** Congenital malformations are twice as common in twin pregnancies compared with singletons and four times more common in triplets. The rate of congenital anomalies in twins is estimated at approximately 4% compared with 2% in singletons. Monozygotic twins have twice the incidence of congenital abnormalities compared with dizygotic twins.
  The anomalies include NTD, hydrocephalus, cardiac anomalies and Down's syndrome.
- **Abortions:** Increased rate of both first and second trimester abortions. More in monozygotic twins.
- **Prematurity** is the most dangerous complication and contributes to morbidity and mortality.
- **IUGR:** Intrauterine growth restriction (IUGR) and discordant growth contribute to adverse outcomes in multiple gestations. Growth restriction in multiple gestations is likely secondary to uteroplacental insufficiency but can also be secondary to structural anomalies, umbilical cord abnormalities, infections, genetic abnormalities or due to twin-to-twin transfusion syndrome. Approximately 14–25% of twin gestations are affected by growth restriction. One or both babies can be IUGR.

- **Asphyxia and stillbirth:** Due to prematurity, preeclampsia, gestational diabetes, cord prolapse, cord entanglement, abruption, malpresentation, and operative interference. The second baby is more at risk. Complications are more in monochorionic twins.
- **IUFD of one fetus.** More in monozygotic twins. If the loss happens in first trimester, the affected fetus '**vanishes**' by resorption. If the death occurs in second trimester, a fetus papyraceous or compressus may form. If the death occurs in late pregnancy, the other fetus may develop acute hypotension, cerebral palsy or even death. Mother may develop DIC.
- Cord prolapse, cord entanglement and interlocking of twins.
- Increase perinatal mortality (PNM).

Best prognosis is seen in dichorionic (DC), diamniotic (DA) variety (10–20% PNM).

Worst prognosis is with conjoint twins (70–90% PNM) followed by monochorionic (MC), monoamniotic (MA) (58–60% PNM).

Special Complications

Twin-to-twin transfusion syndrome (TTTS)
- It occurs only in monochorionic-diamniotic twins
- In this, blood is transfused from a donor twin to its recipient sibling which causes the donor to become anemic and oligohydramniotic and its growth may be restricted, whereas the recipient has polyhydramnios and becomes polycythemic and may develop circulatory overload manifest as hydrops. Similarly, one portion of the placenta often appears pale compared with the rest of the placenta
- This is due to deep arteriovenous anastomosis
- Antenatal criteria recommended for defining the twin-to-twin transfusion syndrome include the following:
  - Same sex fetuses
  - Monochorionicity with placental vascular anastomoses
  - Weight difference between twins greater than 20%
  - Polyhydramnios in the larger twin
  - Oligohydramnios in donor twin
  - Hemoglobin difference greater than 5 g/dL
  - The donor twin has better prognosis.

■ MANAGEMENT

Diagnosis is made with USG and color Doppler.
- Repeated amniocentesis to control polyhydramnios in the recipient. This also improves circulation in donor twin
- Septostomy
- Laser photocoagulation of the anastomotic vessels
- Selective feticide/reduction of one twin done as last resort when survival of both the fetus is at risk.
- **Acardiac twin: Twin reversed arterial perfusion (TRAP) sequence** is a rare (one in 35,000 births) but serious complication of monochorionic, monozygotic multiple gestation. In the TRAP sequence, there is usually a normally formed donor twin that

has features of heart failure as well as a recipient twin that lacks a heart (acardius) and various other structures.
- **Discordant growth** (can occur in DZ and MZ twins): There is difference in weights of twins and is expressed as percentage of larger twin's weight:
  - Grade 1 = difference of 15–25%
  - Grade 2 = difference >25%

Q. Etiology of twins and types/varieties of twins.

INTRODUCTION

When more than one fetus simultaneously develops in uterus, it is called multiple pregnancy.

INCIDENCE

- Incidence of monozygotic twins is constant throughout the world. It is one in 250
- The incidence of dizygotic twins varies from one in 20 in Nigeria to one in 80 in India
- With the advent of ART/IVF, the incidence is on rise.

ETIOLOGY

- **Twins can be of two varieties:** Dizygotic (DZ) and monozygotic (MZ). DZ variety = 80% and MZ = 20% of all twins.
- All dizygotic twins are dichorionic (DC) and diamniotic (DA).
- MZ twins are of following varieties depending upon the time of twinning:
  - Within 72 hours of fertilization = DC, DA (around 30% of MZ twins and 6–7% of all twins)
  - Between 4th and 8th day = Monochorionic (MC), DA (66% of MZ twins and 13–14% of all twins)
  - Between 8th and 12th day = MC, monoamniotic (MA) (1–3% of MZ twins and <1% of all twins)
  - After 12 days = conjoint/Siamese twins (<1% of MZ twins and 0.002–0.008% of all twins).

For Monozygotic (MZ) Twins

Unknown for MZ twins.

For Dizygotic (DZ) Twins

- *Increasing age and increasing parity:* The rate of natural twinning rises from zero at puberty, a time of minimal ovarian activity, to a peak at 37 years of age, when maximal hormonal stimulation increases the rate of double ovulation. This is in accordance with the first consistently observed sign of reproductive aging, an isolated rise in serum FSH. The fall in incidence after 37 years of age probably reflects depletion of the Graafian follicles.
- Incidence increases from 5th gravida onwards

- Personal/family history of twinning. If the patient's mother or sister has twins, there is more chance of twins. Past history of twins also contributes
- *Ovulation induction agents:* **3–8% risk** of twins with clomiphene citrate and **15–30%** with gonadotropins
- *IVF:* **20–45% risk of twins**. It depends on the patient's age and the number of embryos transferred
- Negroes have the highest risk and Mongols have the least risk.

For Conjoined Twins (in Descending Order of Frequency): Remember 'TOPIC'

- **T**horacopagus (joined at thorax), most common variety
- **O**mphalopagus (joined at the abdomen)
- **P**ygopagus (joined at the buttocks)
- **I**schiopagus (joined by ischium)
- **C**raniopagus (joined at the head), least common variety.

Q. Clinical features and management of twin pregnancy.

Q. Intrapartum management of twins.

INTRODUCTION

Twin pregnancy belongs to a high-risk category as twins and higher order multiple pregnancies are at a risk of various complications as compared to singleton pregnancy.

CLINICAL FEATURES

History

- Advanced maternal age and parity
- History of ovulation induction/ART
- Family/personal history of twins.

Symptoms

- **Exaggerated symptoms of normal pregnancy:** Increase in nausea and vomiting and sometimes hyperemesis.
- **Symptoms due to over distended uterus:**
  - Cardiorespiratory embarrassment—dyspnea, palpitation
  - Swelling of legs, varicose veins and hemorrhoids
  - Unusual rate of abdominal enlargement and excessive fetal movements.

On Examination

General Examination

- Pallor (more risk of anemia) may be present
- Excessive weight gain
- Edema feet

Chapter 24: Twins

- High blood pressure (more risk of preeclampsia)
- Proteinuria.

Abdominal Examination

Inspection
Undue enlargement of the abdomen, 'barrel shape'.

Palpation
- Height of uterus and will be more than period of amenorrhea
- Abdominal girth more than normal average at term (100 cm)
- Presence of polyhydramnios
- Palpation of **too many fetal parts**
- Finding of two fetal heads, or three fetal poles.

Auscultation
Simultaneously hearing two distinct FHS with a silent area in between by two observers with a difference in heart rate of 10 beats/min.

INVESTIGATIONS

- Routine ANC investigations to be carried out
- To keep in mind that there is more chance of anemia, preeclampsia and gestational diabetes
- **USG:** Very useful for:
  - *Confirmation of diagnosis:* Count the number of gestational sacs and yolk sacs in first trimester
  - Dating the pregnancy
  - Viability of fetuses, vanishing twin in second trimester
  - Chorionicity establishment.

Signs for Chorionicity on USG

Dichorionicity	Monochorionicity
• The 'twin-peak' sign/lambda sign (placenta intervenes between the membranes) • Intervening membrane is >2 mm thick	• 'T' sign/inverted T sign (right angle relation between the placenta and fetal membranes) • Intervening membrane is <2 mm

- **Twin peak sign/Lambda sign indicates two fused placenta**
  - Detailed nuchal translucency (NT) scan at 11–13 weeks and anomaly scan at 18–20 weeks
  - Fetal growth at 3–4 weeks interval for IUGR/discordant growth
  - To detect malpresentations
  - Color Doppler in cases of IUGR and TTTS
  - Placental localization and AFI
- **Dual marker and triple marker test can also be carried out in twins as there is more risk of Down's syndrome.**

MANAGEMENT

Antenatal Management

Early diagnosis is very important to detect chorionicity, amnionicity and fetal anomalies.

Diet

Increase in dietary requirement. **Extra 300 Kcal/day** is needed over and above that needed for singleton pregnancy. Also increase in proteins needed.

Supplements

- Iron increased to 100–200 mg/day. Additional vitamins, calcium and folic acid (4 mg instead of 400 μg) are also needed
- Adequate rest to the mother
- To watch for preterm labor. Corticosteroids can be given to accelerate lung maturity
- Fetal surveillance by USG for fetal growth at 3–4 weeks interval. **NST, BPP and color Doppler for fetal well-being**
- **More frequent antenatal visits** to detect anemia, preeclampsia, preterm labor and gestational diabetes.

Intrapartum Management

- **Multidisciplinary team approach** (obstetrician, anesthetist, neonatologist and NICU facilities).
- **Skilled obstetrician should be present**
- **Presence of USG is very helpful and should be there**
- Secure IV line (as urgent IV therapy may be needed), **send blood for cross match** and RL drip can be started.
  - Patient is put to bed to prevent early ROM
  - Adequate pain relief (epidural analgesia preferred)
  - Careful fetal monitoring (**preferably continuous EFM**)
  - **PV examination after rupture of membranes to rule out cord prolapse**
  - Neonatologist and a trained assistant to be present for delivery
  - NICU backup.

Delivery

- Route of delivery is decided by the position of first baby
- Only if the first fetus is in vertex position, then normal vaginal delivery is possible
- **Twins with first fetus in nonvertex position** (breech, transverse, oblique, etc.) are to be delivered by LSCS
- **Monochorionic (MC), monoamniotic (MA) variety twins are always to be delivered by LSCS** (even if the first fetus is in vertex position) because of very high risk of **cord prolapse and cord entanglement (Flowchart 24.2)**.

The only indication of IPV in modern day obstetrics is transverse lie in second baby of twins.

Indications of LSCS for Second Baby

- Fetal distress
- Cord prolapse

Flowchart 24.2: Management of twins.

```
                              Twins
         ┌───────────┬──────────┴────────┬──────────────┐
    First baby    First baby         MC, MA       Conjoint twins
    nonvertex      vertex                │              │
        │            │                   │              │
     EL, LSCS  (Wait for spontaneous    EL, LSCS      LSCS
                      labor)
              IV drip │ Epidural analgesia
                      │ fetal monitoring (EFM)
                      ▼
              Deliver 1st baby vaginally
                      ▼
              Cord clamped and divided
                      ▼
                Avoid AMTSL now
                      ▼
         Note the lie of 2nd baby with USG or clinically
                ┌────────┴─────────┐
          Transverse lie      Longitudinal lie
                │                   │
   Delivery ◄ External version   ARM + Oxytocin
      │           │               if needed
   AMTSL       Fails → LSCS          │
                │                 Delivery
                IPV → Fails → LSCS   │
                │                 AMTSL
         Breech extraction
                │
              AMTSL
```

(EL: elective; AMTSL: active management of third stage of labor)

- Abruption (due to sudden decompression) after delivery of the first baby
- Larger second twin with noncephalic presentation
- Prompt closure of cervix after delivery of first baby
- Failed ECV or IPV done for second baby in transverse lie.

Management of Third Stage

- **Active management of third stage of labor (AMTSL) to be done after the delivery of the second baby to prevent postpartum hemorrhage (PPH)**
- Advisable to **continue oxytocin drip** for at least one hour after delivery of second baby
- Closely monitor the patient in postpartum period.

Mother to be given encouragement and support to manage both babies.

Contraception

Contraceptive advice to be given to mother on discharge.

CHAPTER 25

Induction of Labor and Operative Delivery

Q. What is induction of labor? What are the indications and methods for IOL?
Q. Contraindications for IOL.

■ INTRODUCTION

Induction of labor (IOL) needs to be considered when the risk-benefit analysis indicates that **delivering the baby is a safer option for the baby, the mother, or both, rather than continuing the pregnancy,** and when there are no clear indications for cesarean section and no contraindications for vaginal delivery.

DEFINITION

Induction of labor means initiation of uterine contractions by medical, surgical or combined for the purpose of vaginal delivery.

■ INDICATIONS

Maternal and Fetal Conditions

Maternal

- ❖ Gestational hypertension, preeclampsia, eclampsia
- ❖ Premature rupture of membranes
- ❖ Postdatism, post-term
- ❖ Abruptio placentae
- ❖ Chorioamnionitis
- ❖ Maternal medical conditions (e.g., diabetes mellitus, renal disease, chronic pulmonary disease, chronic hypertension, cholestasis of pregnancy)
- ❖ Polyhydramnios
- ❖ Maternal request.

Fetal

- ❖ Fetal demise [intrauterine fetal death (IUFD)]

- Fetal compromise (e.g., severe fetal growth restriction, isoimmunization, oligohydramnios)
- Major congenital anomaly.

CONTRAINDICATIONS

All cases where vaginal delivery is not possible or contraindicated.
- Contracted pelvis, severe cephalopelvic disproportion (CPD)
- Transverse lie, oblique lie, footling breech
- Umbilical cord prolapse
- Active genital herpes infection
- Placenta previa
- Vasa previa
- Previous classical cesarean section, hysterotomy
- Previous myomectomy entering the endometrial cavity
- Cervical cancer
- Fetal distress, severe fetal compromise
- Previous two or more lower segment cesarean section (LSCS).

Bishop Scoring System Used for Assessment of Inducibility (Asked as short note)

Score	Factor				
	Dilatation (cm)	Effacement (%)	Station	Cervical consistency	Cervical position
0	Closed		−3	Firm	Posterior
1	1–2	40–50	−2	Medium	Midposition
2	3–4	60–70	−1	Soft	Anterior
3	≥5	>80	+1 to +2	–	–

In modified Bishop's scoring system, effacement has been replaced by **cervical length in cm**, with scores as follows:
- 0 for >4 cm, 1 for 3–4 cm, 2 for 1–2 cm, 3 for <1 cm.
- Cervical length may be easier and more accurate to measure and has less inter-examiner variability.
- A score of **8 or more conveys a high likelihood for a successful induction**. Score of 4 or less identifies unfavorable cervix and needs for cervical ripening.

METHODS OF INDUCTION OF LABOR

- Medical
- Surgical
- Combined.

Medical

- Oxytocin
- Prostaglandins (PGE1 tablets, PGE2 gel, tablets, inserts)
- Mifepristone.

Oxytocin

- As pregnancy progresses, the number of oxytocin receptors in the uterus increases (by 100-fold at 32 weeks and by 300-fold at the onset of labor).
- Oxytocin activates the phospholipase C-inositol pathway and increases intracellular calcium levels, stimulating contractions in myometrial smooth muscle.
- **Oxytocin is the preferred pharmacologic agent for inducing labor when the cervix is favorable or ripe.**
- **2.5–5 units oxytocin** in 500 mL RL is used. The drip is generally started at 8–10 drops/minute and titrated as required.

Prostaglandins (PGE1, PGE2)

- Alter the extracellular ground substance of the cervix, and **PGE2 increases the activity of collagenase in the cervix.**
- They cause an increase in elastase, glycosaminoglycan, dermatan sulfate and hyaluronic acid levels in the cervix and facilitate the dilatation.
- Increase in intracellular calcium levels, causing contraction of myometrial muscle.
- Slow-release formulations are also available. In general, PGEs are the **drug of choice when cervical ripening is needed in the presence of an unfavorable cervix**.

Dinoprostone

For the purpose of cervical ripening and induction, dinoprostone gel (**PGE2** = 0.5 mg), tablets and dinoprostone inserts (10 mg) are available.

The gel can be repeated **every 6 hourly for 2–3 doses as required**.

Misoprostol

Misoprostol is a synthetic **PGE1** analog that has been found to be a safe and inexpensive agent for cervical ripening and IOL. It can be used by **vaginal, oral, sublingual and buccal route.** Generally 25 μg intravaginally every 4–6 hours is used. Higher doses or shorter dosing intervals are associated with a higher incidence of side effects, especially hyperstimulation.

Finally, uterine rupture in women with previous cesarean section is also a possible complication, limiting its use to women who do not have a uterine scar.

Risks associated with the use of prostaglandins include:
- **Uterine hyperstimulation (tachysystole)** and subsequent fetal distress
- Meconium-stained amniotic fluid (MSAF)
- Very rarely rupture uterus
- Maternal side effects such as nausea, vomiting, diarrhea and fever.
  PGF2 alpha cannot be used for induction of labor.

Mifepristone

Mifepristone (200 mg orally or vaginally) is an antiprogesterone agent. Progesterone inhibits contractions of the uterus, while mifepristone counteracts this action.

Surgical Methods

Stripping of the Membranes

- Stripping of the membranes causes an **increase in the activity of phospholipase A2 and prostaglandin as well as causing mechanical dilation of the cervix, which releases prostaglandins.**
- The membranes are stripped by inserting the examining finger through the internal cervical os and moving it in a circular direction to detach the inferior pole of the membranes from the lower uterine segment.
- Risks of this technique include infection, bleeding, accidental rupture of the membranes and patient discomfort.

Amniotomy/ARM (Artificial Rupture of Membrane) (Short Note)

Mechanism of Action

- It is hypothesized that amniotomy increases the production of, or causes a release of, prostaglandins locally
- It can be combined with oxytocin.

Advantages

- High success rate
- Chance to observe the **amniotic fluid**, blood stained or MSAF and hence helps in further management
- Access to use fetal scalp electrode, fetal scalp blood and intrauterine pressure catheter.

Limitations

It cannot be done in an unfavorable cervix (long, firm and os closed). The cervix should be at least one finger dilated.

Contraindications

- Maternal human immunodeficiency virus (HIV) infection
- Active genital herpes infection
- Floating/unengaged head (can lead to cord prolapse)
- Polyhydramnios (sudden decompression leads to abruption, so in these cases controlled ARM should be done).

Complications

Risks associated with this procedure include:

- Umbilical cord prolapse or compression
- Maternal or neonatal infection
- Fetal heart rate (FHR) deceleration
- Bleeding from low-lying placenta or vasa previa
- Possible fetal injury (rare)
- Abruption due to sudden decompression in cases of polyhydramnios
- Amniotic fluid embolism (AFE) (very rare).

Mechanical Modalities

All mechanical modalities have a similar mechanism of action. Some form of local pressure that stimulates the release of prostaglandins.

- Hygroscopic dilators **(very rarely used)** absorb endocervical and local tissue fluids, causing the device to expand within the endocervix and providing controlled mechanical pressure. The products available include natural osmotic dilators (e.g., Laminaria japonicum) and synthetic osmotic dilators (e.g., Lamicel). The main advantages of using hygroscopic dilators include outpatient placement and no FHR-monitoring requirements.
- Balloon devices provide mechanical pressure directly on the cervix as the balloon is filled.
- A Foley catheter (26 Fr) or specifically designed balloon devices can be used.

The risks associated with these methods include infection, bleeding, membrane rupture and placental disruption.

Q. Prerequisites for forceps application.

The prerequisites for successful application of forceps are:
- The head must be engaged
- The fetus must present as a vertex or by the face with the chin anterior
- The position of the fetal head must be precisely known
- **As per the ACOG guidelines station should be more than or equal to +2**
- The cervix must be completely dilated (10 cm)
- The membranes must be ruptured
- There should be no suspected cephalopelvic disproportion (pelvis deemed adequate)
- Bladder must be empty
- Informed consent (verbal or written)
- Experienced operator, a valid indication and neonatologist
- Backup plan in case of failure (LSCS facilities)
- Adequate maternal analgesia
- Willingness to abandon the procedure when difficulties faced.

Generally, the indications and prerequisites for the use of the vacuum extract or for delivery are the same as for forceps delivery.

Q. Indications for LSCS.

INDICATIONS

- Absolute
- Relative
- Maternal
- Fetal.

Absolute

- Central placenta previa
- Placenta accreta
- Contracted pelvis (severe CPD)
- Pelvic mass (cervical fibroid, broad ligament fibroid)
- Previous classical cesarean section

- ❖ Previous two or more LSCS
- ❖ Advanced carcinoma cervix
- ❖ Vasa previa
- ❖ Cord presentation.

Relative

Complications of labor and factors impeding vaginal delivery, such as:
- ❖ Prolonged labor, obstructed labor or a failure to progress (dystocia)
- ❖ Fetal distress
- ❖ Cord prolapse
- ❖ Malpresentation (breech, brow, transverse lie, oblique lie)
- ❖ Abruption
- ❖ Failed labor induction
- ❖ Failed instrumental delivery by forceps or ventouse (sometimes atrial of forceps/ventouse delivery is attempted, and if unsuccessful, it will be switched to a cesarean section)
- ❖ Macrosomia
- ❖ Triplets and higher order pregnancy
- ❖ Severe IUGR (as normal labor would be stressful or difficult for the severely underweight fetus)
- ❖ Previous myomectomy scar
- ❖ Other complications of pregnancy, pre-existing conditions and concomitant disease, such as:
  - ➢ Preeclampsia, hypertension
  - ➢ Certain heart disease (Marfan's syndrome)
  - ➢ HIV infection of the mother
  - ➢ Sexually transmitted diseases, such as genital herpes (which can be passed on to the baby if the baby is born vaginally)
  - ➢ Precious pregnancy [bad obstetric history (BOH), in vitro fertilization (IVF) conception, elderly primigravida, long standing infertility conception, etc.]
  - ➢ Previous uterine rupture
  - ➢ Rare cases of posthumous birth after the death of the mother.

Q. Episiotomy

■ DEFINITION

An episiotomy (perineotomy) is a **planned, surgical incision** on the perineum and the posterior vaginal wall during second stage of labor. The incision is actually a second degree perineal injury, and is sutured closed after delivery. It is the **most common obstetric procedure performed on women,** and although its routine use in childbirth has steadily declined in recent decades.

■ OBJECTIVES

- ❖ To prevent or **minimize overstretching and tearing of perineal muscles,** episiotomy is done as prophylaxis (tears can involve the perineal skin or extend to the muscles and the anal sphincter and anus).

❖ To enlarge the introitus so as to reduce the strain and stress on fetal head and facilitate easy and safe delivery of the fetus.

INDICATIONS

As per the **ACOG and RCOG guidelines, routine use of episiotomy is not indicated**. It should be done in selective cases such as:
- When perineal muscles are excessively rigid/inelastic perineum
- Instrumental delivery: Forceps, ventouse
- There is a serious risk to the mother of second- or third-degree tearing in cases like:
  - The baby is very large
  - Face to pubis delivery
  - Face delivery
  - After coming head of breech
  - Short perineum (distance between fourchette and anus is <3 cm)
- When a woman has undergone female genital mutilation (FGM) or perineal reconstructive surgery
- Prolonged late decelerations or fetal bradycardia during active pushing
- Shoulder dystocia. Episiotomy does not directly resolve this problem, but it is indicated to allow the operator more room to perform maneuvers to free shoulders from the pelvis.

TIMING

Bulging thin perineum during contraction just prior to or at the time of **crowning** (when 3–4 cm of the head is visible).

ANESTHESIA

1% lignocaine, local anesthesia.

TYPES

There are four main types of episiotomy (**Fig. 25.1**):

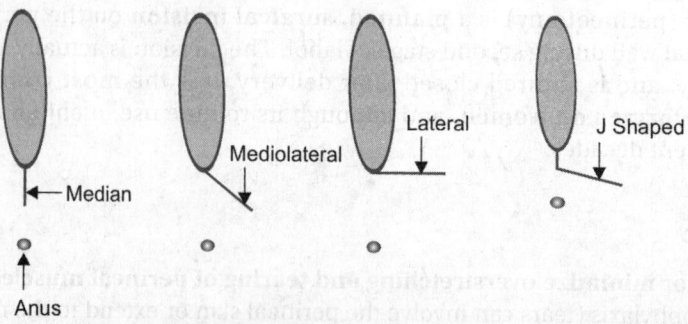

Fig. 25.1: Types of episiotomy.

Mediolateral (Most Common Type)

The incision is made downward and outward from midpoint of fourchette either to right or left. It is directed diagonally in straight line which runs about 2.5 cm away from the anus (midpoint between anus and ischial tuberosity).

An episiotomy performed at 40 degrees results in a post-delivery angle of 22 degrees, which is too close to the midline. A **60-degree episiotomy from the center of the introitus results in a post-delivery angle of 45 degrees.**

Median

The incision commences from center of the Fourchette and extends on posterior side along midline for about 2.5 cm.

Lateral

The incision starts from about 1 cm away from the center of Fourchette and extends laterally. Drawback includes chance of injury to Bartholin's duct; thus some practitioners have totally condemned it.

J-shaped (Very Rarely Done)

The incision begins in the center of the fourchette and is directed posteriorly along midline for about 1.5 cm and then directed downward and outward along 5 or 7 O'clock position to avoid the anal sphincter.

Structures cut are:
- Posterior vaginal wall
- Superficial and deep transverse perineal muscles bulbospongiosus, and part of levator ani and fascia covering those muscles
- Transverse perineal branches of pudendal vessels and nerves
- Subcutaneous tissue and skin.

■ REPAIR

Perfect hemostasis, obliteration of dead space and tension free suture are the principles to be followed.

It is done in three layers in the following order with number 0 chromic catgut or polyglactin (vicryl rapide) sutures:
1. *Vaginal mucosa:* Sutured by continuous/continuous interlocking sutures.
2. *Perineal muscles:* Interrupted sutures.
3. *Skin and subcutaneous tissue:* Interrupted or vertical mattress.

■ WOUND CARE

- The wound is to be kept open, dry and clean. Antiseptic ointment or cream to be applied 2–3 times a day and each time following urination and defecation.
- Analgesics and anti-inflammatory tablets and oral antibiotics for 3–5 days.
- The stitches need not be removed as they are absorbable.

COMPLICATIONS

Immediate and Late

Immediate

- **Extension:** Extension to rectum. More likely in median episiotomy
- Forniceal tear
- Vulval hematoma
- Infection
- Wound dehiscence
- Injury to rectal sphincter
- Rectovaginal fistula
- Necrotizing fasciitis (very rare).

Late

- **Dyspareunia:** This is due to faulty repair technique leading to narrow introitus and perineal scar.
- **Scar endometriosis (rare).**

CHAPTER 26

Previous Lower Segment Cesarean Section/Vaginal Birth After Cesarean

Q. Clinical features of previous cesarean section scar rupture/dehiscence. Mention the rupture rates of various scars.

■ INTRODUCTION

Pregnancy with a previous cesarean delivery belongs to a high-risk category and is quite prevalent today due to liberal use of primary cesarean section.

The dictum has changed from 'once a cesarean always a cesarean' to **'mandatory hospital delivery and individualization of the case'.**

■ CLINICAL FEATURES OF SCAR RUPTURE/DEHISCENCE

The scar begins to rupture from inside-out. In dehiscence, the serosa is intact. Rupture is complete thickness, involves all layers and peritoneal cavity of the mother communicates with amniotic cavity of the baby.

Impending scar rupture (scar dehiscence)	Ruptured uterus
Unexplained tachycardia	Weak thready fast pulse
Hypotension	Shock
Fetal tachycardia	Persistent fetal bradycardia/IUFD
Uterine scar tenderness/suprapubic pain especially in between contractions	Hematuria
Bleeding PV	Bleeding PV
Hematuria	Cessation of uterine contractions
	Recession of presenting part (loss of station)

Change in fetal heart rate (tachycardia/loss of beat to beat variability/decelerations) is the **earliest and the most consistent sign** of impending scar dehiscence, followed by maternal tachycardia.

Estimated Risks for Uterine Rupture in Women with a Prior Cesarean Delivery

Prior uterine incision	Estimated rupture (%)
Classical	4–9
T shaped	4–9
Low vertical	1–7
Low transverse	0.2–1

Q. Criteria/guidelines for vaginal birth after cesarean section (VBAC).

Q. How will manage a case of previous LSCS?

■ INTRODUCTION

Pregnancy with a previous cesarean delivery belongs to a **high-risk category** and is quite prevalent today due to liberal use of primary cesarean section.

The dictum has changed from 'once a cesarean always a cesarean' to **'mandatory hospital delivery and individualization of the case'.**

Recommendations of the ACOG useful for the selection of candidates for vaginal birth after cesarean delivery **(trial of scar):**

- ❖ No more than one prior low-transverse cesarean delivery **(only 1 previous LSCS)**
- ❖ Clinically adequate pelvis [no cephalopelvic disproportion **(CPD)**]
- ❖ No other uterine scars or previous rupture
- ❖ Physician immediately available throughout active labor who is capable of monitoring labor and performing emergency cesarean delivery
- ❖ Availability of resources (anesthesia, OT, blood) for emergency cesarean delivery
- ❖ Patient consent.

■ MANAGEMENT OF A CASE OF PREVIOUS CESAREAN SECTION

- ❖ **It is important to take note in the first visit itself whether the previous cesarean section was LSCS (lower segment transverse) or classical cesarean**
- ❖ Regular antenatal checkup and build up Hb
- ❖ To enquiry about **pain/tenderness over the scar area** or vaginal bleeding at every visit
- ❖ Patients with previous classical scar or hysterotomy scar: **Admit at 36 weeks** (as chance of rupture of such scar is more in last few weeks of pregnancy)
- ❖ **Formulate the route of delivery:** The most important decision is to whether go for repeat elective cesarean section or VBAC
- ❖ **Previous classical cesarean section or hysterotomy: Elective repeat cesarean section at 38 weeks of gestation or even earlier if required**
- ❖ Patients with previous LSCS, enquiry about:
  - ▷ Indication of prior cesarean section (recurrent or nonrecurrent)
  - ▷ Number of previous LSCS **(patients with previous 2 or more LSCS → elective repeat LSCS** at 38–39 weeks of gestation or even earlier if required)
  - ▷ Whether it was elective or emergency
  - ▷ Any intraoperative or postoperative complications and wound healing of the previous scar. Any infection or prior wound gape may weaken the scar.

Chapter 26: Previous Lower Segment Cesarean Section/Vaginal Birth After Cesarean

  ➢ **Ideally go through the previous cesarean section notes or discharge summary, if available**.
- Fetal weight estimation: Clinically and USG
- **Clinical pelvimetry:** For VBAC, the pelvis should be adequate, there should not be any CPD
- Patients with **previous LSCS and having CPD/contracted pelvis** → **elective repeat LSCS** at 38–39 weeks of gestation or even earlier if required
- Patient to be explained about the risk and benefits of VBAC.

The following important points are to be kept in mind:
- In patients with uterine malformations who have undergone cesarean delivery, the risks for uterine rupture in a subsequent pregnancy may be as high as with a classical incision.
- Patients who have previously sustained a uterine rupture are at increased risk of recurrence. Those with a rupture confined to the lower segment have been reported to have a 6% recurrence risk in subsequent labor, whereas those whose prior rupture included the upper uterus have a 32% recurrence risk.
- The rate of uterine rupture is increased nearly fivefold in patients with two previous cesarean deliveries compared with that in those only with one—3.7% versus 0.8%.
- **Any previous vaginal delivery, either before or following a cesarean birth, significantly improves the prognosis for a subsequent successful VBAC.**
- The success rate for a trial of scar depends to some extent on the indication for the previous cesarean delivery. Generally, about **60–80%** of trials after prior cesarean birth result in vaginal delivery, with **success being maximum if previous cesarean section was because of breech presentation.**
- In patients attempting VBAC who had no previous vaginal deliveries, the relative risk of uterine rupture is more than doubled when the birth weight is at least 4,000 g.
- As maternal weight increases, the rate of VBAC success decreases.

■ MANAGEMENT OF LABOR

Team Approach

Senior obstetrician, pediatrician and anesthetist and OT backup.
- Spontaneous onset of labor is desired
- Induction with PG increases the risk of scar rupture and hence ACOG discourages the use of prostaglandin cervical ripening agents
- IV line with RL drip
- Collect blood for grouping and cross-matching
- Closely monitor labor
- Vital parameters (pulse, BP)
- **To watch for scar tenderness** (in between contractions, if we palpate the lower uterine segment the patient winces with pain)
- Fetal heart rate monitoring (electronically preferred)
- **To watch for progress of labor, chart a partogram**
- Attempts to induce cervical ripening or to induce or augment labor increases the risk of uterine rupture in women undergoing a trial of scar
  ➢ ACOG states that oxytocin may be used for both labor induction and augmentation with close patient monitoring, in women undergoing a trial of scar

- ❖ **Epidural analgesia is not contraindicated**
- ❖ Prophylactic forceps or vacuum to **cut short second stage of labor**
- ❖ If the progress is unsatisfactory or evidence of scar tenderness/dehiscence → emergency LSCS
- ❖ Postpartum routine exploration of the scar is not advised. It should only be done in cases where there is excessive vaginal bleeding or maternal hypotension in spite of well-contracted uterus
- ❖ During 3rd time, LSCS patient is to be counseled and **tubal ligation should be offered**.

Q. Differences between LSCS scar and classical cesarean section scar.

Q. Merits/advantages of lower segment operation over classical cesarean section.

Differences between LSCS scar and classical cesarean section scar:

	Lower segment	*Classical*
Techniques	• Operative field less bloody because of less vascularity • The wall is thin, and as such apposition is perfect	• More bloody because of increased vascularity • The wall is thick, and coaptation of the margins is not perfect
Postoperative	• Hemorrhage and shock—less • Peritonitis is less even in infected uterus because of perfect peritonization and, if occurs, localized to pelvis • Peritoneal adhesions and intestinal obstruction are less • Convalescence is better • Mortality is much lower	• More • Chance of peritonitis is more in presence of uterine sepsis • More because of imperfect peritonization • Relatively poor • Mortality is high

Wound healing	The scar is better healed because:
	• Perfect apposition of the thin margins
	
	• Chance of blood collection in the wound is less
	• The wound remains quiescent during healing process
	
	• Chance of gutter formation is unlikely as placental implantation is usually fundal
		The scar is weak because:
		• Imperfect apposition because of thick margins
		• Chance of blood collection in the wound is more, which hinders union
		• The wound is in a state of tension and due to contraction and relaxation of the upper segment. As a result, the knots may slip or the sutures may become lax
		• Chance of gutter formation on the inner aspect is likely because of:
		  ▪ Inclusion of the deciduous or
		  ▪ Inadequate coaptation of the friable inner part when the placenta is anteriorly situated

During future pregnancy	Scar rupture is less **(mainly in labor)**: 0.2–1%	More risk of rupture **(mainly in third trimester)** 4–9%
Following rupture	• Maternal death: Less • Perinatal death 1 in 8	• Maternal death: 5% • Perinatal death 6 in 8

CHAPTER 27

Miscellaneous

Q. Define maternal death and MMR. What are the causes of maternal mortality?

DEFINITION

Maternal death is defined as 'The death of a woman **while pregnant or within 42 days** of termination of pregnancy, irrespective of the **duration and the site of the pregnancy**, from any cause related to or aggravated by the pregnancy or its management, but not from accidental or incidental causes.'

- **Maternal mortality ratio (MMR) is maternal deaths per 1,00,000 live births**
- It varies from 4–40/1,00,000 live births in developed countries and 100–700 in developing countries. In India, it is **97 per 1,00,000 live births**
- Maternal mortality rate indicates maternal deaths divided by number of women of reproductive age (15–49) and expressed per 1,00,000 women of reproductive age per year.
- Every day, approximately 800 women die from preventable causes related to pregnancy and childbirth
- 99% of all maternal deaths occur in developing countries
- Maternal mortality is higher in women living in rural areas and among poorer communities
- Young adolescents face a higher risk of complications and death as a result of pregnancy than older women.

CLASSIFICATION OF CAUSES

- **Direct (75–80%)**
- **Indirect (20–25%)**
- Nonobstetric.

Direct deaths are those resulting from complication of pregnancy/delivery or its management. The most common causes are:

- Hemorrhage [antepartum hemorrhage (APH) and postpartum hemorrhage (PPH)] (20–25%)
- Unsafe abortion (10–13%)
- Hypertensive disorders of pregnancy (preeclampsia, eclampsia) (12%)
- Postpartum infections (puerperal sepsis) (10–15%)

- ❖ Obstructed labor (8%)
- ❖ Ectopic gestation.

Indirect deaths include conditions present before or developed during pregnancy but aggravated by physiological effects of pregnancy and strain of labor:
- ❖ Anemia
- ❖ HIV/AIDS
- ❖ Cardiovascular disease
- ❖ Diabetes
- ❖ Viral hepatitis.

All of these may complicate pregnancy or be aggravated by it.

Nonobstetric causes include:
- ❖ Accidents

Hemorrhage (mainly PPH) is the most common cause of maternal mortality in India.

Hypertensive disorders of pregnancy (preeclampsia, eclampsia) are the most common cause of maternal mortality in developed countries.

Anemia is the most common indirect cause of maternal mortality.

CONCLUSION

- ❖ **Skilled care** before, during, and after childbirth, **good family planning services,** and **education** can save the lives of women and newborn babies.
- ❖ Between 1990 and till to date, maternal mortality worldwide dropped by almost 50%.

Q. Lochia.

INTRODUCTION

It is the vaginal discharge for the first fortnight during puerperium. The discharge originates from the uterine body, cervix, and vagina.

It has got a peculiar offensive fishy smell. Its reaction is alkaline tending to become acid toward the end.

COLOR

Depending upon the variation of the color of the discharge, it is named as:
- ❖ **Lochia rubra** (red): 1–4 days
- ❖ **Lochia serosa** (5–9 days): The color is yellowish or pink or pale brownish
- ❖ **Lochia alba** (pale white): 10–15 days.

COMPOSITION

- ❖ **Lochia rubra** consists of blood, shreds of fetal membranes and decidua, vernix caseosa, lanugo, and meconium.
- ❖ **Lochia serosa** consists of less RBC but **more leukocytes,** wound exudate, mucus from the cervix and microorganisms (anaerobic streptococci and staphylococci). **The presence of bacteria is not pathognomonic unless associated with clinical signs of sepsis.**

Chapter 27: Miscellaneous

❖ **Lochia alba** contains plenty of decidual cells, leukocytes, mucus, cholesterin crystals, fatty and granular epithelial cells, and microorganisms.

AMOUNT

The average amount of discharge for the first 5–6 days, is estimated to be 250 mL.

NORMAL DURATION

The normal duration may extend up to 3 weeks. The red lochia may persist for longer duration especially in women who get up from the bed for the first time late. The discharge may be scanty, especially following premature labor or may be excessive in twin delivery or hydramnios.

CLINICAL IMPORTANCE

The character of the lochial discharge gives useful information about the abnormal puerperal state. **The vulval pads are to be inspected daily to get information:**
❖ **Odor:** If malodorous, indicates infection. **Retained plug or cotton piece inside the vagina should be kept in mind**
❖ **Amount:** Scanty or absent—signifies infection or lochiometra. If excessive—indicates infection
❖ **Color:** Persistence of red color beyond the normal limit signifies subinvolution or retained bits of conceptus
❖ **Duration:** Duration of the lochia alba beyond 3 weeks suggests local genital lesion.

Q. Cause of IUFD.

INTRODUCTION

Intrauterine fetal death (IUFD) includes all deaths of fetus weighing 500 g or more, occurring during pregnancy (antepartum) or during labor (intrapartum). For all practical purpose, antepartum death occurring beyond the period of viability is termed as intrauterine fetal death.

ETIOLOGY

❖ Maternal (5–10%)
❖ Fetal (25–40%)
❖ Placental (25–35%)
❖ Unexplained (25–35%).

Maternal (5–10%)

❖ **Antiphospholipid antibodies** (lupus anticoagulant and ACL-anticardiolipin antibodies)
❖ **Diabetes**
❖ **Hypertensive disorders** (preeclampsia, eclampsia)
❖ Thrombophilias (factor V Leiden, protein C and S deficiency)
❖ Abnormal labor (prolonged, obstructed labor, uterine rupture)

- Sepsis
- Acidosis/hypoxia
- Post-term pregnancy
- Drugs.

Fetal (25–40%)
- **Chromosomal anomalies**
- Nonchromosomal birth defects
- Nonimmune hydrops
- Infections.

Placental (25–35%)
- **Abruption**
- **Cord accident**
- **Placental insufficiency**
- Intrapartum asphyxia
- Previa
- Twin-to-twin transfusion
- Chorioamnionitis.

Unexplained (25–35%)

Q. Ultrasonography (USG) in obstetrics.

INTRODUCTION

Ultrasounds are sound waves with frequencies higher than the upper audible limit of human hearing (>2 MHz). The clinical application of ultrasound in obstetrics was introduced and popularized by **Ian Donald**. Ultrasonography (USG) is an essential tool in managing almost every pregnancy.

The commonly used frequency range in obstetrics is **3–5 MHz for abdominal transducers and 5–7 MHz for vaginal transducers**.

In clinical practice USG images are:
- B mode: 2 D images are obtained routinely
- M mode: To study motion, e.g., fetal heart rate
- Doppler ultrasound: To study the blood flow.

INDICATIONS/USES OF USG IN OBSTETRICS

First Trimester

In the first trimester, a standard ultrasound examination typically includes:
- Diagnosis of pregnancy
- Gestational sac size, location, and number

Chapter 27: Miscellaneous

- Fetal cardiac activity (viability)
- **Diagnosis of ectopic pregnancy**
- Measurement of **crown rump length (dating of gestational age)**
- Fetal number, including number of amnionic sacs and **chorionicity for multiple gestations**
- Diagnosis of molar pregnancy
- Assessment of embryonic/fetal anatomy appropriate for the first trimester **(nasal bone, anencephaly)**
- CVS is always done USG guided
- Embryo reduction in cases of multiple pregnancy
- Nuchal translucency (NT) assessment
- Evaluation of the maternal uterus, ovaries, pelvic mass.

Second Trimester

In the second trimester, a standard ultrasound examination typically includes:
- Detailed fetal anatomical survey/anomaly scan
- Cervical incompetence/cervical length assessment
- Placental localization
- Baseline record of biometry
- Amniocentesis and cordocentesis are done USG-guided
- Amniocity and chorionicity for multiple gestations if not done in first trimester.

Third Trimester

- Assessment of growth/monitoring intrauterine growth restriction (IUGR)
- Estimation of fetal weight
- Lie and presentation
- Placental localization/bleeding in 3rd trimester
- Diagnosis of IUFD
- AFI (oligohydramnios/polyhydramnios)
- Fetal well-being/**BPP**
- **Intrauterine transfusion (IUT)** is always done USG-guided
- Before and after ECV.

■ COLOR DOPPLER

Indications

- **Intrauterine growth restriction (IUGR)** (most important investigation for management) (details in IUGR answer)
- **Rh isoimmunization management**. Peak systolic velocity (PSV) in the middle cerebral artery (MCA) is increased with fetal anemia because of increased cardiac output and decreased blood viscosity. PSV in MCA is now used in management of Rh isoimmunized fetuses and timing of IUT
- Prediction of PIH
- Diagnosis of **placenta accreta/percreta, vasa previa**
- In cases of ectopic pregnancy **(ring of fire appearance)** of ectopic sac.

Recent Advances

3D and 4D USG

- 3D USG creates a **3-dimensional** image of the fetus. It is considered better than 2D USG for detecting **facial clefts**, CNS and CVS defects, and also a **life-like photo** improves antenatal parental bonding
- **4D allows a 3-dimensional picture in real time**, rather than delayed, due to the lag associated with the computer constructed image, as in classic three-dimensional ultrasound.

Q. Shoulder dystocia.

■ DEFINITION

Shoulder dystocia is an uncommon obstetric complication of cephalic vaginal deliveries during which the **fetal shoulders do not deliver after the head has emerged** out of the introitus. A head-to-body delivery time **exceeding 60 sec** is used to define shoulder dystocia.

It occurs when one or both **shoulders become impacted against the bones** of the maternal pelvis.

■ INCIDENCE

- Incidence is 0.2–1%

■ RISK FACTORS

These include: **D, O, P, E.**
  D = Diabetes mellitus
  O = Obesity
  P = Postdatism and previous history
  E = Excessive weight gain during pregnancy (mother or fetus).

■ COMPLICATIONS

Maternal

- **PPH:** Usually from uterine atony, but also from vaginal and cervical lacerations
- Increase in operative delivery.

Fetal

- Significant **fetal/perinatal morbidity and even mortality**
- Asphyxia
- Transient **Erb or Klumpke brachial plexus palsies** are the most common injury
- Clavicular fractures and humeral fractures and sternocleidomastoid hematoma.

■ DIAGNOSIS

- Definite recoil of head back against perineum **(turtle neck sign)**
- Fetal face becomes plethoric.

MANAGEMENT OF SHOULDER DYSTOCIA

- **Call for extra help**
- To involve anesthetist and pediatrician (for neonatal resuscitation)
- Extend the episiotomy, remove the lithotomy position
- Never give fundal pressure (as it causes further impaction of shoulder)
- **Moderate suprapubic pressure** should be applied by an assistant while downward traction is applied to the fetal head. This will reduce the bisacromial diameter
- Check if it is a unilateral shoulder dystocia (posterior shoulder is in hollow of sacrum, anterior is above pelvic brim) or a bilateral shoulder dystocia (both shoulders above pelvic brim)
- If it is **bilateral shoulder dystocia,** directly proceed to perform lower segment cesarean section (**LSCS**) after doing the **Zavanelli** maneuver (cephalic replacement back into the vagina and then cesarean delivery)
- The rest of the maneuvers can be tried for unilateral shoulder dystocia, and if they fail, then proceed for **Zavanelli maneuver** and LSCS
- The **McRoberts maneuver**: The maneuver consists of removing the legs from the stirrups and sharply flexing them up onto the abdomen. This procedure causes straightening of the sacrum relative to the lumbar vertebrae, rotation of the symphysis pubis toward the maternal head, and a decrease in the angle of pelvic inclination
- Woods reported that, by progressively rotating the posterior shoulder 180° in a corkscrew fashion, the impacted anterior shoulder could be released. This is frequently referred to as the **Woods corkscrew maneuver**
- Delivery of the posterior shoulder
- **Rubin's maneuver: Posterior pressure on the anterior shoulder**
- **Gaskin maneuver:** Involves moving the mother to an **all fours position** with the back arched, widening the pelvic outlet
- Cleidotomy consists of cutting the clavicle and is usually used for a dead fetus. Symphysiotomy has also been applied successfully.

As per ACOG guidelines, planned cesarean delivery is to be considered for the nondiabetic woman carrying a fetus with an estimated fetal weight exceeding **5,000 g** or the diabetic woman whose fetus is estimated to weigh more than **4,500 g** to avoid the risk of shoulder dystocia.

Q. Uterine inversion.

INTRODUCTION

It is an extremely rare and a life-threatening complication in the 3rd stage in which the **uterus is turned inside out partially or completely**.

INCIDENCE

Incidence is about **1 in 20,000 deliveries**.

CAUSES AND RISK FACTORS

These include:
- It is well-established that *mismanagement of the third stage of labor* (combination of premature traction on umbilical cord and fundal pressure before separation of placenta) is the most **common cause of acute uterine inversion**

- Uterine atony
- Fundal implantation of a **morbidly adherent placenta**
- Manual removal of the placenta
- Precipitate labor
- Short umbilical cord
- Connective tissue disorders (Marfan syndrome, Ehlers-Danlos syndrome)
- Sudden emptying of a distended uterus
- Spontaneous inversion of unknown etiology: Localized atony on placental site over fundus and associated sharp rise of intra-abdominal pressure.

However, in up to 50% of cases, no risk factors are identified and there is no mismanagement of the third stage. This condition can, therefore, be unpredictable.

CLASSIFICATION ACCORDING TO SEVERITY OF UTERINE INVERSION

- **First degree** (incomplete): The inverted fundus extends down but remains above the cervical ring (internal os).
- **Second degree** (incomplete): The inverted fundus extends through the cervical ring but remains within the vagina.
- **Third degree** (complete): The inverted fundus extends out of the introitus so the endometrium (with or without the placenta) is visible outside the vulva.
- **Fourth degree** (total): The vagina is also inverted.

CLASSIFICATION ACCORDING TO TIMING OF THE EVENT

- **Acute** occurs within 24 hours of birth
- **Subacute** occurs after 24 hours, within 4 weeks
- **Chronic** occurs after 4 weeks, rare.

CLINICAL FEATURES

Symptoms

Acute severe lower abdominal pain with bearing down sensation.

Signs

- **Shock (neurogenic)** thought to be due to the parasympathetic effect caused by tension on the nerves due to stretching of the ligaments supporting the uterus and ovaries
- Cupping or dimpling on fundal surface in mild degrees
- Uterine **fundus is not palpable** abdominally
- Bimanual examination can confirm the diagnosis and degree of inversion
- In complete variety a **pear-shaped mass reddish purple in color, protrudes outside the vulva, broad end pointing downward**
- PPH.

TREATMENT

Delay in treatment increases the mortality rate. It is necessary that a number of steps be taken immediately and simultaneously **(Flowchart 27.1)**:
- Call for help, including an anesthesiologist immediately.

Chapter 27: Miscellaneous

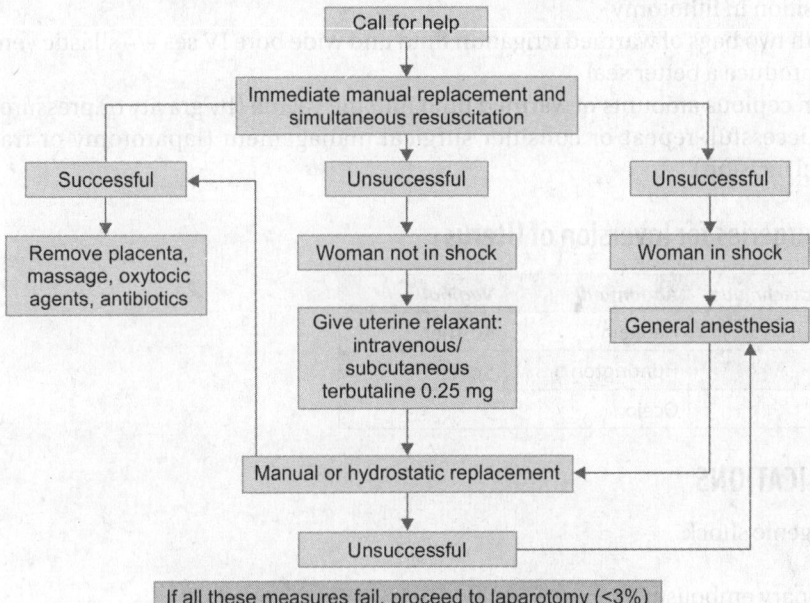

Flowchart 27.1: Management of uterine inversion.

- Administer oxygen
- Insert two wide bore IV cannulas
- Group and cross-match four units of blood
- Resuscitate with rapid infusion of crystalloids
- Monitor vital signs.

Manual Replacement (Johnson Maneuver)

- Immediately push up on the fundus with the palm of the hand and fingers toward umbilicus in the direction of the long axis of the vagina to replace the freshly inverted uterus **(to replace that part first which has inverted last)**
    - Do not remove the placenta if it is adherent
    - Maintain hand in place until a sustained contraction
- Anesthesia (preferably halothane or enflurane) and tocolytics have been used successfully for uterine relaxation and repositioning
- As soon as the uterus is restored to its normal configuration, **oxytocin drip started to contract the uterus** while the operator maintains the fundus in normal position
    - Once uterine inversion corrected, perform manual removal of placenta in theatre under anesthesia if still attached
    - Give stat dose oxytocin 10 IU IV
    - Commence oxytocin infusion (oxytocin 40 IU in 500 mL sodium chloride 0.9%) at 125 mL/hr over 4 hours.

O'Sullivan's Hydrostatic Technique

- If initial uterine replacement unsuccessful:
    - O'Sullivan's hydrostatic repositioning can be done in theater or in labor ward +/− anesthesia

- Exclude uterine rupture first
- Position in lithotomy
- With two bags of warmed irrigation fluid and wide bore IV set +/– silastic ventouse cup to produce a better seal
- Run copious amounts of warmed fluid into the vagina (by gravity or pressure)

❖ If unsuccessful, repeat or consider surgical management (laparotomy or transvaginal cervical incision).

Various Surgeries for Inversion of Uterus

Hydrostatic technique	Abdominal	Vaginal
O'Sullivan	Haultain	Kustner
Ogueh	Huntington	Spinelli
	Ocejo	

■ COMPLICATIONS

- ❖ Neurogenic shock
- ❖ PPH
- ❖ Pulmonary embolism
- ❖ Maternal mortality
- ❖ If left uncared for: Infection, sloughing and chronic inversion.

Q. Hyperemesis gravidarum.

■ DEFINITION

It is a severe type of vomiting of pregnancy which has got deleterious effect on the health of the mother and/or incapacitates her in day to day activities.

■ INCIDENCE

There has been marked fall in the incidence during the last 30 years. **Less than 1 in 1,000 pregnancies**.

■ ETIOLOGY

Obscure but the following are the known facts:
- ❖ It is mostly limited to the first trimester
- ❖ It is more common in **first pregnancy**, with a tendency to recur again in subsequent pregnancies. It has got a **familial history**
- ❖ More prevalent in **hydatidiform/vesicular mole and multiple pregnancy**
- ❖ More common in unplanned pregnancies.

■ THEORIES

- ❖ *Hormonal*
  - Excess of human chorionic gonadotropin (hCG) is associated: Frequency of vomiting at the peak level of hCG and also increased association with vesicular mole and twins.

- High serum level of estrogen
- Progesterone excess leading to relaxation of the cardiac sphincter and impaired gastric motility.

Other hormones involved are:
- Thyroxin, prolactin, leptin, and adrenocortical hormones
- *Psychogenic:* Neurogenic element sometimes plays a role, as evidenced by its subsidence after shifting the patient from the home surroundings. Conversion disorder, somatization are the other theories
- *Dietetic deficiency*: Probably due to low carbohydrate reserve
- *Allergic* or *immunological basis*.

METABOLIC, BIOCHEMICAL AND CIRCULATORY CHANGES

The changes are due to the combined effect of **dehydration and starvation** consequent upon vomiting.

Metabolic

- There is incomplete oxidation of fat and accumulation of ketone bodies. The acetone is ultimately excreted through the kidneys and in the breath.
- Glycogen depletion will occur and the fat reserve is broken down.

Biochemical

- Decrease in Na, K, and Cl
- Ketoacidosis
- Increase in blood urea and uric acid
- Hypoglycemia; hypoproteinemia; hypovitaminosis; and rarely hyperbilirubinemia.

Circulatory

- Hemoconcentration leading to rise in hematocrit values
- Slight increase in the WBC count with increase in eosinophils.

CLINICAL COURSE

- Early
- Late (moderate to severe).

The patient is usually a nullipara, in early pregnancy. The onset is insidious.

Early: Vomiting occurs throughout the day. Normal day-to-day activities are curtailed. **There is no evidence of dehydration or starvation.**

Late: Evidences of dehydration and starvation are present.

Symptoms

- Vomiting is increased in frequency with retching
- Urine quantity is diminished even to the stage of oliguria
- Epigastric pain, constipation may occur. Complications may appear if not treated.

Signs

Features of dehydration and ketoacidosis.

Dry coated tongue, sunken eyes, acetone smell in breath, tachycardia, hypotension, rise in temperature may be noted, jaundice is a late feature.

Such late cases are rarely seen these days.

INVESTIGATIONS

- **Urinalysis**:
  - Quantity—small
  - Dark color
  - High specific gravity with acid reaction
  - Presence of acetone, occasional presence of protein, and rarely bile pigments
  - Diminished or even absence of chloride
- **Biochemical and circulatory changes**: Mentioned previously
- **Ophthalmoscopic examination** is required if the patient is seriously ill. Retinal hemorrhage and detachment of the retina are the most unfavorable signs
- **ECG** when there is abnormal serum potassium level.

DIAGNOSIS

- **The pregnancy is to be confirmed first**.
- **Ultrasonography** is useful not only to confirm the pregnancy but also to exclude other obstetric (hydatidiform mole, multiple pregnancy), gynecological, surgical or medical causes of vomiting.

COMPLICATIONS

- Ketoacidosis
  The following complications may occur which are fortunately rare nowadays.
- Neurologic complications
  - Wernicke's encephalopathy due to thiamine deficiency
  - Pontine myelinolysis
  - Peripheral neuritis
  - Korsakoff's psychosis.
- Stress ulcer in stomach
- Esophageal tear (Mallory-Weiss syndrome)
- Jaundice
- Convulsions and coma
- Renal failure.

MANAGEMENT

The principles in the management are:
- To control vomiting
- To correct the fluids and electrolytes imbalance

Chapter 27: Miscellaneous

- To correct metabolic disturbances (acidosis and alkalosis)
- To prevent the serious complications of severe vomiting.

Hospitalization

Surprisingly the patient improves rapidly (with the same diet and drugs used at home)
NBM: Till at least 24 hours after the cessation of vomiting.

IV Fluids

- **3 liters/24 hours** (half is 5% dextrose and half is Ringer's solution)
- Extra amount of 5% dextrose equal to the amount of vomitus and urine in 24 hours, is to be added
- Serum electrolyte to be corrected if there is any abnormality
- Enteral nutrition through nasogastric tube may also be given.

Drugs

- **Antiemetic drugs: Promethazine** 25 mg or **prochlorperazine** 5 mg may be administered twice or thrice daily intramuscularly.
  - Trifluoperazine 1 mg twice daily intramuscularly is a potent antiemetic therapy.
  - **Vitamin B_6 and doxylamine** are also safe and effective.
  - **Metoclopramide** stimulates gastric and intestinal motility without stimulating the secretions. It is found useful.
- **Hydrocortisone** 100 mg IV in the drip is given in a case with hypotension or in intractable vomiting. Prednisolone is also used in severe cases.
- **Nutritional support**—with vitamin B_1, vitamin B_6, vitamin C, and vitamin B_{12} are given.

Nursing Care

- **Sympathetic but firm handling** of the patient is essential. Social and psychological support should be extended.
- **Hyperemesis progress chart** is helpful to assess the progress of patient while in hospital.
- **Daily record** of pulse, temperature, blood pressure at least twice daily, intake-output, **urine** for acetone, protein, bile, blood biochemistry, and ECG (when serum potassium is abnormal) are important.

Evidence of Improvement

Clinical features of improvement are evidenced by:
- Subsidence of vomiting
- Feeling of hunger
- Better look
- Disappearance of acetone from the breath and urine
- Normal pulse and blood pressure
- Normal urine output.

Diet

Before the intravenous fluid is omitted. At first, dry carbohydrate foods like biscuits, bread, and toast are given. Small but frequent feeds are recommended. Gradually full diet is restored.

Termination of Pregnancy

It is rarely indicated. Intractable hyperemesis gravidarum in spite of therapy is rare these days.

Q. Management of Rh-isoimmunized pregnancy. Add a note on prevention of isoimmunization (anti-D).

INTRODUCTION

Rh-isoimmunized pregnancy means that the Rh-negative mother has already been sensitized **(positive indirect Coombs' test)** to Rh positive cells and **developed antibodies** against them. Antibodies once formed remain lifelong.

These antibodies are of two types:
1. **IgM:** Cannot cross the placenta and are not harmful to the fetus
2. **IgG:** Cross the placenta and will cause fetal RBC hemolysis (of Rh-positive fetus).

It can lead to development of:
- Hydrops fetalis (most serious form) and even IUFD
- Icterus gravis neonatorum (intermediate variety)
- Congenital anemia of newborn (least severe and mild variety).

MANAGEMENT (FLOWCHART 27.2)

Rh isoimmunized patients should be managed in centers with special **'fetal medicine unit'** and facilities for **intrauterine blood transfusion**.

Also NICU, facilities for exchange transfusion and expert neonatologist would be needed to tackle the affected babies.
- In case of first affected pregnancy, Rh isoimmunized women should undergo determination of their anti-D antibody titers or quantitative estimation of antibody levels
- These are usually performed monthly until 24 weeks of gestation, after which time titers should be repeated every 2 weeks
- If titers remain below the critical titer, delivery can happen at term
- A critical titer is defined as the titer associated with a significant risk for fetal hydrops
- Usually, pregnancies in which antibody titers are **1:8** or lower can be managed by serial monitoring of maternal antibody titers
- But if the titer is **1:16 or higher**, fetal wellness assessment is mandatory by ultrasonography evaluation of middle cerebral artery peak systolic velocity **(MCAPSV)** or **serial amniocentesis for delta OD450** if the former is not available.

Management of Women with a History of a Previous Anemic Fetus or Infant

- When there is a history of a previous anemic fetus or newborn, the probability of subsequent affected Rh D-incompatible fetus is more than 80%
- In these cases, maternal antibody titers are not predictive for the severity of fetal anemia and fetal clinical surveillance, by assessment of middle cerebral artery peak systolic velocity (MCA-PSV) or serial amniocentesis for delta OD450 should be started at **18–20 weeks or 10 weeks prior to the date of previous IUFD or hemolytic manifestation of the fetus**.

Chapter 27: Miscellaneous

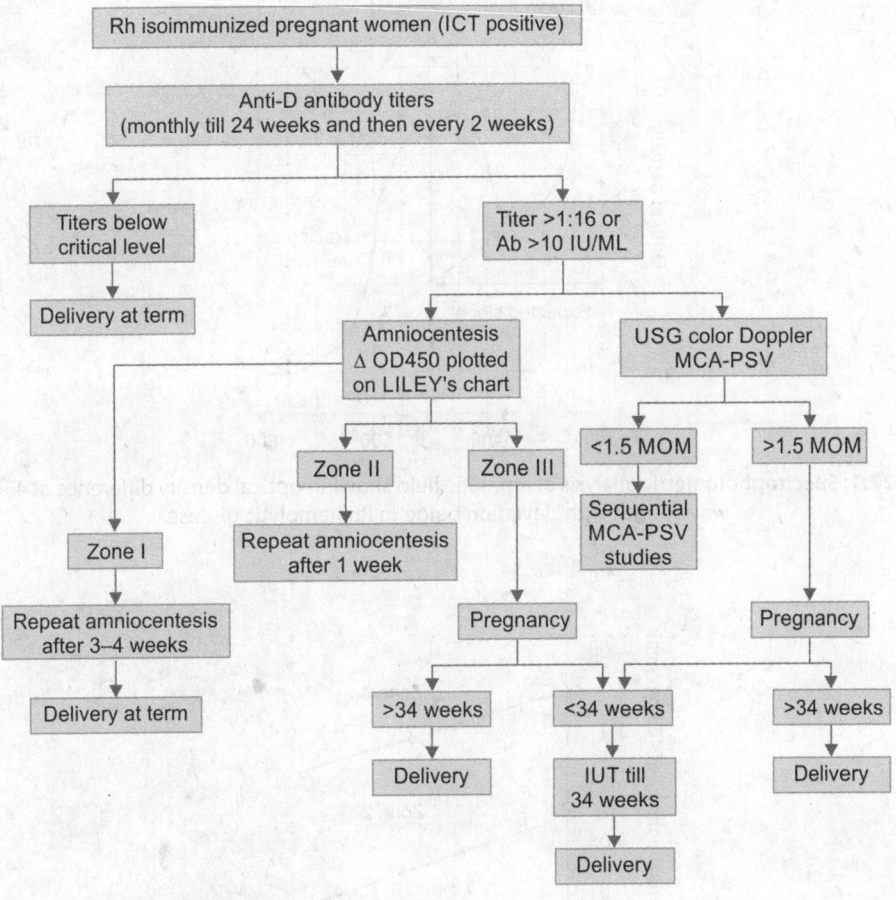

Flowchart 27.2: Management of Rh isoimmunized pregnancy.

Amniocentesis and Amniotic Fluid Evaluation

❖ When fetal blood cells undergo hemolysis, breakdown pigments, mostly bilirubin, are present in amniotic fluid
❖ The amount of amniotic fluid bilirubin correlates roughly with the degree of hemolysis and thus indirectly predicts the severity of the fetal anemia
❖ The concentration is measured by a continuously recording spectrophotometer and is demonstrable as a change in absorbance **(deviation bulge) at 450 nm**, referred to as **ΔOD450**, and the value is plotted on **Liley's chart (Figs. 27.1 and 27.2).**
❖ Optical density values in **zone 1** indicate a fetus that will have only **mild disease** or unlikely to be affected. Amniocentesis should be repeated in **3–4 weeks.**
❖ In **zone 2,** the fetus is at moderate risk. In low zone 2, the expected fetal hemoglobin concentration is between 11.0 g/dL and 13.9 g/dL, whereas in upper zone 2, the anticipated hemoglobin level ranges from 8.0 g/dL to 10.9 g/dL. Amniocentesis should be repeated **after 1 week.**
❖ **Values in zone 3 indicate a severely affected fetus with a hemoglobin level of less than 8.0 g/dL,** and, without therapy, death is predicted within **7–10 days.** A value in zone 3

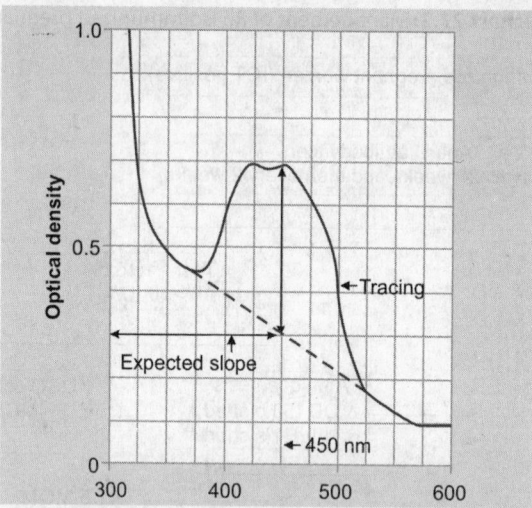

Fig. 27.1: Spectrophotometric analysis of amniotic fluid showing optical density difference at 450 nm wavelength with 'deviation bulge' in Rh hemolytic disease.

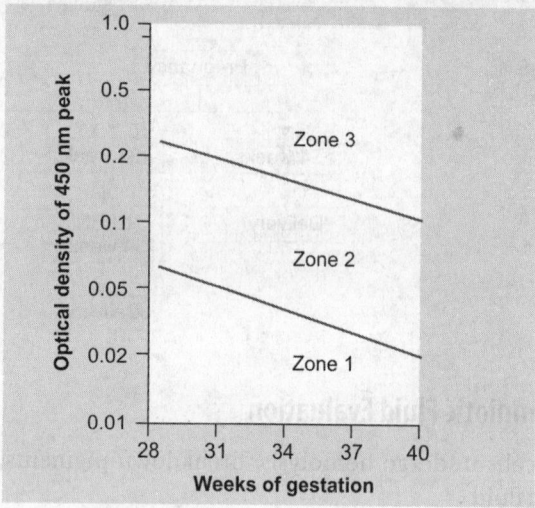

Fig. 27.2: Plotting of the 'deviation bulge' in Liley's prediction chart at different periods of gestation.

demands immediate **fetal red blood cell transfusion (intrauterine transfusion) or delivery depending on weeks of gestation.**

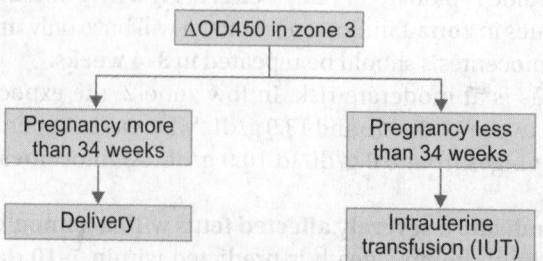

RECENT ADVANCES

❖ Fetal anemia can be predicted noninvasively using middle cerebral artery (MCA) color Doppler. The anemic fetus shunts blood preferentially to the brain to maintain adequate oxygenation. **Peak systolic velocity (PSV) in the MCA is increased with fetal anemia because of increased cardiac output and decreased blood viscosity.**
❖ Nowadays this method is preferred over amniocentesis (which is an invasive procedure). If the PSV is above the cutoff (**more than 1.5 MOM** for the corresponding gestational age) it indicates moderate to severe fetal anemia. Cordocentesis and IUT or delivery is indicated depending upon the weeks of gestation.

METHODS OF DELIVERY

Vaginal

PG gel can be used for cervical ripening.

Lower Segment Cesarean Section (LSCS)

❖ For obstetric indications
❖ In cases of preterm fetus with unfavorable cervix
❖ Cases where IUT has been done, LSCS is safer and preferred.

CARE DURING DELIVERY

❖ **Early cord clamping** (as soon as possible) to prevent further antibody transfer
❖ **Cord to be kept long 15–20 cm** for exchange transfusion, if needed
❖ Avoid manual removal of the placenta (MROP) at LSCS and minimize the spillage of blood in peritoneal cavity
❖ Cord blood investigations: Hb, ABO and Rh grouping, DCT, and bilirubin.
   As the mother is already sensitized there is no role of anti-D and hence it is not to be given after delivery.

TRANSFUSION THERAPY

Types of Therapy

Intrauterine Transfusion (IUT)

❖ IUT continues to be the mainstay of therapy for severe Rh isoimmunization.
❖ It is indicated in cases where there is **severe affection of the fetus prior to 34 weeks of gestation.**
❖ The purpose of intrauterine transfusion is to:
  ▹ **Treat hydrops fetalis and severe fetal anemia** (and thereby preventing IUFD) and maintain the fetal hemoglobin value at more than 9 g/dL
  ▹ Prolong/allow pregnancy **to complete 34 weeks** of gestation.

When to Perform

Nicolaides has recommend that transfusions be started when the hemoglobin is at least 2 g/dL below the mean for normal fetuses of corresponding gestational age. Another recommendation is to perform transfusions when the **fetal hematocrit (Hct) is below 30%,** which is 2 standard deviations below the mean at all gestational ages. **Hydropic changes occur when Hct is <15%.**

Serial intrauterine transfusions, if required, are usually performed until 34 weeks of gestation, because after this time the risk of the procedure is greater than benefits and so delivery should be done.

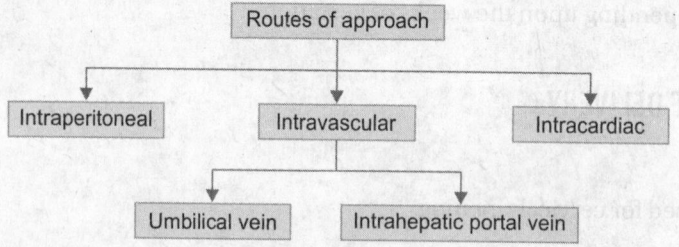

- Fresh **O-negative** double packed cells (with Hct 70–80%) crossed match with mother is to be transfused
- **The procedure is done in sterile room or OT under strict aseptic precautions with antibiotic cover under USG guidance**
- Tocolytics are given to prophylactically. Also steroids are given to enhance lung maturity
- **Temporary fetal paralysis is achieved by injection pancuronium/atracurium or vecuronium**
- It is given IM into fetal thigh, gluteal or deltoid
- Fetal paralysis last for 3–4 hours
- Fetal surveillance with USG and NST to be done in post-transfusion period.

Intravascular Transfusion

- Cordocentesis is done and blood is transfused into umbilical vein under USG guidance
- The amount of blood required to be transfused is calculated by various formulas depending upon fetal Hct and donor Hct
- Goal is to achieve a Hct of 50%
- **Multiple transfusions may be needed 10–14 days as fetal Hct drops at the rate of 1%/day.**

Intraperitoneal Transfusion

- It is done if vascular access is not available
- Blood is transfused in fetal peritoneal cavity which is taken up by subdiaphragmatic lymphatics
- The amount of blood transfused is calculated as number of weeks of gestation over 20, multiplied by 10 (e.g., at 30 weeks: 10 × 10 = 100 mL).

Complications of Therapy

- Umbilical cord hematoma
- Fetal bradycardia

Chapter 27: Miscellaneous

- Chorioamnionitis
- Preterm labor
- Abruption
- Fetal injury
- Volume overload
- IUFD (procedure related fetal loss is 4–5%).

Advantages of Therapy

- Correction of fetal anemia and improved oxygenation
- Improved fetal hepatic function
- Helps to prolong pregnancy thereby avoiding birth of an extremely preterm fetus.

Overall neonatal survival is 90–100% for nonhydropic fetus and about 50–70% for hydropic fetus.

Other Therapies

For the rare patient with very early (≤18 weeks) severe isoimmunization, **plasma exchange (plasmapheresis) and administration of high dose intravenous immunoglobulin G (IVIG)** may maintain the fetal hematocrit above life-threatening levels long enough to achieve a gestational age when IUT is technically feasible.

■ PREVENTION OF ISOIMMUNIZATION

Anti-D

- It is an IgG antibody that is given by IM route
- Monoclonal and polyclonal varieties are available.

Mechanism of Action

It binds to fetal RBCs and blocks the Rh antigens of fetal cells, so that they cannot stimulate the maternal immune system and hence prevents the antibody formation.

To prevent maternal Rh sensitization, **women who are Rh negative** (and not yet sensitized/ICT negative) should receive anti-D injections in the following situations:

- **At 28 weeks of gestation to all unsensitized Rh-negative mothers** (married to Rh-positive partner). This reduces the risk of sensitization from 1.2% to 0.2 %
  - Postpartum within 72 hours (as early as possible) **if the baby's blood group is Rh positive**
- After abortion, MTP, ectopic pregnancy, molar pregnancy
- After amniocentesis, CVS, cordocentesis
- After ECV
- After manual removal of placenta (in any situation where fetomaternal hemorrhage is expected).

When the mother is already sensitized (positive indirect Coombs' test or positive Rh titer), there is no role of anti-D.

300 µg will protect the mother from fetal hemorrhage of up to **15 mL of D-positive red cells or 30 mL of fetal whole blood.**

The amount of fetal blood entering maternal circulation may be calculated by **Kleihauer-Betke (KB) test. It is not done routinely but to be done in cases when large FMH is suspected.**

Indications and Recommended Dose of Anti-D

Indications	Recommended dose (µg)
First trimester abortion/MTP	50
First trimester ectopic pregnancy	50
Second trimester abortion/MTP	300
Second trimester amniocentesis	300
Prophylaxis at 28 weeks	300
After delivery	300

Q. Anencephaly.

INTRODUCTION

The incidence of neural tube defects (NTDs) is **1–2 per 1,000 live births**, and they are second only to cardiac anomalies, which are the most frequent structural fetal malformation.

- Anencephaly is a lethal NTD characterized by **absence of the brain and cranium above the base of the skull and orbits** but the facial portion is normal.
- It can be diagnosed as early as the **first trimester on USG**.
- 70% of fetuses are female.
- Face presentation is the most common presentation.
- Recurrence risk is 5% after one affected fetus and 13% after two affected fetuses.
- Frog eyes are seen.

Polyhydramnios is commonly seen due to the following reasons:
- Transudation of fluid across the membranes
- Absence of swallowing
- Absent fetal pituitary (absence of ADH hormone implies that the baby passes more urine)
  - Postdatism is seen as fetal pituitary plays an important role in initiation of labor.
  - However preterm labor can also be there due to polyhydramnios.
  - **Pseudoshoulder dystocia** is seen as the soft head/face can slip through incompletely dilated cervix.

MANAGEMENT

- If diagnosed before 20 weeks of gestation, MTP should be offered and done after counseling patient, as it is a lethal anomaly.
- If diagnosed later, legally MTP is not allowed. Labor may be induced. The uterus is often refractory to oxytocin and hence PGs may be required.

PREVENTION

- Some NTDs are associated with a specific mutation in the methylenetetrahydrofolate reductase gene, the adverse effects of which can be largely overcome by **periconceptional folic acid supplementation**.
- More than half of NTDs could be prevented with daily intake of **400 µg of folic acid throughout the periconceptional period** (1 month before pregnancy and the first trimester of pregnancy).

- In patients with **past history of NTDs, 4 mg folic acid** is recommended throughout the periconceptional period.

Q. Dilatation and evacuation/suction evacuation.

INTRODUCTION

In this operation, the cervix is dilated and the products of conception are evacuated from the uterine cavity.

Nowadays, **always one stage operation is performed, where both dilatation and evacuation are done in one sitting.**

Two-stage procedure (slow dilatation of cervix followed by rapid dilatation and evacuation) **is almost never performed** nowadays due to availability of misoprostol (PGE1).

INDICATIONS

- Incomplete abortion
- Inevitable abortion
- MTP (up to 12 weeks)
- Hydatidiform/vesicular mole.

PROCEDURE

- **Anesthesia:** Short general anesthesia (TIVA)/IV sedation
- **Position:** Lithotomy.

STEPS

- **Vulva, vagina swabbed with antiseptic solution**
- **Cervix cleaned with povidone iodine solution**
- **Bladder emptied**
- Internal examination to note the size and position of uterus
- Sim's posterior vaginal wall speculum is introduced
- Anterior lip of cervix held with vulsellum/Allis forceps
- Cervix is gradually dilated up to desired extent by graduated metal dilators (Hegar's dilators). (Misoprostol 400 µg can be introduced in the vagina 3-4 hours prior to dilatation to facilitate this step)
- The products removed by ovum forceps.
- In suction evacuation, the suction cannula of appropriate size is introduced in the uterus such that the tip of cannula is in the middle of the cavity. The pressure is raised to 400-600 mm Hg. The cannula is moved up and down and rotated 360 degree in the cavity. Alternately manual vacuum aspiration (MVA) syringe can also be used.
- Vacuum is stopped and cannula is withdrawn
- The end point of suction:
    - No more material is sucked out
    - Gripping of cannula by uterus
    - Grating sensation
    - Appearance of bubbles

- Use of curette post-evacuation is discouraged nowadays (risk of Asherman's syndrome and perforation)
- Uterotonic agent like methergin 0.2 mg IM/IV may be given
- Instruments removed, uterus massaged bimanually
- USG, if available in the OT, can confirm if the cavity is completely empty.
- If the uterus is remaining firm and bleeding is stopped/minimal, vagina and perineum are tioleted, sterile vulval pad is placed and patient shifted out of theater
- Use of USG during the procedure shortens operative time and decreases complications

POSTOPERATIVE CARE

- NBM for few hours
- Antibiotics (doxycycline and metronidazole)
- Contraceptive advise
- Anti-D injection in cases of Rh-negative mother (if the partner is Rh-positive)

COMPLICATIONS

Immediate

- **Excessive bleeding** (incomplete evacuation or atonic uterus)
- **Injury:** Cervical laceration, broad ligament hematoma (rare), uterine perforation, bowel and bladder.
- **Sepsis, hematometra**
- Complications of anesthesia

Late

- PID and subsequent infertility
- Cervical incompetence (excessive forceful dilatation) and preterm labor
- Uterine synechiae (Asherman syndrome).

SECTION 3

Pediatrics
Short Notes

Section Outline

- APGAR Score
- Asphyxia Neonatorum
- Care of the Newborn at Birth
- Causes of Convulsion in Neonate
- Down Syndrome
- Kernicterus
- Neonatal Jaundice

CHAPTER 28

Pediatrics Short Notes

Q. APGAR score.

INTRODUCTION

APGAR score, introduced by *Dr Virginia Apgar* (American Anesthesiologist at Columbia Presbyterian Medical Center, 1952) is a quantitative method for assessing the infant's respiratory, circulatory and neurological status.

APGAR SCORE SYSTEM

	0	1	2
Color of the body (**A**ppearance)	Blue/pale	Body pink Extremities blue	Pink completely
Heart rate/min (**P**ulse)	Absent	<100	>100
Reflex stimulation (**G**rimace)	No response	Grimace	Cries, coughs or sneezes
Muscle tone (**A**ctivity)	Flaccid	Some flexion	Actively moving the extremities
Respiratory effort (**R**espiration)	None	Slow, irregular	Good crying

- 8–10: Normal
- 5–7: Moderately asphyxiated
- <4: Severe distress.

Note: The ideal score at 1 minute is **9 as the periphery is always blue (acrocyanosis) and score is not 10 at 1 minute**.

TIMING OF THE SCORE

- At first cry
- After regular respiration has been established
- Delayed to detect any neurological deficit.

To satisfy the above criteria, the Apgar score is taken at 1 minute, 5 minutes and 10 to 20 minutes (extended APGAR, if required).

■ IMPORTANCE

Apgar score is a **'monitoring score'** to determine the **efficacy of resuscitation** and gives an overall view of condition of newborn
- As the score declines, it indicates drop in arterial pH (acidosis)
- Prognostic value: If score is **<4 at 20 minutes**, it indicates a very bad prognosis
- Five minutes score is more useful indicator to the status of newborn
- If the score is low, it may indicate any of the following:
  - Birth asphyxia
  - Drugs given to mother during labor
  - Congenital malformations
  - Intrauterine infections/septicemia.

■ FALLACIES

- It is a subjective scoring (except heart rate)
- It ignores the time of first cry of newborn
- 1 minute score is not useful in deciding upon the intervention necessary for resuscitation as action must be initiated before that
- Apgar scoring cannot be used in:
  - Preterm baby
  - Neurologically floppy infant
  - Severely sedated infant
  - Infant with Erb's palsy
- Respiration cannot be judged if the newborn is on IPPR
- It does not give any idea of the duration of asphyxia
- It does not give the severity of the asphyxia; 1 and 5 minutes scores cannot tell the progression.
  Hence 10 and 20 minutes scores are done to tell about possible neurological deficit.

Q. Asphyxia neonatorum.

■ INTRODUCTION

Asphyxia neonatorum is the consequence due to lack of oxygen and/or lack of perfusion to various organs resulting from nonestablishment of satisfactory pulmonary respiration at birth.

■ ETIOLOGY

Continuation of Intrauterine Hypoxia (90%)

Functional Failure of Placenta as Respiratory Organ

- Anatomical changes in the placenta: Thin small placenta, circumvallate placenta
- **Uteroplacental insufficiency**
  - Premature separation of placenta/abruption
  - Extensive infarcts with/without postdatism

- Hypertensive disorders in pregnancy
- Supine hypotensive syndrome
- Cord compression/prolapse, true knot in the cord, vascular anomalies in the cord, etc.

Maternal Hypoxic States

- Anemia
- Eclampsia
- Cyanotic cardiovascular disorders
- Status asthmaticus
- Shock.

Birth Trauma to the Neonate

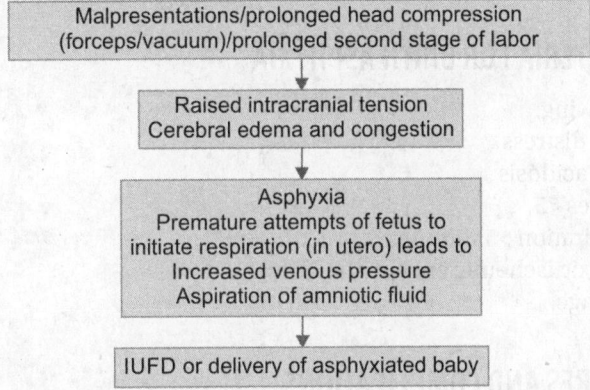

Prenatal and Intranatal Medications to the Mother

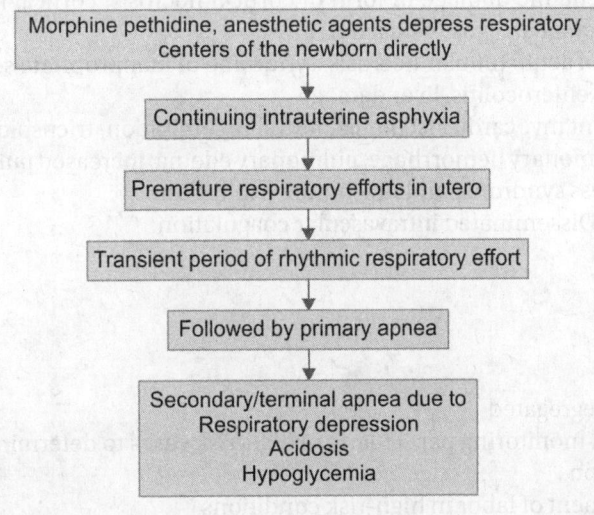

PATHOPHYSIOLOGY OF HYPOXIC ISCHEMIC ENCEPHALOPATHY

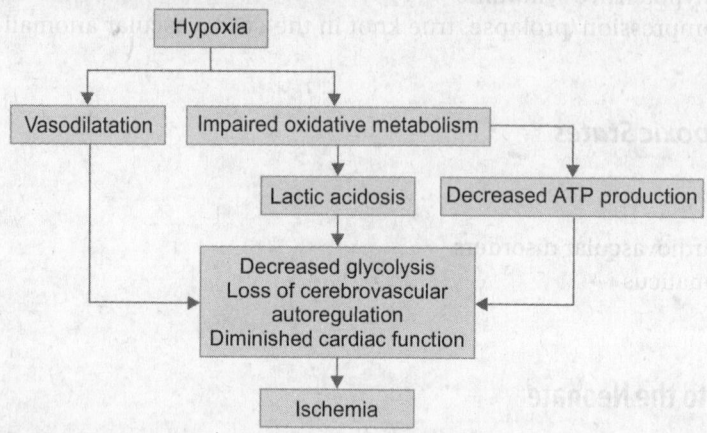

DIAGNOSTIC CRITERIA FOR BIRTH ASPHYXIA

Any four of the following:
1. Evidence of fetal distress
2. Acute metabolic acidosis
3. Apgar at 5 minutes <5
4. Initiation of respiration >5 minutes
5. Features of hypoxic ischemic encephalopathy
6. Multiorgan damage.

CLINICAL FEATURES AND COMPLICATIONS

Depend on: Etiology, intensity and duration of O_2 lack, plasma CO_2 excess and subsequent acidosis.
- **CNS:** Hypoxic ischemic damage in form of cortical necrosis, cortical infarcts, necrosis of thalamus/basal ganglia. Signs of raised ICT
- **Renal:** Features of acute tubular necrosis, syndrome of inappropriate secretion of ADH
- **GIT:** Necrotizing enterocolitis, liver damage
- **Cardiac:** Transient myocardial ischemia, mitral regurgitation, tricuspid regurgitation
- **Respiratory:** Pulmonary hemorrhage, pulmonary edema, increased pulmonary resistance, respiratory distress syndrome and meconium aspiration
- **Hematological:** Disseminated intravascular coagulation.

MANAGEMENT

Prophylactic

- High-risk cases segregated
- Intrapartum fetal monitoring particularly in high-risk cases to determine fetal distress and timely intervention
- Careful management of labor in high-risk conditions

- Judicious administration of anesthetic agents and depressant drugs during labor
- Proper care of newborn at the time of birth.

Definitive
- Maintain hydration IV fluids
- Maintain temperature
- Symptomatic treatment of hypoglycemia, hypocalcemia, convulsions, etc.
- Treatment of cerebral edema.

POOR PROGNOSTIC FACTORS
- Severe prolonged asphyxia
  - Seizures of early onset, especially difficult to treat
  - Raised intracranial pressure
- Abnormal neurological signs at the time of discharge
  - Sarnat stage 3
  - Hypodensities on CT brain
  - Persistent oliguria.

Q. Care of the newborn at birth.

PRINCIPLES
- Maintenance of temperature and asepsis
- Initiation of respiration
- Diagnosis of severe congenital malformations.

STEPS OF NEONATAL CARE

Preparation
- Temperature of the labor room to be kept at about **30°C to prevent hypothermia**. Exposure to cold may lead to metabolic acidosis, hypoglycemia and increased renal losses of solute and water
- Prewarm towels are kept ready
- **Radiant warmer** of receiving trolley are kept on.

Reception
- Keep under warmer (at a distance of 80 cm)
- Air passage suctioned after the baby's head comes out. **Air passages cleared by suction of oral cavity, oropharynx and nose (in the same order)**
- The baby should be received in a sterile prewarmed towel and then kept on warm surface in a head low position
- Wipe and **clean dry the baby**, special care should be taken to **dry the head**, which forms a large part of surface area in a newborn.

Apgar Scoring

Apgar scoring to be done at 1 minute and 5 minutes.

Resuscitation

Resuscitation if required: Four cardinal principles of neonatal resuscitation:
1. Minimize immediate heat loss
2. **Ensure open airway**
   - Proper position
   - Suction of mouth followed by nose (to prevent aspiration)
   - If thick meconium, endotracheal intubation and suction
3. **To initiate breathing**
   - Tactile stimulation (gentle rubbing on back/flicking soles of feet)
   - Face mask and AMBU bag positive pressure breathing
   - Endotracheal intubation and mechanical ventilation if required
4. **To maintain circulation**
   - Chest compression
   - Medication.

Physical Examination of the Baby

To be conducted:
- Soon after birth
- Within 24 hours of birth
- Before discharge from the nursery.

First examination is done to determine:
- Any congenital anomalies
- To categorize the baby in the birth weight, gestational age groups
- To detect other disorders which may affect neonatal course
  - *Umbilical cord:* Look for single umbilical artery
  - *Ears:* Low set ears, preauricular tags of sinus which are associated with congenital renal malformations
  - *Mouth:*
    - Cleft palate/lip
    - Tracheoesophageal fistula
  - *Nose:* Choanal atresia
  - *Neck:*
    - Branchial/thyroglossal cysts, neonatal goiter, cystic hygroma
    - Webbed neck in Turner's syndrome
  - *Chest:* Auscultate for murmur
  - *Arms:* Erb's palsy, Klumpke's palsy
  - *Genitalia:*
    - Imperforate hymen with hydrocolpos
    - Hypospadias/epispadias
    - Cryptorchidism
    - Ambiguous genitalia

- *Feet:* Talipes equinovarus
- *Rectum:*
  - Record initial temperature
  - Exclude imperforate anus

Gestational Age Estimation

Plantar creases, descent of testes
Preterm   <37 weeks
Post-term   >42 weeks

Maintenance of Body Temperature

- Environmental temperature around 25°C
- Preterm and sick-thermo-neutral environment
- Larger and older babies –32°C with 40–60% relative humidity
- Warm, woolen clothes
- Radiant warmer/incubator/servo controller.

Identification Tag

To prevent accidental exchange of babies. Also footprint of the baby is taken on the case paper to confirm identification.

Transfer to Nursery/Mother's Room and Care in the Nursery

- **Baby bath:** Not routinely favored to prevent cross infection vernix, blood and meconium wiped off using sterile moist swabs and skin is kept dry using soft towel. Baby bath may be given day prior to discharge. Use of bland soap, soft towel and separate bath tub for each baby.
- **Weight:** Baby should be weighed naked.
- **Care of umbilical cord:**
  - Inspect for slippage of ligature
  - Watch for foul smell, delayed separation, periumbilical redness (suggestive of sepsis)
  - Cord stump falls by 5–10 days.
- **Eye care:** Clean with normal saline
- **Medications:**
  - Vitamin K_1 mg IM to minimize hemorrhagic tendency
  - Prophylactic antibiotic therapy required if:
    - Premature rupture of membranes
    - Instrumentation (laryngoscopic intubation)
- **Close observation:**
  - Excessive mucus secretion
  - Bleeding from umbilical cord stump
  - Hourly temperature till it stabilizes above 36°C
- **Rooming in as early as possible:** Even within half hour after delivery, baby is given to the mother. Advantages are easy establishment of breastfeeding and emotional bond development.

Q. Causes of convulsion in neonate.

Neonatal seizures are epileptic fits occurring from birth to the end of the neonatal period. The neonatal period is the most vulnerable of all periods of life for developing seizures, particularly in the **first 1–2 days to the first week from birth**.

The prevalence is approximately 1.5% and overall incidence approximately 3 per 1,000 live births.

	Frequency
Hypoxia-ischemia/birth asphyxia • Prenatal (toxemia, fetal distress, abruptio placentae, cord compression) • Perinatal (iatrogenic, maternal hemorrhage, fetal distress) • Postnatal (cardiorespiratory causes such as hyaline membrane disease, congenital heart disease, pulmonary hypertension)	+++++++
Hemorrhage and intracerebral infarction • Intraventricular and periventricular (mainly preterm neonates) • Intracerebral (spontaneous, traumatic) • Subarachnoid • Subdural hematoma • Cerebral artery and vein infarction	++++
Trauma • Intracranial hemorrhage • Cortical vein thrombosis	++++
Infections • Encephalitis, meningitis, brain abscess • Intrauterine (rubella, toxoplasmosis, syphilis, viral—such as cytomegalovirus, herpes simplex virus, human immunodeficiency virus, coxsackie virus B) • Postnatal (beta-hemolytic streptococci, *Escherichia coli* infection, herpes simplex virus, *Mycoplasma*)	++++
Metabolic • Hypoglycemia (glucose levels <20 mg/d in preterm and <30 mg/d in full-term babies indicating hypoglycemia; mainly associated with prenatal or perinatal insults) • Neonates of diabetic mothers • Pancreatic disease • Glycogen storage disease (idiopathic) • Hypocalcemia (early, in first 2–3 days, mainly in preterm neonates with prenatal or perinatal insults; late, at 5–14 days, is mainly nutritional; maternal hyperparathyroidism; DiGeorge's syndrome) • Hypomagnesemia (may accompany or occur independently of hypocalcemia) • Hyponatremia (mainly associated with prenatal or perinatal insults; inappropriate secretion of antidiuretic hormone) • Hypernatremia (mainly nutritional or iatrogenic) • Inborn errors of metabolism (amino acid and organic acid disorders, hyperammonemias; they usually manifest with peculiar odors, protein intolerance, acidosis, alkalosis, lethargy, or stupor) • Pyridoxine dependency • Kernicterus	++
Malformations of cerebral development: All disorders of neuronal induction, segmentation, migration, myelination and synaptogenesis such as polymicrogyria, neuronal heterotopias, lissencephaly, holoprosencephaly and hydranencephaly	++

Contd...

Contd...

	Frequency
Neurocutaneous syndromes: Tuberous sclerosis, incontinentia pigmenti	++++
Drug withdrawal and toxic: Withdrawal from narcotic-analgesics, sedative-hypnotics and alcohol; heroin- and methadone-addicted mothers; barbiturates	+++
Inadvertent injections of local anesthetics during delivery	++
Idiopathic benign neonatal seizures (familial and nonfamilial)	

Q. Down syndrome.

■ INTRODUCTION

Down syndrome is the **most common autosomal trisomy.** In Down syndrome, the chromosome number 21 is present in triplicate. Down syndrome is a common cause of mental retardation.

■ GENETIC BASIS

- ❖ *Nondysjunction* **(95% of patients):** Meiotic separation does not occur for number 21 chromosome. One of the gamete carries an extra chromosome. On fertilization of this gamete, it leads to trisomy 21.
- ❖ *Translocation* **(4% of cases):** When part of chromosome 21 becomes translocated onto another chromosome usually a D group (number 13, 14 or 15) or a G-group (number 21 or 22) chromosome. Affected people have two normal copies of chromosome 21 plus extra material from chromosome 21 attached to another chromosome, resulting in three copies of genetic material from chromosome 21.
- ❖ *Mosaicism* **(1% of cases):** Some cells having 46 chromosomes and two number 21 chromosomes and some cells having 47 and three number 21 chromosomes.

■ INCIDENCE

Down syndrome occurs in 1 in 600 to 1 in 800 live births **(50% of cases abort in early pregnancy).**

■ RISK IN RELATION TO INCREASING MATERNAL AGE

Age of mother	Approximate risk of Down syndrome
20 years	1 in 2,000
30 years	1 in 1,000
40 years	1 in 100
45 years	1 in 30

■ CLINICAL FEATURES

Mosaic Down syndrome children have milder clinical presentation as compared to other two types.

Dysmorphic Features

Dysmorphic Facial Features
- Flat facial profile
- Short, upslanting palpebral fissures
- Brushfield spots on iris
- Flat nasal bridge with *epicanthal folds*
- Small, mouth with protruding tongue
- *Short ears* with abnormal ear lobes
- Cataract and squint is common
- High arched palate with small teeth
- *'Scrotal'* (Furrowed) tongue.

Other Dysmorphic Features
- Microcephaly, brachycephaly
- Skin: Excess posterior neck skin
- Short stature/short 'long' bones
- Clinodactyly with hypoplastic middle phalanx
- Single palmar crease *(Simian crease)*
- Sandal gap.

Functional and Structural Abnormalities
- **Hypotonia:** Frequent accompaniment. Most noticeable in the newborn (poor Moro's reflex and hyperflexibility of joints, hip dysplasia)
- **Mental retardation** and developmental delay. The mean IQ is 50%
- **Cardiac defects:**
  - Endocardial cushion defects
  - Septal defects (VSD/ASD)
  - Patent ductus arteriosus
- **Abdomen and pelvis**
  - Duodenal atresia and Hirschsprung disease
  - Omphalocele, congenital diaphragmatic hernia
  - Small penis
  - Cryptorchidism
  - Renal pyelectasis
- **Hypothyroidism** and **leukemia** occur at higher frequency
- **Social aspects:** Behave as good babies, happy children and tend towards mimicry, are friendly and have a good sense of rhythm and enjoy music.

■ MANAGEMENT

Counseling
- To be given after confirmation of diagnosis
- Both the parents should be present
- Counseling given by a team of pediatrician, geneticist and psychiatrist

- ❖ Explain the parents about the disease that the child is going to be mentally retarded, require special schooling
- ❖ Explain about congenital heart diseases, other abnormalities.

Counseling about the Recurrence Risk

Chromosome constitution			Risk of offspring	
Affected child	Father	Mother		
Trisomy 21 (nondisjunction)	N	N	Mother <30 years in present pregnancy	2–3%
			Mother >30 years; had Down baby before 30 years of age	Risk at mothers age +1%
			Mother >30 years; had Down baby after 30 years of age	Risk at mother's age
Translocations 14/21, 15/21, 13/21, 21/22	N C	C N		11.9% 2–3%
Translocations 21/21	N C	C N		100% 100%
Mosaic	N	N		2–3%

C = Carrier, N = Normal

In Future Pregnancy

The only 100% confirmatory test for Down syndrome is karyotyping, the sample for which can be obtained by chorionic villus sampling (CVS) or amniocentesis. Hence, in a patient who has a past history of fetus with Down syndrome, **fetal karyotyping should be done in all future pregnancies.**

■ PREVENTION

Early Detection of Down's Syndrome and MTP

Antenatally NT scan and dual marker test (hCG + PAPP A) at **11–13 weeks** of gestation or **triple marker test**, should routinely be offered to all patients as **a screening test.**

Triple Marker Test

This is a **screening** test done between **16 and 18 weeks of gestation**, mainly to identify a mother who is at a high-risk of having a fetus with trisomy 21. It involves estimation of 3 hormones: hCG, AFP, and unconjugated estriol (uE3).

Interpretation

	hCG	AFP	uE3
Down syndrome (T 21)	↑	↓	↓

In following cases, **confirmatory test (karyotyping) should be done** and if abnormal MTP should be offered:
- ❖ Maternal age >35 years

- Previous autosomal trisomy birth
- Major fetal structural defect identified by ultrasound/increase NT
- High-risk detected by dual/triple marker test.

Q. Kernicterus.

■ DEFINITION

Unconjugated hyperbilirubinemia in the neonatal period can cause bilirubin encephalopathy with necrosis of neurons in the basal ganglia, hippocampus, and subthalamic nuclei. This *'nuclear staining'* with bilirubin is called **'Kernicterus'** (*Bilirubin brain damage/Bilirubin encephalopathy*).

■ PATHOPHYSIOLOGY

- Unconjugated bilirubin can be bound to albumin or exist as free bilirubin if albumin is exhausted.
- 3 gm of albumin binds with 21–24 mg indirect bilirubin.
- A newborn has about 3 g% of albumin in blood. **If the indirect bilirubin goes above 24–25 mg%** then albumin is not available for binding and the excess indirect bilirubin accumulates.
- The bilirubin bound to albumin cannot cross the blood-brain barrier. However, the indirect bilirubin not bound to albumin can do so.
- Once bound to the neurons, *the free indirect bilirubin* acts as a mitochondrial toxin. This leads to *mitochondrial damage*. Once the free indirect bilirubin binds to mitochondria, it is almost irreversible change but the bilirubin can still be dissociated and hence this effect can be considered partly reversible.
- It is also said that bilirubin reversibly *inhibits phosphorylation* of 'synapsin' which is believed to regulate neurotransmitter release. After initial entry into the neurons, the bilirubin departs leaving behind neuronal atrophy and gliosis.
- Also, several other cytoplasmic proteins such as ligandin, fatty acid binding protein and lipoprotein show high affinity for bilirubin. As the bilirubin binding capacity of the tissue proteins is exhausted, the free bilirubin seeps into the neurons.

■ HIGH-RISK FACTORS

Prematurity and Preterm Infants

- Blood-brain barrier is weak
- Capacity of albumin to bind to bilirubin is also low.

Neonates Suffering from the Following Conditions

- Hypoglycemia
- Hypothermia
- Acidosis
- Serious metabolic illnesses.
  All these lead to a fall in blood pH and uncouple bilirubin from bilirubin-albumin complex.

Pathological States

- Hypoxia
- Hemolysis
- Septicemia
- Ketoacidosis.
  All these conditions can lead to increased levels of free bilirubin in the blood.

Drugs

- Salicylates
- Sulfonamides
- Nonesterified fatty acids.
  These decrease bilirubin binding with albumin.

Others

- Hypocalcemia
- Hypomagnesemia
- Birth asphyxia
- Respiratory distress syndrome
- Hyaline membrane disease.
  All these cause a decreased threshold for bilirubin brain damage.

PARTS OF BRAIN AFFECTED BY HYPERBILIRUBINEMIA

- Eighth nerve nucleus
- Basal ganglia
- Cerebral cortex (if free indirect bilirubin levels are very high).

CLINICAL FEATURES

- Appear between 3 to 7 days of life
- Lethargy, refusal of feeds, shrill cry
- Icterus, bulging fontanelle, setting sun sign, dampened reflexes, convulsions, rigidity, opisthotonos, abnormal Moro's reflex
- In very mild type, there may just be deafness and hearing loss [detected by brainstem evoked response audiometry (BERA) on follow-up].

STAGES

- **Stage 1:** Hypotonia, poor Moro's reflex, lethargy, vomiting, high pitched cry
- **Stage 2:** Seizures, rigidity, opisthotonos, fever, oculogyric crisis, paralysis of upward gaze
- **Stage 3:** Decrease in spasticity (one week of age)
- **Stage 4:** Late sequelae.

SEQUELAE

- Deafness (VIII nerve nucleus affected)

- Spastic/athetoid type of cerebral palsy (basal ganglia affected)
- Intellectual retardation and learning disabilities (cortical involvement)
- Paralysis of upward gaze
- Epilepsy
- Dental dysplasia
- Brownish staining to teeth.

INVESTIGATIONS

- Serum bilirubin: Direct, indirect
- Serum albumin
- Blood electrolytes (r/o acidosis), a blood culture (r/o septicemia), a blood sugar (r/o hypoglycemia)
- Hb, CBC, ESR (hemolytic process).

MANAGEMENT

Treating the indirect hyperbilirubinemia:
- Phototherapy
- Exchange transfusion
- Use of tin-metalloporphyrin
  (For details, please refer to note on Neonatal Jaundice)
- Rehabilitation of the patient later on is equally important (in cases of cerebral palsy, MR, deafness, etc.). Proper referrals should be made
- The prime objective has to be preventing the rise of bilirubin to toxic levels which may cause kernicterus.

Q. Neonatal jaundice.

DEFINITION

Physiological Jaundice

Unconjugated hyperbilirubinemia with following characteristics:
- *In full term newborns:* Peak bilirubin level of 6–8 mg/dL by 3 days of life and maximum reached up to 12 mg/dL. Returns to normal by 10th day of life
- *In preterm newborns:* Peak bilirubin level by fifth day of life rising up to 15 mg/dL. Returns to normal level by 15th day.

Pathological Jaundice

Nonphysiological hyperbilirubinemia with any of following characteristics:
- Clinical jaundice prior to 36 hours of age
- Clinical jaundice persisting for >8 days in full term babies or 14 days in preterm newborns
- Serum bilirubin increasing to >5 mg/dL/day
- Total serum bilirubin >15 mg/dL in formula fed term baby or >17 mg/dL in breastfed term baby.

INCIDENCE

- 25–60% of full term newborns develop clinical jaundice
- 70–85% of preterm infants develop clinical jaundice
- 3% of normal term infants show bilirubin levels >15 mg/dL.

Note
- 1 g of hemoglobin produces 34 mg of bilirubin
- Normal newborn produces 6–10 mg of bilirubin/kg body weight/day as compared to 3–4 mg/kg/day in adult.

POSSIBLE MECHANISMS INVOLVED IN PHYSIOLOGIC JAUNDICE

- Increased bilirubin load on liver cells:
  - Increased RBC volume/kg as compared to adult
  - Decreased RBC survival 90 days
  - Increased enterohepatic circulation of bilirubin
  - Defective hepatic uptake of bilirubin from plasma
- *Defective bilirubin conjugation*: Decreased UDP glucuronyl transferase activity and decreased UDP glucose dehydrogenase activity
- Defective bilirubin excretion.

FACTORS EXAGGERATING PHYSIOLOGIC JAUNDICE

- Male sex
- Prematurity
- Maternal diabetes
- Hypoxia
- Cutaneous bruising and cephalohematoma.

CAUSES OF PATHOLOGICAL JAUNDICE

Overproduction

- **Hemolytic Disorders**
  - Extracorpuscular
    - Immunological: Rh incompatibility, ABO incompatibility
    - Nonimmunological: Sepsis, vitamin K induced hemolysis.
  - Intracorpuscular
    - Hemoglobinopathies: Thalassemia
    - Enzyme defects: G6PD deficiency, pyruvate kinase deficiency
    - Membrane defects: Hereditary spherocytosis, elliptocytosis, poikilocytosis.
- **Extravascular blood**
  - Cephalohematoma and other hematomas
  - Pulmonary and cerebral hemorrhage.
- **Polycythemia:** Chronic fetal hypoxia
- **Exaggerated enterohepatic circulation**
  - Mechanical obstruction: Atresia and stenosis, meconium ileus, Hirschsprung's disease
  - Reduced peristalsis: Underfeeding.

Undersecretion

- **Obstructive disorders**
  - Biliary atresia
  - Choledochal cyst
  - Tumor or band
  - Dubin Johnson syndrome
  - Rotor's syndrome.
- **Metabolic and endocrinal disorders**
  - Galactosemia
  - Crigler-Najjar syndrome
  - Gilberts syndrome
  - Hypothyroidism
  - Hypopituitarism
- **Prematurity.**

Mixed

- *Intrauterine infections:* Toxoplasmosis, rubella, herpes zoster, syphilis
- Maternal diabetes
- Respiratory distress syndrome
- Asphyxia
- Erythroblastosis fetalis.

BREAST MILK JAUNDICE

Introduction

In up to 1% breastfed babies, the serum bilirubin levels remain high after the third day instead of the usual fall and may rise up to 20–30 mg% by two weeks of age. With continued breastfeeding, the levels stay elevated and then gradually fall to return to normal by 1 to 3 months of age. If breastfeeding is stopped, the bilirubin level falls rapidly in 48 hours. This is harmless condition and kernicterus does not occur.

Clinical Examination

- **Severity of jaundice (Kramer's rule)**
  - Icterus limited to head and neck   4–8 mg%
  - Icterus involving upper trunk   5–12 mg%
  - Icterus over lower trunk   8–16 mg%
  - Icterus over arms, legs   11–18 mg%
  - Icterus over palms and soles   >15 mg%
- **Color of jaundice**
  - Hemolytic   : Lemon yellow
  - Hepatic   : Bright yellow/orange yellow
  - Obstructive : Green yellow
- **Gestational age:** Prematurity
- **General condition of newborn:** Sepsis, fever, tachycardia, tachypnea, evidence of injuries
- **Umbilical discharge:** Umbilical sepsis
  - Pallor, hemorrhage, petechiae

- ❖ **Hepato/splenomegaly**
  - ➢ Neurological signs
  - ➢ Cry: Shrill cry in kernicterus
  - ➢ Tone
  - ➢ Reflexes: Moro's and sucking reflexes are weak or absent
- ❖ **Features of endocrinal disorders**
- ❖ **Any congenital malformation.**

Investigations

- ❖ Hb, CBC, reticulocyte count
  - ➢ Peripheral smear for RBC morphology
- ❖ ABO and Rh grouping of mother and baby
- ❖ Coomb's test of mother and baby
- ❖ Serum bilirubin: Direct and indirect
- ❖ Blood culture
- ❖ Serum albumin
- ❖ Other liver function tests
- ❖ G-6-PD enzyme studies
- ❖ Ultrasonography of abdomen and liver scans
- ❖ T3, T4, TSH.

Approach to a case of neonatal jaundice has been discussed in **Flowchart 28.1**.

Treatment

- ❖ **Physiological jaundice:**
  - ➢ No specific treatment required
  - ➢ Continue breastfeeding
  - ➢ Watch for any complicating illness or sudden rise in bilirubin levels
  - ➢ Treat/prevent any exaggerating factor.
- ❖ **Pathological jaundice:**
  - ➢ Phototherapy
  - ➢ Exchange transfusion
  - ➢ Phenobarbital
  - ➢ Agar-Agar
  - ➢ Albumin infusion
  - ➢ Tin protoporphyrin.

Phototherapy

Mode of Action

Phototherapy helps by lowering unconjugated hyperbilirubinemia.
- ❖ **Structural isomerization:** Phototherapy modify bilirubin deposited in the skin by photoisomerization process forming bilirubin isomer, which is rapidly excreted in the bile with a half-life of about 2 hours.
- ❖ **Intramolecular cyclization:** To lumirubin, which is rapidly excreted in bile and urine without conjugation.
- ❖ **Photo-oxidation:** Bilirubin absorbs light and get oxidized to polar color less products which are excreted in urine.

Flowchart 28.1: Approach to a case of neonatal jaundice.

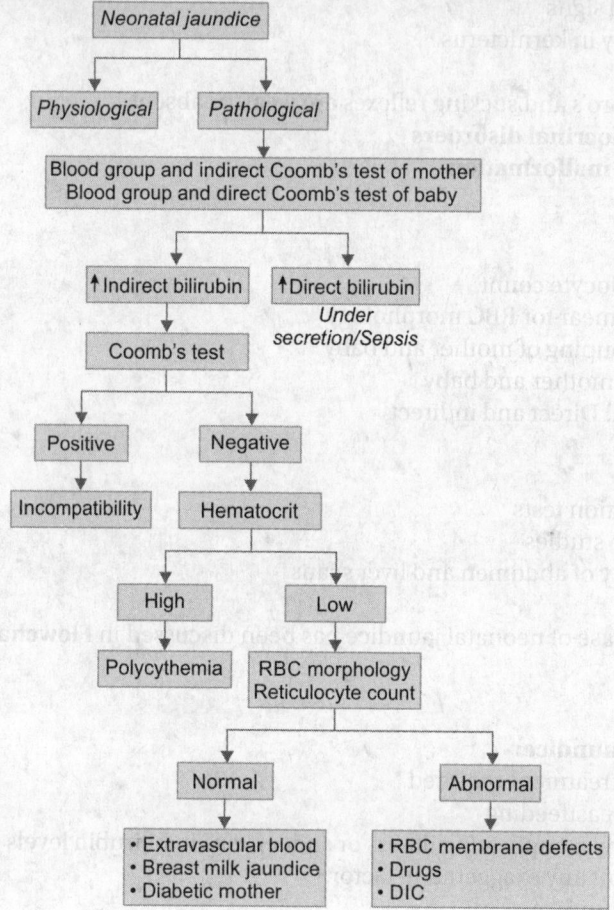

Indications

- Serum bilirubin above 15 mg% for term infants and 10 mg% for preterm infants.
- Serum bilirubin 5 mg% or more in the first 24 hours.
- In hemolytic disease of newborn—immediately after birth.
- Adjunct to exchange transfusion in hemolytic disease of newborn.
- Prophylactically in:
  - Very low birth weight babies who are likely to develop dangerous levels of bilirubin.
  - Severely bruised premature infants.

Contraindications

- Obstructive jaundice—**ineffective in reducing direct hyperbilirubinemia**
- Light sensitive porphyria.

Techniques

- **Light source:** Four blue/green light fluorescent lamps
- **Position of infant:** Placed naked at a distance of 45 cm below light source

- **Protection of infant:** Eye patches to protect from retinal damage and diaper to protect external gonads
- **Duration of phototherapy:** 24–48 hours exposure is generally long enough to bring down serum bilirubin level to safe limit.

Side Effects of Phototherapy

- Dehydration
- Diarrhea
- Skin burns/rash
- Tanning
- Bronze baby syndrome—reduced hepatic excretion of bilirubin photoproduct
- Decreased serum calcium levels
- Hyperthermia
- Hemolysis
- Retinal damage.

Exchange Transfusion

Aims and Objectives

- *Remove* excess bilirubin and other harmful substances and to replace the blood by healthy donor blood
- Correct anemia by replacing blood of low PCV with that of normal PCV avoiding circulatory overload also.

Indications

- **Uncomplicated hemolytic disorders:**
  - Severe anemia Hb <8 g%
  - Serum bilirubin >20 mg% at any time
  - Serum bilirubin rising by >1 mg% per day
  - Cord bilirubin >4.5 mg% and cord Hb <11 g%
  - Serum bilirubin rising >0.5 mg% with hemoglobin level between 11 g% and 13 g%.
- **Complicated hemolytic disorders:**
  - Hydrops fetalis
  - Impending heart failure.

Donor Blood

- Should be fresh (<3 days old)
- Amount required.

Double volume exchange: 160 mL/kg (exchanges 87% of infant's blood volume).

Single volume exchange: 80 mL/kg (exchanges 63% of infant's blood volume).

Blood Group

- In Rh incompatibility: O Rh negative blood, cross-matched against mother's blood.
- In ABO incompatibility: Same ABO and Rh group as of baby.
- Tested for HIV, HBsAg and VDRL.

Techniques

- Strict asepsis
- Cardiac monitor
- Umbilical vein cannulated with umbilical catheter
  - Exchange transfusion done by push-pull method.

Complications

- **Vascular:** Embolization, thrombosis, vasospasm
- **Cardiac:** Arrhythmias, arrest circulatory overload
- **Electrolyte and acid base:** Hyperkalemia, hypocalcemia, acidosis
- **Bleeding:** Thrombocytopenia, deficient dolling factors
- Infections
- **Others:** Hypo/hyperthermia, perforation of vessels, transient maculopapular rash.

Phenobarbital

Mechanism of Action

Induces activity of the enzyme glucuronyl transferase. Increases bilirubin conjugation and excretion.

Dosage and Role in Neonatal Jaundice

Therapeutic: 5–8 mg/kg/day to the newborn: Indicated only in Crigler-Najjar syndrome type II and other conjugated hyperbilirubinemia.

Disadvantages/Side Effects

- Take time (3–4 days) to become therapeutically active.
- Child may become drowsy which is also an early feature of kernicterus. Slow feeding.

Agar

Mechanism of Action

Binds bilirubin in gut and diminishes enterohepatic circulation.

Dosage and Role in Neonatal Jaundice

125 mg every 3 hourly in mild to moderate hyperbilirubinemia as an adjunct.

Albumin Infusion

Mechanism of Action

Raises bilirubin binding capacity.

Dosage and Role in Neonatal Jaundice

1 mg/kg of salt free albumin can be used as an alternative to exchange transfusion in very small infants.

Tin Protoporphyrin

Heme oxygenase enzyme inhibitor.

INDEX

Page numbers followed by *f* refer to figure and *fc* refer to flowchart.

A

Abdomen 114, 334
   lump in 59
Abdominal encerclage operation 195
Abdominal examination 46, 60, 185, 203, 285
Abdominal hysterectomy 70
   total 111
Abdominal mass 72
Abdominal pain
   classic triad of 202
   lower 272
   unilateral lower 139
Abdominal surgeries 245
Abdominal tone 72
Abdominovaginal examination 274
Abnormal uterine
   bleeding 54, 94
      causes of 54
   contraction 185
ABO blood group 276
Abortion 190, 240, 281
   causes of 190, 191*fc*
   first trimester 83
      medical method of 132
   inevitable 197
   missed 195
   recurrent
      first trimester 240
      spontaneous 94
   threatened 198
Abruptio placentae 153, 221
   risk factors for 221
   signs of 221
   symptoms of 221
Abruption
   management of 221, 223, 224*fc*
   prevent 277
   types of 222, 222*f*
Acanthosis nigricans 83
Accrete previa, diagnosis of 305
Acetic acid, visual inspection with 98
Acne 83, 84, 128
   treatment of 86
Acriflavine heals 73
Acute pelvic inflammatory disease, clinical features of 36
Addison's disease 4
Adenocarcinoma 108
Adenomyosis 47, 55, 61, 124
Adenosine deaminase levels 33
Adherent placenta, morbidly 308
Adhesiolysis 27, 56, 90, 91
Adrenal failure, chronic 134
Adriamycin 112
Advanced carcinoma 103
   cervix 293
Airway disease, chronic 72
Albumin 154
   infusion 344
Allen-Master syndrome 56, 88
Alloimmune 191
   disease 191
Alopecia, male pattern 83
Alpha methyldopa 215
Amendment of Act 148
Amenorrhea 52, 83, 84, 89, 124, 197, 202
   cause of primary 56
   period of 271, 272
   primary 56
Amino acids 151
Amniocentesis 315
Amnioinfusion 279
Amnion nodosum 279
Amniotic fluid 152, 291, 316*f*
   evaluation 315
   index 153, 158, 252, 256, 275, 278
   meconium stained 255, 258, 290
Amniotomy 291
Ampicillin 38, 233
Amputation 192
Amsel's criteria 40
Anastrozole 63, 85
Anatomic distortions, correction of 90
Androgen excess, signs of 50
Android pelvis 179, 185, 189
Androstenedione 82, 83
Anemia 128, 225, 234, 249, 280
   case of 234
   cause of 236
   complications of 234
   congenital 314
   degree of 235
   physiological 235
   signs of 50
   type of 235
Anencephaly 275, 305, 320

Anesthesia, complications of 322
Anesthetic complications 93
Anovular menorrhagia 49
Anovulation 4, 26
   chronic 81, 82
Antecubital venous pressure 156
Antenatal care 157, 161
   components of 161
Antenatal management 286
Antepartum 258
   hemorrhage 221, 228, 245, 258
Anthelmintics 237
Anthropoid pelvis 178
Anti-apolipoprotein antibodies 243
Anticardiolipin antibody 191, 243
Anticonvulsant therapy 218
Anti-D gamma globulin 183
Anti-D injection 207
Anti-Koch treatment 33
Antimicrobial regimens 260
Anti-Müllerian hormone 11, 57
   test 11
Antiphospholipid antibody 303
   syndrome 242, 243
Antiseptic 176
   solution 321
Antisperm antibody 24
Antral follicle count 11
Anuria 213, 250
Anxiety 144
Apgar score 325, 326, 330
   system 325
Apnea 248
Appendicitis 140
   acute 245
Arginine donor 253
Aromatase inhibitor 63, 90, 112
Aromatization, defective 82
Arrhythmia 134
Asepsis 176
Asherman's syndrome 95f, 322
Asoprisnil acetate 63
Aspermia 20
Asphyxia 282
   neonatorum 326
   severe prolonged 329
Aspirin, low dose 216, 253
Assisted reproductive technology 24, 201
Asthenospermia 20
Atonic postpartum hemorrhage 60, 229
Atrial natriuretic peptide 156
Atrial septal defect 241
Atrophy 65
Atypia, hyperplasia with 53
Auditory system 249
Auscultation 285

Autoimmune 191
   diseases 4
   factors 191
Autosomal dominant inheritance 243
Autosomal trisomy, common 333
Azoospermia 20, 25
Aztreonam 261

B

Baby
   bath 331
   physical examination of 330
Bacterial vaginosis 40, 244
   complications of 40
Bacteroides 66
   fragilis 35
   species 258
Bad obstetric history 183
Bakri balloon 229
Balloon devices 292
Bandl's ring 264
Bartter's syndrome 276
Basal body temperature 7, 8
Basal endometrium 53
Basal estradiol 10
Basal follicle-stimulating hormone 10
Bayle's sign 19
Beat-to-beat variability 159
   loss of 178
Benson and Durfee cerclage 195
Beta-2 agonist 245
Beta-adrenergic agents 246
Beta-hemolytic streptococci 332
Betamethasone 245
Bicornuate uterus 56, 244
Bilirubin
   brain damage 336
   encephalopathy 336
   free indirect 336
   isomer 341
Biochemical marker 214
Biophysical profile 157, 253, 256
   score 158
Biopsy 98, 103
Birth 247
   injuries 182, 242
   trauma 327
Birth asphyxia 182, 332
   diagnostic criteria for 328
Birth control 119
   device, used 120
   pills 141
Bishop scoring system 289
Bispinous diameter, transverse 188
Bivius 35

Index

Bladder
  care 177
  emptied 321
  tumor invasion of 113
Blastocyst, implantation of 123
Bleeding 142, 344
  breakthrough 128
  control of 172
  disorder, signs of 50
  excessive 322
  expulsion of 172
  irregular 124
  per vagina 165, 197, 202
  postcoital 101
  postmenopausal 94, 110
  slight 196
Blood 37
  coagulation factors 154
  donor 343
  group 343
  investigations 236
  loss, reduction of 124
  pressure 156, 168, 177
  smear, peripheral 235
  urea nitrogen 272
  vessels, atypical 98
Blood transfusion 223, 226, 238
  advantages of 238
  start 269
Bloodstream 29
Body mass index 50, 72
Body temperature, maintenance of 331
Boggy mass 203
Bone density changes 131
Bowel symptoms 71
Brachial plexus stretching 182
Bradycardia 159, 178, 268
  transient 183
Brain 320
  parts of 337
  sparing effect 252
Brandt Andrew's maneuver 174
Breast
  diseases, benign 127
  milk jaundice 340
Breast cancer 129, 146
  premenopausal 263
Breastfeeding 119, 262
  advantages of 262
Breath, acetone smell in 312
Breathing, initiate 330
Breech
  etiology of 180
  footling 184
  preterm 184
  types of 180, 181

Breech presentation 184, 299
  complications in 181
  prevalence of 181
Broad ligament 67
  fibroid 60
  hematoma 322
Bromocriptine 22, 262
Bronchopulmonary dysplasia 248
Bronze baby syndrome 343
Buccal route 290
Burr cells 212

C

Cabergoline 22, 90, 262
Calcareous degeneration 65
Calcium 164, 217
  channel blocker 245
  supplements 162
Caldwell-Moloy classification 178
Calwin cannula 14
Cancer 108
  cervix
    clinical staging of 106
    management of 104
  protection against 127
  treatment 10
Candida vaginitis 42
Caput epididymis 19
Carbetocin 229
Carbohydrate 262
Carboplatin 112, 116
Carcinoma cervix 105
  radiotherapy for 105
  risk factors for 100
  staging for 106, 107
  treatment for 105
Carcinoma endometrium 108
  staging for 112, 113
Carcinoma, progression to 109
Cardiac anomalies 241
Cardiac defects 334
Cardiac failure 234
Cardiac monitoring 233
Cardiac output increases 155
Cardiac patient, intrapartum management of 232
Cardinal ligament 68
Cardiomyopathy 242
Cardiotocography 160
Cardiovascular diseases 134, 163
Cardiovascular system 249
Carneous degeneration 65, 233
Carneous mole 196
Caseation necrosis 31
Caudal regression syndrome 241
Cavity distortion 125
Cefotaxime 39

Cefotetan 38
Cefoxitin 38, 39
Ceftizoxime 39
Ceftriaxone 38, 39
Centimeters 176
Central hemodynamics 156
Central nervous system 241, 250
    injury, signs of 250
Central placenta previa 292
Central venous pressure 156
    monitoring 233
Cephalic prominence 186
Cephalic replacement 307
Cephalic version, external 182, 270
Cephalopelvic disproportion 264, 289, 298
Cephalosporin 39
Cerclage procedure 193
Cerebral artery, middle 252, 314
Cerebral development, malformations of 332
Cerebrospinal fluid 137
Cervical 5
    amputation 75
    atresia 46
    biopsy 98, 103
    canal 37
    caps 122
    cause 44
    cytology 73
    dilatation 168, 176, 193
    dysplasia, rule out 78
    dystocia 195
    ectopic pregnancy 197
    encerclage 192
    factors 28
    injury 134
    laceration 322
    length 193, 247
    ligament, transverse 68
    stenosis 55
    stromal invasion 113
    tear 195
Cervical cancer 129
    clinical features of 100
    diagnosis of 100
    incidence of 97
    management of 100
    screening 97
    staging of 106
Cervical epithelium 97
    life cycle of 97
Cervical erosion 141
    area of 142
    causes of 141
    symptoms of 142
Cervical incompetence 75, 192, 322
    management of 192

Cervical intraepithelial neoplasia
    management of 96
    pathogenesis of 101, 101f
    risk factors for 96
Cervical mucus
    changes in 127
    study 7, 8
    thick 124, 130
Cervix 30, 108, 168, 290
    amputation of 75
    cleaned 321
    dilatation of 46, 168, 197
    effacement of 176
    front of 194
    step amputation of 75
    supravaginal elongation of 73
Cesarean section
    indications for 184
    lower segment 182, 223, 224, 233, 247, 266
    scar, classical 300
Chemotherapy 4, 112, 116
Child, desirous of 85
Childbearing function 75
Chlamydia 120, 244
    trachomatis 35
Chocolate cystectomy 56
Chorioamnionitis 153, 195, 245
Chorioangioma 276
Chorionicity, signs for 285
Chromopertubation 12, 15, 16f, 91, 92f
Chromosomal abnormalities 148
Chromosomal anomalies 304
Chromosome constitution 335
Chromosome
    copies of 333
    deletions in 58
Cilastatin 261
Cisplatin 112
Clean dry baby 329
Clear cell variety 110
Clindamycin 38, 261
Clomiphene citrate 23, 85
    challenge test 11
Clostridium species 258
Clotrimazole 43
Clotting function 272
Clue cells 40
Coccobacilli 40
Coital problems 6
Coitus dependent 121
Collapsed follicle 9
Colloid 226, 229
    oncotic pressure 156
Colon malignancy 115
Color Doppler 205, 226, 252, 305

Index

Colpocleisis 80
   complete 78
   partial 78
Colpoperineorrhaphy 74
Colporrhaphy 74
Colposcope 98
Columnar epithelium 141
Combined oral contraceptive pills,
     contraindications for 129
Complete blood
   cell 212
     count 272
     count 260
Concealed abruption, severe variety of 223
Condom 120, 122
   disposal of 121
   female 121, 121f
   tamponade 121
Conduplicato corpore 185
Congenital anomalies 183, 241, 278, 281
Congenital malformations 56, 126, 148, 341
Congenital weakness 69
Connective tissue disorders 69, 308
Continue oxytocin drip 287
Continuous combined hormone replacement
     therapy 145
Continuous electronic fetal monitoring 178
Contraception 35, 119, 287
   failure 200
   harmless method of 120
   long acting reversible 136
   natural 263
Contraceptive advice 239
Contraceptive failure, grounds of 134
Contraceptive implants 136
Contracted pelvis 183, 264, 289, 292
Coombs' test, positive indirect 314, 319
Copper-releasing intrauterine device 123
Cord
   blood 151
   compression, prevent 279
   traction, controlled 174
Cord prolapse 182, 277, 281, 291
   high risk of 184
Cornual catheterization 95
Cornual endometrium 30
Coronary artery disease 146
Corticosteroids 212
Cough, chronic 69
Cranium 320
Crown rump length 305
Cryocautery 143
Cryptomenorrhea 45
Crystalloids 226, 229
Cuff salpingostomy 27
Culdocentesis 205

Cullen's sign 203
Cyclophosphamide 112
Cyproterone 126
Cyst
   chocolate 88, 90
   dermoid 137, 139
   ovarian 55, 185
   theca lutein 273
Cystic degeneration 64
Cystocele 70, 72
   presence of 71
Cystoscopy 103
Cystourethrocele 72
Cytoreductive surgery 115, 116

D

Danazol 52, 89
Decidua basalis, deep spongy layer of 171
Deep vein thrombosis 130, 242
Dehydration, evidence of 311
Dehydroepiandrosterone 26, 84
Delivery
   expected date of 162
   methods of 216, 317
Dental caries 244
Depot medroxyprogesterone acetate 63, 116, 130, 239
Depression 144
Dermoid plug 138
Desmopressin acetate 52
Desogestrel 126
Destruction, techniques of 99
Detorsion 141
Diabetes 303
   complications of 239
   effects of 240
   insipidus 276
   mellitus 22, 109, 130, 163, 191, 256, 258
Diagnostic cone biopsy 98, 103
Diagnostic hysteroscopy, indications for 94
Diaphragm 121f
Diathermy 143
Dienogest 89
Dietary advice 165
Dietetic deficiency 311
Diminished ovarian reserve 4, 26
Dimorphic anemia 234
Dinoprostone 290
Disseminated intravascular coagulation 212, 223, 224, 273
Distant metastasis 113
Diverticulitis 140
Dizygotic twins 283
Doderlein's bacilli 40
Dominant follicle 9, 85
Dot-dash pattern 138
Double decidual sign 198

Index

Down's syndrome 333, 335
   early detection of 335
   risk of 285
Doxycycline 38, 39, 125
Doxylamine 313
Drospirenone 86, 126
Drug
   antiandrogen 18
   antiemetic 313
   uterotonic 174
   withdrawal and toxic 333
Dual marker test 164
Ductus venosus 252
Duncan mechanism 171
Dydrogesterone 55, 144, 199
   norethisterone 89
Dyschezia 87
Dysfunctional uterine bleeding 47, 48, 49, 62
   management of 48
Dysmenorrhea 54, 59, 62, 87, 124, 125, 130
   primary 54
Dysmorphic facial features 334
Dyspareunia 144, 296
   deep 87
Dyspnea, progressive 232
Dysuria 102

E

Early cord clamping 317
Early pregnancy
   abort in 333
   features of 203
Ears 330
Ecchymosis 50
Eclampsia 208, 209, 245, 273, 302, 303
   actual 213
   impending 213
   management of 217, 217fc
   treatment for 217, 220
Ectocervix 141
Ectopic minded 203
Ectopic pregnancy 47, 92, 126, 127, 200, 206, 305
   acute 202, 204
   chronic 204
   diagnosis of 305
   etiology of 200
   old 203
   presumed 205
   primary treatment of 206
   protects against 124
   ruptured 140
   unruptured 205
Ectopy 141
Edema feet 163
Eespiratory organ 326
Ehlers-Danlos syndrome 69, 308

Eisenmenger's syndrome 132
Ejaculation, retrograde 22
Ejaculatory ducts, transurethral resection of 24
Elagolix 90
Electronic fetal monitoring 256
Embryo transfer 25
Emergency contraception 131
   methods of 131
Emotional bond 262
Emotional support 175
End organ changes, evaluation of 8
Endocervical curettage 98
Endocervix replaces, columnar epithelium of 142
Endocrinal disorder 340
   features of 341
Endocrine 6
   disorders 191
   function 151
Endometrial ablation 53
Endometrial biopsy 7, 9, 37, 50
Endometrial cancer 108, 125
   grading of 112
   hormone treatment for 112
   management of 108
   surgical staging for 112
Endometrial destruction 31
Endometrial hyperplasia
   development of 51
   prevention of 124
   treatment of 124
Endometrial implants 90
Endometrial polyps 108
Endometrial sampling 50
Endometrial thickness 17
Endometrioma 90
   ovarian surgery for 10
Endometriosis 16, 27, 55, 61, 81, 87, 89, 91, 92, 124, 128, 140
   clinical features of 87
   development of 87
   laparoscopy in 88f, 92f
   management of 87
   medical management of 130
Endometriotic implants, electrocoagulation of 90
Endometritis especially tuberculosis 4
Endometrium 9, 108
   ablation 95
   alteration of 127
   biochemical changes in 123
   causes cellular changes in 123
   histopathological examination of 110
   hyperplasia of 47
   irregular shedding of 48
Endopelvic fascia 68
End-organ damage, signs of 208
Enterocele 72, 76

Index

Enzymatic function 151
Epicanthal folds 334
Epidermal cells 153
Epididymal obstruction 19
Epididymis 24
Epidural analgesia 177, 233, 300
Episiotomy 247, 293
　infection 261
　routine use of 294
　types of 294f
Epispadias 5
Epithelial cancer 113
Epithelial ovarian cancer 113
　clinical features of 113
　detecting 114
　increased risk of 86
Epithelial ovarian malignancy 113
Equine estrogen, conjugated 51
Erb's palsy 326, 330
Erectile dysfunction 6
Erythrocyte sedimentation rate 154
Escherichia coli 258
　infection 332
Estradiol 82
Estrogen 52, 131, 144, 145
　cream 73
　decreases collagen strength 69
　deficiency 143
　dependent
　　cancer 109
　　tumor 58
　level, excess 141
　progestogen, combined 89
　receptor modulators 145
　therapy 147
Estrone 82
Ethambutol 33
Ethinyl estradiol 126
Eugenic grounds 132
Exfoliative cytology 97, 102
Exogenous factors 192
External cephalic version, contraindications of 183
Extraperitoneal insufflation 93
Eye
　care 331
　sunken 312

F

Face, compressed 278
Fallopian tube 29, 36, 37, 108
　ostia, cannulation of 27
Falloposcopy 12, 16
Fat 262
Fatty degeneration 65
Feeding vessel sign 50
Feinberg-Whittington media 41

Femoral venous pressure 156
Fenticonazole 43
Ferric salts 237
Fertility, surgery for restoration of 34
Fertilize ova, capacity to 123
Fertilized ovum, prevent implantation of 123
Fetal anemia, severe 317
Fetal breathing 157
Fetal circulation
　amniotic compartment to 152
　transudation of 152
Fetal complications 241
Fetal compromise 289
Fetal deaths, number of 157
Fetal distress 160, 178, 222
Fetal heart
　action, undetectable 268
　beat 160
　sound 224, 266, 276
　structures, auscultation of 163
　surveillance 183
Fetal heart rate 168, 220, 256, 291
　change in 297
　deceleration 160
Fetal hematocrit 318
Fetal hyperglycemia 240
Fetal karyotyping 335
Fetal lung
　fluid 152
　maturity 245
Fetal medicine unit 314
Fetal membranes 168
Fetal movement 157, 159, 272
　absent 165
Fetal neuroprotection 247
Fetal shoulders 306
Fetal skin 153
Fetal surveillance 158
Fetal tachycardia 269
Fetal tone 158
Fetal vessels 252
Fetal well-being 158, 177
　antenatal tests for 157
　test for 253
Fetus
　dead 222
　detecting sex of 147
　protect 153
　swallows 152
Fibroid 17, 18, 28, 55, 58-61, 91, 95, 125, 185, 233
　classification for 66
　clinical features of 58
　degenerations in 64
　effects of 60
　etiology of 58
　management of 58

protective for 58
relationship of 66
secondary changes in 64
signs of 58
size of 59
surgery in asymptomatic 63
symptoms of 58
Filariasis 5
Fimbrial expression 207
Fimbrioplasty 27
Fine latex rubber 120
Fire appearance, ring of 205
First fetus, twins with 184, 286
Fluconazole 43
Fluid transit, obstruction of 275
Flutamide 86
Foley catheter 229
Folic acid 162, 164, 237, 320
deficiency 221
supplementation, periconceptional 320
Follicle-stimulating hormone 82, 147
Forceps application, prerequisites for 292
Foreign body reaction 123, 124
Fothergill's operation 75
Foul-smelling lochia 259
Four-quadrant technique 278
Fractures 182
Fragile X syndrome 4
Fusobacterium species 258
Future pregnancy
prevention of hypertension in 216
repeat in 193

G

Galactogogues 262
Galactokinetic hormone 261
Galactopoiesis 261
Galactorrhea 18, 50
Galactosemia 4
Gardnerella vaginalis 40, 258
Gaskin maneuver 307
Gastroesophageal reflux 248
Gastrointestinal system 248
Gastrointestinal tract lining 248
Genetic abnormality 23
Genetic analysis 21
Genetic basis 333
Genetic transmission 242
Genital herpes 293
infection, active 289, 291
Genital infections, female 258
Genital lesion 303
Genital mutilation, female 294
Genital prolapse
clinical features of 71
signs of 71

symptoms of 71
types of 70
Genital tract 228
infections 244
Genital tuberculosis 29, 32f
treatment of 29
Genitalia 330
Genitofemoral nerve 78
Genitourinary fistula 265
Gentamicin 38, 233
Germ cell tumor, benign 137
Gestation
limit, increase in 134
period of 162, 316f
weeks of 213, 216
Gestational age
dating of 305
estimation 331
Gestational diabetes mellitus 86, 239, 242, 281
Gestodene 126
Gestrinone 52, 63, 89
Glycerin 73
Glyceryl trinitrate transdermal patches 55
Gonadotropin 85
Gonadotropin-releasing hormone 144
analogs 51, 52, 63, 89, 112
secretion 6
Gonadotropin-resistant ovary syndrome 4
Gonococcus ascends 35
Goodell and Powell surgery 78
Gram-negative bacteria 258
Granulosa cells 11
Great vessels, transposition of 241
Growth hormone 147
Gunshella sutures 231
Gynecoid pelvis 178

H

H1N1 vaccination 165
Halban's disease 48
Hanging drop preparation 41
Hayman sutures 231
Head
compression 160
descent of 168
Hearing disorder 249
Heart disease 232, 293
Metcalfe's criteria for 232
signs of 232
symptoms of 232
Heart rate 156
HELLP syndrome 211, 213, 216, 228
diagnosis of 211
Helmet cells 212
Hematocolpos 46f
Hematologic system 249

Index

Hematological changes 154
Hematological indices 236
Hematometra 46f, 322
Hematuria 102
   cyclical 87
Hemodynamic changes 155
Hemodynamic instability 226
   causes 228
Hemodynamically stable 206
Hemoglobin
   electrophoresis 164
   level of 315
Hemoglobinopathy 148
Hemolysis 211
Hemolytic disorders 339
   complicated 343
   uncomplicated 343
Hemorrhage 273, 302, 332
   postpartum 221, 228, 258, 265, 277
   prevent postpartum 287
Hemostasis, living ligature principal of 172
Hereditary thrombophilia 242
Herpes simplex virus 96, 332
High-intensity focused ultrasound 64
Hirsutism 83, 84, 86, 128
   antiandrogens for 86
Homogeneous 9
Hormonal emergency contraception, types of 131
Hormonal estimation 7, 8
Hormonal evaluation 21
Hormonal therapy 112
Hormone 89
Hormone replacement therapy 141, 144, 145
   contraindications of 145
   types of 145
Human chorionic gonadotropin 310
Human epididymis protein 114
Human immunodeficiency virus 25, 96, 258
   infection 291
Human menopausal gonadotropin 85
Human papillomavirus 96, 97
   deoxyribonucleic acid test 98, 103
   infection 96, 117
Hyaline degeneration 64
Hyaline membrane disease 242
Hydatidiform 310
Hydralazine 215
Hydramnios 303
Hydrocortisone 313
Hydronephrosis 60
Hydrops fetalis 314, 317
Hydroureter 60, 102
Hygroscopic dilators 292
Hymen 46
   imperforate 45, 46, 46f
Hyperandrogenism 81, 82
Hyperbilirubinemia 242, 337
   reducing direct 342
   unconjugated 336, 338
Hyperemesis 280
   gravidarum 310
   progress chart 313
Hypergonadotropic hypogonadism 23
Hyperhomocysteinemia 191, 243
Hyperinsulinemia 82, 85
Hyperplasia, type of 109
Hyperprolactinemia 6, 18, 50
Hypertension 109, 208
   chronic 209
   residual 214
   severe 208
   treatment of 279
Hypertensive disorders 208, 228, 302, 303
   diagnosis of 208
Hyperthecosis 82
Hyperthyroidism 137
   manifestations of 50
Hypertrophic obstructive cardiomyopathy 241
Hyperviscosity syndrome 242
Hypocalcemia 242, 337
Hypoechoic masses 61
Hypoglycemia 242
Hypogonadotropic hypogonadism 23
Hypomagnesemia 242
Hypoplastic left ventricle 241
Hypospadias 5, 6
Hypotension 249, 312
Hypothalamus 144
Hypothermia 248
Hypothyroidism 47, 50, 334
Hypotonia 334
Hypotonic myometrium 228
Hypoventilation 93
Hypovolemia 223
Hypoxia 160
Hypoxia-ischemia 332
   encephalopathy, pathophysiology of 328
Hysterectomy 53, 63, 269
   simple 99, 104
Hysterolaparoscopy 91
Hysterosalpingo contrast sonography 12, 15
Hysterosalpingography 13f, 32, 32f
   defects detected on 94
Hysteroscopy 28, 51, 61
   indications of 94
Hysterotomy scar 268

I

Ibuprofen 55
Iceberg sign, tip of 138
Icterus gravis neonatorum 314
Iliac artery ligation, internal 230

Imipenem 261
Immediate postpartum hemorrhage, causes of 228
Immune system 249
Immunization 165
Immunological basis 311
Immunological disorder 191
Immunological function 152
Immunotherapy 116
In utero transfer 246
In vitro fertilization 25, 86
    conception 293
    embryo transfer 90
Indomethacin 55, 246, 277
Infant
    prematurity 336
    preterm 336
    protection of 343
Infection 6, 29, 66, 120, 125, 142, 191, 244, 249, 332
    higher risk of 240
    polymicrobial ascending 35
Infective endocarditis prophylaxis 233
Infertile couple, male partner in 18
Infertility 3, 34, 58, 59, 83, 85, 87, 91, 94
    causes of 3, 5
    female 17
    treatment for
        female 26
        male 22
    types of 3
    unexplained 28
    uterine factors of 17
Influenza vaccination 165
Inguinal lymph nodes 113
Inherited thrombophilias 191
Inhibits ovarian function 119
Inhibits phosphorylation 336
Insufflation test 12
Insulin 82
    like growth factor 241
    resistance 81, 83, 240
    sensitizers 85, 86
Interceptive agents 131
Interconceptional period 193
Interleukin 244
Internal iliac arteries, ligation of 230
Interval cytoreduction 116
Interval cytoreductive surgery 116
Intra-abdominal pressure 91
Intracerebral infarction 332
Intracranial hemorrhage 182
Intracytoplasmic sperm injection 25
Intramolecular cyclization 341
Intranatal medication 327
Intrapartum 163, 234, 258
Intrauterine
    adhesions 55, 95, 95f

blood transfusion 314
hypoxia, continuation of 326
infections 340
insemination 24, 34
transfusion 305, 317
Intrauterine contraceptive device 35, 47, 56, 120, 274
    misplaced 94, 125
Intrauterine device
    and failure rates, mechanism of action of 123
    complications of 125
    contraindications of 125
    pearl index of 123
Intrauterine fetal death 153, 183, 223, 224, 245, 266, 269
    cause of 303
Intrauterine growth restriction 60, 157, 183, 281, 305
    asymmetric 252
    causes of 251
    etiology of 250
    management of 253fc
    symmetric 252
    types of 250
Intravascular transfusion 318
Intravenous
    fluids 269
    glucocorticoids 213
    immunoglobulin G, high dose 319
Invasive carcinoma 101, 101f
Iron 164
    deficiency 235, 236
        anemia, management of 234
    sucrose 238
Irregular periods 84
Ischemic heart disease 146
Isoimmunisation, prevention of 319
Isoniazid 33
Isoxsuprine 245
Itraconazole 43

J

Jaundice
    causes of pathological 339
    dosage and role 344
    neonatal 338, 342fc
    pathological 338, 341
    physiologic 339
    physiological 338, 341
    severity of 340

K

Kadar's rule 205
Kallmann's syndrome 6, 18
Kartagener syndrome 5
Karyotype 56, 335
Kernicterus 336
Ketoacidosis 265, 312, 337

Index

Khanna's sling 76
Kielland forceps 189
Klebsiella 258
Kleihauer-Betke test 319
Klinefelter's syndrome 6, 19, 21
Klumpke brachial plexus palsies 306
Klumpke's palsy 330
Knee presentation 181
Kramer's rule 340
Krustner's sign 138
Kupferberg's media 41

L

Labetalol 215
Labor 167
    abnormal 303
    and operative delivery, induction of 288
    cardiac patient in 233
    complications of 293
    contraindications for induction of 288
    course of 186
    diagnosis and mechanism of 185
    false 168
    first stage of 167
    fourth stage of 168
    induction of 256
    management 187, 299
        during 239
        of third stage of 168, 170, 172, 173fc, 174, 287
    mechanism of 186
    methods of induction of 289
    mismanagement of third stage of 307
    onset of 176
    physiology of third stage of 170
    preterm 240, 280, 322
    progress of 176, 299
    risk of induction of 255
    scheme of mechanism of 187fc
    second stage of 167
    stages of 167
    third stage of 168, 174
    true 168
Lactation
    stimulation of 262
    suppression 262
Lactational amenorrhea method 119
Lactic acid wash 40, 42
Lactobacilli 40, 42
Lactogenesis 261
Laminaria japonicum 292
Langhan's cells, infiltration of 31
Laparoscopic hysterectomy 70
Laparoscopic ovarian cystectomy 90
Laparoscopic presacral neurectomy 55
Laparoscopic surgery, advantages of 92
Laparoscopic uterine nerve ablation 55, 90

Laparoscopy 9, 12, 15, 16f, 33, 37, 61, 84, 87, 92f
    advantages of 91
    complications of 91
    contraindications of 91, 93
Laparotomy 204, 269
    exploratory 114
Laproscopic sacrocolpopexy 80
Lax perineum 72
Le Forte's operation 78
Leishman stain 235
Lesions, intracavitary 94
Letrozole 85, 90
Leukemia 334
Leukocytosis 37
Leukomalacia, periventricular 245, 250
Leukoplakia 98
Leukorrhea 43
Leuprolide 89
Levator ani muscle 68, 69
    neuromuscular damage of 69
Levonorgestrel-releasing intrauterine
    device 51, 52, 89
    system 144
Ligament 68
    round 67
    uterosacral 68
Liley's chart 315
Limb contractures 278
Linear salpingectomy 204, 207
Lipid profile 84
Lipoproteins, low-density 84
Liquid-based cytology 97, 102
Liquor
    disorder 271
    sudden escape of 221
Liver
    diseases, severe 134
    enzymes, elevated 211
    failure 47
    function test 272
    tumor 129
Local anesthesia and sedation 78
Local estrogen vaginal cream 145
Lochia 302
    alba 302, 303
    rubra 302
    serosa 302
Low platelet count 212
Lowenstein-Jensen media, culture in 32
Lumirubin 341
Lung
    and respiratory system 248
    disease, chronic 248
Lupus anticoagulant 191, 243
Luteal phase defect 4, 26, 191
Luteinized unruptured follicle 4

Luteinizing hormone 82, 147
Lycopene 216
Lying down adrenal sign 278

M

Mackenrodt's ligament 68
Macrosomia 244
Magnesium sulfate 216, 246, 247
Malabsorption syndrome 238
Malnutrition 128
Malpresentations 281
Mammary murmur 155
Mammogenesis 261
Manchester operation 75
Mandatory hospital delivery 270
Manipulative delivery 269
Manning's score 157
Marfan's syndrome 69, 233, 293, 308
Maternal adaptation, phenomenon of 153
Maternal age, increasing 333
Maternal death 301
Maternal diabetes 159
Maternal distress 178, 240
    evidence of 178
Maternal health factors, chronic 192
Maternal hypoxic states 327
Maternal injury, prevent 217
Maternal medical illness 192
Maternal morbidity, causes of 264
Maternal mortality 265, 310
    cause of 301, 302
    ratio 301
Maternal serum, transudation of 152
Maternal uterine artery velocimetry, increased impedance of 252
Maternal vasculopathy 242
Matthews Duncan method 171f
Mayer-Rokitansky-Küster-Hauser syndrome 56
McCall culdoplasty 80
McDonald's cerclage 194, 194f
McRoberts maneuver 307
Medical and surgical
    disorders 232
    illness 245
Medical termination of pregnancy
    indications of 132
    methods of first trimester 133
Medical Termination of Pregnancy Act 134
    recent changes in 134
Medical Termination of Pregnancy Rules 135
Medroxyprogesterone 89
    acetate 51, 89
Mefenamic acid 55
Megaloblastic anemia 235, 236
Membrane
    artificial rupture of 254, 256, 291

controlled artificial rupture of 277
    premature rupture of 165, 195, 221, 245, 258, 276
    prolonged rupture of 258
    stripping of 291
Memory
    aid 172
    loss 144
Mendelson's syndrome, prevent 177
Meningitis 249
Menopause 143
Menorrhagia 46, 48, 59, 94, 125, 130
    causes of 46, 47
    control 62
    following prolonged amenorrhea 83
Menstrual abnormalities 59
Menstrual blood, reflux of 36
Menstrual cycle 43
    day 10 11
Menstrual disorders 45
    cure of 127
Menstrual history 7, 255
Menstrual period, last normal 162
Mental abnormalities 132
Mental retardation 334
Metabolic disorders 4, 148, 340
Metabolic disturbances, correct 313
Metabolic syndrome 83
Metformin 85, 86
Methergine 233
Methotrexate 206
    therapy 206
Methylene blue dye 15
Metoclopramide 313
Metritis following cesarean delivery,
    pathogenesis of 259fc
Metronidazole 38-40, 42
Metropathia hemorrhagica 49
Metroplasty, lateral wall 18, 28, 95
Metrorrhagia 59
Miconazole 43
Micronecrothrombosis 65, 233
Microsurgical reconstructive surgery, results of 28
Middle cerebral artery, blood flow in 252
Mifepristone 63, 290
Milk ejection reflex 261, 261f
Mirror syndrome 276
Miscarriage 190
    incomplete 197
    threatened 199
Misoprostol 229, 290
    medical management with 198
    tablets 133
Mitochondrial damage 336
Mitral stenosis 232
Mobiluncus species 258
Modern day obstetrics 267

Index

Molar pregnancy
  complications of 271
  incidence of 271
Moniliasis 42
Monitoring score 326
Monochorionicity 285
Monophasic pills 126
Monozygotic twins 283
Mosaic down syndrome 333
Mosaic pattern 98
Mosaicism 333
Moschcowitz operation 80
Mother's room 331
Müllerian agenesis 56
Müllerian anomalies 91
Müllerian fusion defects 192
Müllerian inhibiting factor 57
Multidisciplinary team approach 247, 254, 286
Multigravida 198
Multiparity 184
Multiphasic pills 126
Multiple gestation 244
  chorionicity for 305
Multiple pregnancy 86, 185, 310
Multivitamins 164
Mumps orchitis 18
Mycoplasma 244
  hominis 35
Myocardial infarction 128
Myohyperplasia 62
Myoinositol 85, 86
Myomectomy 28, 56, 63
Myotamponade 172

N

Nafarelin 89
Narcotic-analgesics, withdrawal from 333
Nasal bone 305
Natural osmotic dilators 292
Nausea 280
Neck 163
Necrotizing enterocolitis 245, 248
Necrozoospermia 20
Neisseria gonorrhoeae 35
Neoadjuvant chemotherapy, cycles of 116
Neodymium-doped yttrium aluminum garnet 53
Neonatal care, steps of 329
Neonatal complications 242
Neonatal death 184
Neonatal intensive care unit 246, 253
Neonatal seizures, idiopathic benign 333
Neural tube defects, incidence of 320
Neurocutaneous syndromes 333
Neurologic complications 312
Neurological anomalies 69
Neurological development 262

Newborn, care of 329
Nifedipine 215, 245, 246
Night sweats 144
Nitric oxide 156
  donor 253
Nodular surface 60
Nonabsorbable suture 194
Nondysjunction 333
Nongravid women 54
Nonsteroidal anti-inflammatory drugs 62
Non-stress test 157, 158, 253
  reactive 159f, 182
Norethisterone 51, 126
  enanthate 130
Norgestimate 126
Noristerat 130
Normal labor, management of first stage of 175
Norplant system 136
Nose 329
Nulliparity 58, 125
Nulliparous patients 75
Nursery
  care in 331
  transfer to 331
Nutritional support 313
Nystatin 43

O

O'sullivan's hydrostatic technique 309
Obesity 22, 50, 58, 83, 85, 109
Obscure 310
Obstetric hysterectomy 231
Obstetric management 220
Obstetric procedure, common 293
Obstructed labor 264
  management of 264
Obstructive disorders 340
Obstructive rupture 268
Occipitoposterior position, management of 188fc
Oil-based dye, advantages of 14
Oligoasthenoteratospermia 20
  severe 25
Oligohydramnios 153, 214, 254, 277-279
  etiology of 277
  sequence 278
Oligomenorrhea 48, 83, 124
Oligo-ovulation 4
Oligozoospermia 20
Oliguria 213, 250
Omega 3 fatty acids 217, 262
Omental emphysema 93
Oocytes, number of 11
Operative delivery 281
  increase risk of 213
Operative hysteroscopy 18, 95
Ophthalmic system 249

Index

Ophthalmoscopic examination 312
Optimal cytoreduction, evidence of 115
Oral cavity, suction of 329
Oral contraceptive pills 35, 120, 127
    combined 51, 52
    low dose 62
    risks of 128
    side effects of 128
    use of 116
Oral iron 237
Oral pill 89
Ormeloxifene 53
Oropharynx 329
Orthopnea 232
Osteoporosis 144
Otitis media 249
Ovarian cancer 108, 146, 263
    diagnosis of 114
    reducing risk of 116
Ovarian cystectomy 139
Ovarian cysts, complications of benign 139
Ovarian dysgenesis 56
Ovarian failure
    causes of premature 4
    premature 4, 143
Ovarian functional cysts 127
Ovarian hyperstimulation syndrome 86
Ovarian malignancy 113, 114
Ovarian metastasis 115
Ovarian reserve
    concept of 10
    ultrasound evaluation of 11
Ovarian torsion 137
    management of 139
Ovarian tumor 62, 91, 139
Ovarian volume 11
Ovary 16, 92, 108
    normal 28
Ovulation induction
    agents 85, 284
    side effects of 86
    surgery for 86
Oxygen 233
Oxytocin 170, 261, 290
    drip, injection 229
    use of 267
Oyster ovaries 84

P

P450C17 enzyme dysfunction 82
Paclitaxel 112, 116
Pain 87, 197
    abdomen 60, 202
    back 222
    cramp like 126
    mid-menstrual 7
    ovulation 7
    pelvic dragging 71
    relief of 177
Palpable cystic distention 19
Palpation, abdominal 177
Pap smear 78, 97, 102
Pap test 97
Parametritis 260
Parenteral iron 238
    dose of 238
    indications for 238
Partogram 168, 299
Patent ductus arteriosus 249
Patent fallopian tube 24
Pearl index 124, 127
Pedersen's hypothesis 241
Pelvic abscess 260, 261
Pelvic adhesions 201
Pelvic cellular tissue 68
Pelvic congestion syndrome 56
Pelvic disease 180
Pelvic examination 137
Pelvic floor
    muscle training 80
    trauma 240
Pelvic grip 186
Pelvic infection 134
    following cesarean delivery 260
    management of acute 34
    reduce risk of 126
Pelvic inflammatory disease 15, 34, 47, 55, 61, 128, 200
    acute 35
    oral regimens for 39
    parenteral regimens for 38
    risk of 124
    stages of 37
    treatments of 38
Pelvic inlet 185
Pelvic lesions, acute 91
Pelvic mass 91, 292
Pelvic organ
    pathology of 29
    prolapse 72
        quantitative scoring 70
Pelvic pain 87, 91
Pelvic peritoneum 30
Pelvic peritonitis 260
Pelvic tuberculosis 125
Pelvic tumors 58, 180, 185
Pelvic ultrasound 138
Pelvis 334
    types of 178
Penicillins, extended-spectrum 261
Penile examination 19
Percreta previa, diagnosis of 305
Percutaneous estrogen gel 145

Index

Pericervical ring 68
Perinatal morbidity 306
    causes of 264
    increase 277
Perinatal mortality 181
    increase 242, 277, 282
Perineal injury, reason for 187
Perineal muscles 295
    tearing of 293
Peripheral smear 212
Perisalpingitis 30
Peritoneal factors 4, 12
Peritonitis, unresponsive 261
Pfannenstiel incision 77
Phospholipase, activity of 291
Photo-oxidation 341
Phototherapy 341
    duration of 343
    side effects of 343
Pinch test 73
Pituitary tumors 18
Placenta
    accreta 292
    cornu-fundal attachment of 180
    delivery of 168
    fetal surface of 152
    functional failure of 326
    functions of 151
    low-lying 225, 227
    periphery of 171
    previa 183, 185, 224, 227, 258
        degree of 225, 225f
        diagnosis of 226, 305
        management of 224
        marginal 225
        partial 225
        total 225
        types of 224
    removal of 163
    types of separation of 171f
Placental expulsion, mechanism of 171
Placental implantation site 228
Placental membranes 152
Placental separation
    methods of 171
    signs of 172
Placental site 170
Placental thrombosis 191
Plasma
    exchange 319
    protein
        changes 154
        concentration 154
Plasmapheresis 319
Platelets 272
    count with 212

Platypelloid pelvis 179
Plus ampicillin 261
Pneumonia 249
    congenital 248
Polycystic ovarian syndrome 4, 58, 81, 86, 128
    pathophysiology of 82f
Polycythemia 242
Polyhydramnios 185, 221, 240, 244, 275, 280, 291
    management of 274
Polymenorrhagia
    perimenopausal 110
    premenopausal 110
Polymenorrhea 48
Polypectomy 28, 56
Polyps 17, 18, 28, 51, 95
Polyurethane 120
    sponge made of 122
Postdatism 159
    complications of 254
    management of 254, 256fc
Post-hysterectomy vault prolapse 79
Postmenopausal atrophy 69
Postmenopausal bleeding, causes of 107
Postpartum pituitary necrosis 223
Potter syndrome 278
Pouch of Douglas 9, 37, 76
Povidone iodine solution 321
Precious pregnancy 293
Pre-Conception and Pre-Natal Diagnostic
    Techniques Act 147
Preeclampsia 157, 208, 273, 280, 302, 303
    etiopathology of 209
    features of 226
    management of 213, 215fc
    mild 211
    pathogenesis of 210fc
    risk factors of 209
    severe 211, 216, 245
Pregnancy 9, 126
    and fertility treatment 147
    antihypertensives in 215
    complications 47
        anticoagulation prevents 243
    continuation of 134
    diabetogenic state 240
    first 310
    high-risk 157
    management 158
    post-term 255, 278
    renal changes in 155
    second trimester of 65, 234
    specific syndrome 209
    symptoms, subsidence of 196
    termination of 135, 314
    third trimester of 267
    uncomplicated 161

Premenstrual syndrome 128
Pre-Natal Diagnostic Techniques (Regulation and Prevention of Misuse) Act 147, 148
Presacral neurectomy 90
Preterm labor
　etiology of 244
　etiopathogenesis of 244fc
　idiopathic 222
　management of 244, 247
Previous cesarean section
　management of 298
　scar rupture, clinical features of 297
Previous pregnancy, postpartum complications of 163
Primordial oocyte pool, size of 11
Pritchard's rule 223
Probenecid 39
Probiotics 40
Prochlorperazine 313
Proctoscopy 103
Progesterone 52, 62, 63, 82, 124, 144, 156
　gels 26
　micronized 144
　natural micronized 26
　receptor modulator 63, 132
　side effects of 144
　supplementation 247
Progestin 51, 112
Progestogen
　only methods, users of 129
　oral 89
　pills 129-131, 239
Prolactin 261
Prolapse 67
　degrees of 70
　etiology of 69
　stages of 70
　surgeries for 74
　surgical treatment for 74
　type of 70, 74
Promethazine 313
Prominent ischial spines 189
Prophylactic forceps, use of 233
Prostaglandin 156, 244, 290, 291
　use of 267
Protein 262
　C and S deficiency 191
　growth factor-binding 82
　hormones 151
Proteinuria 208
Proteus species 258
Pseudo sac 205
Pseudomenopause regimen 89
Pseudopregnancy 89
　regimen 89, 130
Pseudoshoulder dystocia 320
Pubocervical ligament 68

Puerperal pyrexia 257
　causes of 257
Puerperal sepsis 125, 257
　predisposing factors of 258
Puerperium 240
　period 234
Pulmonary blood flow 156
Pulmonary capillary wedge pressure 156
Pulmonary embolism 242, 310
Pulmonary hypertension 132
Pulmonary hypoplasia 278
Pulmonary insufficiency, acute 273
Pulmonary metastasis 104
Pulmonary tuberculosis 257
Pulmonary vascular resistance 156
Pulse
　daily record of 313
　oximeter monitoring 233
　rate 170
Punch biopsy 103
Purandare's cervicopexy 76
Purandare's sling operation 76
Purpura 50

R

Radiation therapy 4
Radical hysterectomy 105
　modified 111
Radical trachelectomy 105
Rectal examination 46
Rectocele 71, 72
Rectovaginal fistula 265
Renal agenesis 278
Renal blood flow 156
Renal disease
　chronic 163
　severe 134
Renal failure 47, 213, 223
Renal function test 272
Renal system 250
Reproductive aging, female 9
Reproductive tract infections 163
Respiratory diseases
　severe 134
　syndrome 212, 242, 248
Respiratory function 151
Respiratory system changes 154
Resuscitation 204, 330
　efficacy of 326
Retinopathy of prematurity 249
Rh
　blood group 276
　hemolytic disease 316f
　incompatibility 153, 343
　isoimmunization 276, 314
　　management 305
　isoimmunized pregnancy, management of 314, 315fc

Index

Rifampicin 33
Ring pessary 79
   indications of 79
Ringer's lactate 269
Ritodrine 245
Rokitansky nodule 138
Rokitansky protuberance 137
Rubin's cannula 14
Rubin's maneuver 307
Rubin's test 12
Rupture 261
   phase of 269
   spontaneous 267
   uterus
      causes of 267
      etiology of 268fc
      management of 267
Ruptured ectopic pregnancy, management of 200

S

Sacral agenesis 241
Sacral promontory 77
Sacrocolpopexy, abdominal 80
Sacrospinous fixation 80
Saline infusion
   sonography 12, 14, 61
   sonohysterography 12
Salpingectomy 206
Salpingitis isthmica nodosa 30
Salpingo-oophorectomy
   bilateral 111
   unilateral 116
Salpingo-ovariolysis 27
Salpingoscopy 12, 17
Salpingostomy 27
Sampson's theory of retrograde menstruation 87
Sandwich therapy 89
Sarcoma 66
Savage syndrome 4
Scar
   classical 268
   endometriosis 296
   rupture
      clinical features of 297
      rates of 297
   tenderness, watch for 299
   trial of 298
Schiller's test 98, 102
Schistocytes 212
Schroeder's disease 49
Schroeder's ring 264
Schultze mechanism 171
Schultze method 171f
Scrotal temperature 5
Scrotal ultrasonography 21
Sebaceous material 137

Sedative-hypnotics and alcohol 333
Semen
   analysis 19
      abnormal 20
      values 20
   collection, methods of 19
Seminal fluid
   errors in 6
   fructose content in 21
Sengstaken-Blakemore tube 229
Sepsis 249, 273, 322
Septal resection 18, 28, 95
Septate uterus, hysteroscopy in 94f
Septic pelvic thrombophlebitis 259
Sertoli-cell-only-syndrome 6
Serum estradiol 8
Serum fasting insulin 84
Serum luteinizing hormone 9
Serum progesterone 8, 198, 205
Serum testosterone 83
Serum thyroid stimulating hormone 84
Serum uric acid 214
Sex chromatin 147
Sex hormone binding globulin 82, 83
Sex-linked disorders 148
Sexual characters, secondary 56
Sexually transmitted
   diseases 35, 120, 293
   infections 163
Sheehan's syndrome 223, 265
Shirodkar's cerclage 194
Shirodkar's modification 75
Shirodkar's sling 76, 77
Shirodkar's uterosacral ligaments advancement 75
Shivkar's pack 121, 121f, 229, 230f
Shock 308
   early pregnancy 204
   neurogenic 310
   severe emotional 191
Shoulder dystocia 240, 306
   management of 307
Sibai protocol 219
Sickle cell anemia 130
Sigmoid mesentery 78
Sildenafil 22, 253
Simpson's pain 110
Skin and subcutaneous tissue 295
Sling operations
   fertility 76
   types of 76
Sperm
   deposit 6
   function tests 22
   killing of 122
   retrieval techniques 25
   transport, impeding 123

Spermicides 122
Spina bifida
    occulta 69
    open 275
Spinal anesthesia, use of 220
Spinal vertebra 144
Spines, level of 188
Spironolactone 86
Squamocolumnar junction 100
Squamous cell carcinoma 100
Squamous epithelium 142
Stallworthy's sign 226
Staphylococcus aureus 258
Starvation, evidence of 311
Status eclampticus 219
Sterilization procedures 28
Steroidal hormones 151
Stillbirth 282
Stitch, removal of 195
Stress 162
    urinary incontinence 144
Strict asepsis 176
Stroke 128
    volume 156
Sturmdorff suture 75
Submucous fibroid 51, 61, 95f
Submucous polyp 61, 95f
Suction evacuation, complications of 134
Sugars, control of 22
Sulbactam 38
Suprapubic pressure, moderate 307
Swine flu vaccination 165
Symphysis-fundal height 251
Synapsin 336
Syncopal attack 126, 202
Synthetic osmotic dilators 292
Systemic lupus erythematosus 192

T

Tachycardia 159, 178, 269, 312
Tachysystole 290
Tadalafil 22
Tamoxifen 85
Tdap vaccine 165
Teratospermia 20
Terbutaline 245
Testicular biopsy 21
Testicular failure 23
Testis, undescended 5
Testosterone 82, 145
Tetanus 165
Therapeutic hysteroscopy 95
Thrombophilias 303
    disorder 191, 146, 242
    obstetric complications of 243

treatment of 243
types of 242
Thyroid
    disorders 191
        correction of 22
    enlargement 50
    stimulating hormone 19
    tissue 137
Thyroiditis 4
Thyroxine 272
Tibolone 145
Tin protoporphyrin 344
Tocolytic agents 245
    potential complications of 246
Tongue, dry coated 312
Torsion of ovarian tumor
    clinical features of 139
    management of 139
Toxic shock syndrome, development of 122
Toxins 4
Transfusion therapy 317
Transrectal ultrasound 21
    indications for 21
Transvaginal ultrasonography 84, 196
Transverse lie, etiology of 184
Trauma 191, 332
Traumatic operative delivery 258
Trichomoniasis 41
Trifluoperazine 313
Triple marker test 285, 335
Trophoblast lymphocyte 152
Trophoblastic disease, malignant 125, 273
Trophoblastic invasion
    abnormal 211
    incomplete 211
Tubal adhesions 91
Tubal factor 4, 12, 27
    evaluation 91
Tubal ligation 91, 270, 300
    reversal of 27
Tubal lumen 17
Tubal obstruction 4
Tubal patency 12
    tests for 12
Tubal pregnancy, unruptured 203
Tubal surgery 201
Tuberculosis 32, 163
Tuberculous endometritis 47
Tubocornual anastomosis 27
Tubo-ovarian mass 30, 62
Tuboplasty
    corrective 34
    operation 27
Tubotubal anastomosis 27
Tubular necrosis, acute 223

Index

Tumor 55
    necrosis factor 244
    protection against benign 127
Turner's syndrome 4, 56, 146, 330
    features of 146
Turtle neck sign 306
Twin 174, 280
    acardiac 282
    delivery 303
    interlocking of 281
    intrapartum management of 284
    management of 287fc
    peak sign 285
    pregnancy
        complications of 280, 280fc
        management of 284
    reversed arterial perfusion 282
    second baby of 286
    to-twin transfusion syndrome 282

U

Ulcer
    decubitus 73
    tropic 73
Ulipristal acetate 63, 132
Ultrasonography 304, 312
Umbilical artery 252, 254
Umbilical cord 152, 330
    care of 331
    prolapse 289, 291
Umbilical discharge 340
Umbilical grip 185
Unruptured ectopic pregnancy, management of 200
Ureaplasma urealyticum 40
Uremia, hydronephrosis leading to 102
Urethral meatus 19
Urinalysis 19, 312
Urinary incontinence 92
Urinary luteinizing hormone 9
Urinary tract 244
    infections 144, 249
Urine
    analysis 170
        routine 164
    for proteins 214
    output 177
    routine 245
    sample, postejaculatory 22
Urogenital atrophy 144
Uterine
    anomalies 17, 125, 185, 192, 244
    artery embolization 64, 231
    atony 281
    bleeding 48, 271
    compression sutures 230
    contractions 160, 168, 177, 264
    fibroid 180
        management protocol of 62fc
    fundus 308
    hemorrhage 134
    hyperstimulation 290
    inversion 307
        cause of acute 307
        management of 309fc
        severity of 308
    layers 267
    malformations 184
    massage 174
    perforation 91, 134
    polyps 55
    prolapse 73
    relaxants 194
    rupture 195, 298
    sarcoma 108
    scar tenderness 269, 297
    spiral arteries 211
    synechiae 192, 322
        formation 31
    tenderness 222
    thermal balloon 53
Uterocervical length 73
Uteroplacental blood flow 156
Uteroplacental insufficiency 160, 245, 278, 326
Uterus 16, 30, 53, 92, 108, 124, 197
    absent 28
    cardinal support of 68
    conserve 99
    couvelaire 223
    feel of 226
    fibromyoma of 127
    height of 226
    ligamentous supports of 68f
    massage 174
    over distended 228, 244
    prolapse of 72
    rupture 264, 265
    septate 17
    size of 197
    supports of 67f
    surgeries for inversion of 310

V

Vagina 30, 40, 42, 108
    support of 68
    swabbed 321
    transverse septum of 46
Vaginal birth, guidelines for 298
Vaginal bleeding 202, 222
    abnormal 101

painless 225
suspicious 125
Vaginal breech delivery, complications of 182
Vaginal cytology 7, 8
Vaginal delivery 69, 220, 227, 299
    factors impeding 293
Vaginal discharge 42, 142, 302
Vaginal dryness 144
Vaginal examination 176, 178
    indications of 176
Vaginal hysterectomy 70, 78
Vaginal inflammation 40
Vaginal metastasis 113
Vaginal mucosa 295
Vaginal pessaries 80
Vaginal pH 42
Vaginal prolapse, type of 70
Vaginal septum, transverse 45, 56
Vaginal sponge today 122
Vaginal vault prolapse 79
Vaginitis 40
Vaginoplasty 57
Valvular disease 134
Valvular heart disease 146
Varicocele 5, 23
Vasa previa, diagnosis of 305
Vasogram 21
Venereal disease research laboratory 164
Venous thromboembolic events 128
Ventricular septal defect 241
Vesicovaginal fistula 265
Vesicular mole 271, 273, 310
    disorder 271
Violin string adhesions 37
Virkud's composite sling operation 76, 77
Visceral injuries 182
Visual disturbances 18
Vitamin
    B12 237
    B6 313

C 237
D 262
Vomiting, severe type of 310
Vulva 30, 108, 321
Vulval cancer 108
    etiology of 117
    staging of 117
Vulval examination 46
Vulval hematoma 296
Vulval intraepithelial neoplasia 117
Vulval pads 303

W

Walls of uterus, apposition of 172
Warfarin 243
Water-soluble dye, advantages of 14
Weight
    gain 131
    loss 22
Wernicke's encephalopathy 312
Whiff test 40
Whorl-like appearance, loss of 64
Woods-Corkscrew maneuver 307
Wound
    care 295
    infection 257, 259, 261

X

X-linked placental sulfatase deficiency 254

Y

Young's stitch 75
Young's syndrome 18
Yq11 microdeletion 6, 22

Z

Z technique 238
Zavanelli maneuver 307
Ziehl-Neelsen stain 32